Community Health

Community Health

Edited by

June Clark

BA(Hons) MPhil SRN HVCert Dip Soc Research FRCN

Health Visitor

West Berkshire Health Authority

Jill Henderson

MSc SRN SCM HV RNT

Formerly Lecturer in Charge of Health Visitors' Courses at the University of Surrey

Foreword by

Grace M. Owen

MPhil BSc (Soc Hons) SRN SCM QNS HVTut RNT FRCN

Head of Department of Nursing and Community Health Studies, Polytechnic of the South Bank, London

CHURCHILL LIVINGSTONE

EDINBURGH LONDON MELBOURNE AND NEW YORK 1983

CHURCHILL LIVINGSTONE
Medical Division of Longman Group Limited

Distributed in the United States of America by Churchill Livingstone Inc., 1560 Broadway, New York, N.Y. 10036, and by associated companies, branches and representatives throughout the world.

First published 1983

ISBN 0 443 02000 0

British Library Cataloguing in Publication Data
Community health.
1. Community health services — Great Britain
I. Title II. Clark, June
III. Henderson, Jill
362.1'0425 RA485

Library of Congress Cataloging in Publication Data
Community health.
Includes index.
1. Public health. 2. Community health services.
I. Clark, June. II. Henderson, Jill. [DNLM:
1. Community health services — Essays.
WA 546.1 C7335]
RA425.C75 1983 362.1'2 82-22038

Printed in Singapore by Selector Printing Co Pte Ltd

Foreword

This book is a welcome publication, especially because it comes at a time when primary care and community health are currently issues for debate and discussion.

During the last few decades there has been a growing emphasis on community care as distinct from hospital care. The very fact, however, that there is a recognisable dichotomy between these two approaches to providing care, gives some indication of the nature of the struggle. In Western Society over the last century or so the more dramatic aspects of health care provided within the hospital system have always claimed more attention and therefore greater resources than community care. It is possible that a medical model for the provision of care and curative medicine has been influential, but it should also be taken into consideration that professionals themselves are socialised within their own cultural setting and this must, to some extent, perpetuate this perspective. The public image that health and sickness are somehow related to doctors and hospitals dies hard in public imagination and the desire to allow the professional to hold on to the mystique of health care can sometimes be very tenacious.

In recent years the impetus of social change has accelerated rapidly, with personal and social consequences for individuals and communities, and health care systems have not been immune from these influences. Changing values, economic constraints, political pressures, increased knowledge of social, physical and behavioural sciences, have all combined to reshape many perspectives on health care. Recent trends reflect a growing appreciation of the effects of man's interaction with his environment and the importance of a holistic approach to maintaining health. There is also a surge of interest in alternative medicine and a recognition of the need for individuals to assume more responsibility for their own personal health.

Inevitably the preparation and education of health professionals is affected by the current state of a body of knowledge in health related subjects but it is not often widely appreciated that a medical model can predominate to a considerable extent to preserve the *status quo* and overshadow the importance of personal involvement of individuals and communities concerned.

However, the current constraints in manpower provision and resources may well be pressurising both bureaucrats and professionals to re-examine priorities and concepts that have hitherto been held paramount, and so to re-think some issues in a different light.

Many professionals are responding to the challenge of rapid change and its consequences and asking many pertinent questions. This book could be, therefore, of considerable value to any who seek to re-examine established concepts in a different context and in the light of social change. The writers come from a variety of spheres of work and bring different perspectives to the current situation. New ideas are explored tentatively and questions raised; roles and relationships are re-assessed in the light of prevailing social policy and the organisational framework.

The book should stimulate professional practitioners in many fields to take a new look at themselves, their colleagues and clients and to prepare to adapt to new ideas. It should also be helpful to students who are in the formative stages of developing a professional ethos and who will find it of value in establishing a holistic and questioning approach to health care in the community.

G.M.O.

Preface

This collection of essays brings together the ideas of people whose common purpose is the prevention of illness and the promotion of health. The subject is wide, and one's view of it varies with the perspective one adopts and the personal position from which one starts. Our contributors include people engaged in large scale and long-term planning for community health, as well as field-level health workers whose immediate concern is the relatively small number of individuals in their care; they include doctors and nurses, administrators, teachers and practitioners. Some will be immediately recognised by readers as experts in their speciality; other names will be new. Each contributor, however, was asked to write on a subject about which he or she had particular knowledge and strong personal views.

The essays are loosely grouped into four sections according to their subject matter. In the first section contributors discuss some of the basic concepts which community health workers use every day but rarely question or analyse. The second section considers the environment — cultural, social and political as well as physical — in which health care is sought and delivered. The third section considers some aspects of health care from the perspective of the consumer or client, while the fourth takes the complementary perspective of the professional helper and offers some ideas about the systems by which health care may be delivered both in the United Kingdom and in other countries.

A book of readings is in no sense a textbook, nor can it be completely comprehensive in its coverage. This book does not pretend to be either. Its selections and omissions reflect the biases of the editors as well as the individuality of the contributors. We believe that it will make a useful contribution to the literature which is available to students who are preparing to work in the service of community health — in particular health visitors, district nurses, social workers and general practitioners.

1983

J.C.
J.H.

Contributors

Monica Baly BA SRN SCM HVCert
Lecturer for the Diploma in Nursing. Lately Area Officer for the Royal College of Nursing

Jennifer M. Barnard SRN SCM OHNCert HVCert
Occupational Health Nursing Consultant, Sherborne St John, Basingstoke

Ann Burkitt MSc Dip Health Ed Dip F Ed SNR SRMN(NZ)
Senior Lecturer in Health Education, Department of Nursing and Community Health Studies, Polytechnic of the South Bank, London

Anthony Butterworth MSc RMN SRN DN(Lond) RNT
Principal Lecturer, Manchester Polytechnic, Manchester

June Clark BA (Hons) MPhil SRN HVCert Dip Soc Research FRCN
Health Visitor, West Berkshire Health Authority

Jeremy Cobb MSc MRCP MFCM
District Medical Officer, East Berkshire Health Authority

Mary Coleman SRN NDN(Cert) HV
Health Visitor, South West Herts Health Authority

Peter Coleman MA BD BSc(Econ)
Minister, Leavesden Road Baptist Church, Watford

Caroline Cox BSc(Soc) MSc(Econ) SRN
Director, Nursing Edication Research Unit, Chelsea College, London

John Dennis MSc
Research Assistant, Unit for the Study of Health Policy, Guy's Hospital London

Peter Draper MA MB BChir FFCM
Director, Unit for the Study of Health Policy, Guy's Hospital, London

Cynthia Finlayson BSc SRN Dip HV
Health Visitor, City and East London Area Health Authority, London

Jean Gaffin BSc(Econ) MSc
Organising Secretary, Child Accident Prevention Trust, London

Jenny Griffiths BA
Planning Administrator, South West Thames Regional Health Authority

Alexander D. G. Gunn MRCGP DObst RCOG DPH
Director, University Health Service, Reading Berks

Alix Henley BA(Hons)
DHSS/King's Fund Project, Havelock Centre, Southall, Middlesex

Gwen Hiskins SRN SCM HV FWT
Lately Health Visitor, Harrow

Brian Hodges MSc BA(Hons) SRN RNMS DN(Lond) Teacher's Certificate (Man) RNT
Senior Lecturer in Nursing Studies, Manchester Polytechnic, Manchester

J. Deborah Holroyd SRN SCM Higher Diploma in Health Visiting
Health Visitor, London

Maura Hunt MPhil SRN SCM HV HVTCert
Nursing Research Liaison Officer, South East Thames Regional Health Authority and Reader in Nursing and Community Health Services at the Polytechnic of the South Bank, London

R. H. Jackson MC MRCP
Medical Secretary, Child Accident Prevention Trust, London. Consultant Paediatrician, Royal Victoria Infirmary, Newcastle upon Tyne

Karen Luker BNurs PhD
Lecturer, Department of Nursing, University of Manchester, Manchester

Gaynor Nurse SRN SCM HVTCert RNT Dip in Nursing (London) AIE(Lond) FRCN
Principal Advisory Tutor, Institute of Advanced Nursing Education, Royal College of Nursing, London

Jennie Popay MA
Research Officer, Study Commission on the Family

Sheila Quinn
Family Planning Sister, Margaret Pyke Centre, London

Elizabeth Raymond SRN SCM QN HVTut RNT TCertEd
Senior Lecturer in Nursing Studies, Polytechnic of the South Bank, London

Barry L Reedy MB BS FRCGP DObst RCOG
Senior Lecturer in the Organisation of Health Care, University of Newcastle upon Tyne, Newcastle upon Tyne

Elizabeth Lumsden Rix RGN
Counsellor, Manchester Marriage Guidance Council; Formerly Senior Sister, Professorial Medical Unit, University Hospital of South Manchester, Manchester

Keith J B Rix BMedBiol MB ChB MPhil MIHE MRCPsych
Lecturer in Psychiatry, University of Manchester; Visiting Lecturer, Alcohol Studies Centre, Paisley College of Technology, Paisley

Kate Robinson BA SRN HV
Research Assistant, Department of Nursing and Community Health Studies, Polytechnic of the South Bank London

Christine Sage SRN SCM TCertEd RNT
Lecturer, Department of Nursing and Community Health Studies, Polytechnic of the South Bank, London

Jane Salvage SRN
News Editor, Nursing Times

Muriel Skeet FRCN
Nursing Consultant, World Health Organisation

Patricia Slack SRN SCM HVCert Dip Health Ed
Nursing Management Editor, Nursing Times

Joyce Wiseman MSc SRN SCM HVCert DipN(Lond) Man Studies (Lond)
Research Director for the North West Region Nurse Staffing Levels Project, Blackpool

Marie Wagg MA(Hons) BA(Hons) PhD
Formerly Senior Lecturer in Psychology and Education, Goldsmith's College University of London, London

Contents

Section 3 **Clients**

Section 4 **Professional approaches**

SECTION ONE

Concepts

In the first section of this book the authors have been concerned with the examination of certain fundamental aspects of community health which are more complex than is generally assumed. Words such as health, prevention, education and handicap are abstract ideas which mean different things to different people and it is helpful, also challenging, to have the threads drawn together. Nurses have tended, in the past, to be the passive recipients of other people's ideas, largely because of the medical, and therefore by implication male, domination of the nursing profession. Abstract ideas are not, however, confined to the realms of medicine or even of philosophy; these are as relevant to nursing as to any other discipline. It is with this thought in mind, and with a view to encouraging nurses to conceptualize for themselves, that this section has been written.

Concepts are culturally determined as is illustrated by the following definition of the word community given by a native of New Caledonia: 'A community is a group of people around a fire with their faces in the light, and in order to feel secure I must know the faces of everybody reflected in that light. If there is someone sitting in shadow he threatens me, he threatens the whole group. So I have to recognise each face and only those who live within the group can do this. Those who don't have this experience can never know all the faces. There is always someone sitting in shadow.' (Brake et al, 1979). Betty Raymond looks at the concept of community and how we could, or should, regard community care in this country, with a new perspective on what the term community care really encompasses.

There have been enough definitions of the word health to fill a whole book though it is doubtful whether it would merit publication. Kate Robinson rightly draws our attention away from such deliberations to the more relevant consideration which is the analysis of the concept itself, an important analysis for all, but especially for those who believe, with Plato, that life without health is not worth preserving.

In solving problems we often create new ones and it is perhaps important in considering prevention to reflect on what problems may have been created by reductions in mortality connected with, for example, birth and infancy and the conquest of infectious diseases. Peter Draper and colleagues have entered a most complex field, both in terms of definition and also of viability and he reminds us of the confused thinking of governments in their neglect of the health implications of some of their economic policies.

Ann Burkitt, in her essay on health education, discusses further the concept of health already introduced by Kate Robinson and presents seven models of health with some possible approaches to health education. She also introduces the increasingly important topic of alternative medicine. Tony Butterworth draws our attention to the importance of considering the maintenance of the mental health of the community at large and not just treatment of the mentally disordered. The concept of handicap with its attendant problems is outlined by Brian Hodges with an emphasis on the importance of assessment, yet another aspect of prevention taken in its broadest sense. He stresses the desirability of regarding people with disability first and foremost as people, but people with special needs. This section concludes with a chapter on spiritual care by Peter and Mary Coleman who offer five insights into the nature of care that are derived from a spiritual outlook on life. Again, in recognising that spiritual care is as much concerned with health as with disease, a positive approach is taken.

It will be seen from this introduction that there is an inevitable and, in fact, desirable, overlap between the chapters. This is, of course, because all the individual concepts discussed are parts of a whole, the concept chosen as the title of this book — community health.

1

Into the community

Elizabeth Raymond

Why is a book about community health important? For at least twenty years, reports and legislation have contained elements seeking to shift aspects of health care from institutions into the community. What motives have been responsible for this consistent tendency? Is there significance in the fact that the emphasis on community health care parallels the era of nuclear medicine, urbanisation of society, and the breakown of centuries-old traditional family structures? Toffler (1970) discusses the effect on individuals and society of the ever-accelerating rate of change in the Western world, and the experience of transience which it brings with it. He calls the effect future shock, and suggests that:

> . . .unless intelligent steps are taken to combat it, millions of human beings will find themselves increasingly disoriented, progressively incompetent to deal rationally with their environments. The malaise, mass neurosis, irrationality, and free-floating violence already apparent in contemporary life are merely a foretaste of what may lie ahead unless we come to understand and treat this disease.

In Toffler's view, not only individuals, but whole communities are being shaken to the core, and he calls for deliberate action to devise means of controlling and regulating change, and to restore stability.

Students of physical chemistry will be familiar with Le Chatelier's principle, applicable to chemical reactions. It states that:

> If to a system in equilibrium a constraint be applied, that change will take place in the system which will tend to nullify the constraint.

It may be suggested that this principle has a wider application than to chemistry, and that Toffler's book itself is an example of something being produced within the system of the human race which is tending to nullify the constraint of wildly accelerating change. Many suggest that balance and equilibrium are the natural order of things. Ecologists and environmental conservationists in particular are concerned with what is described as 'the balance of nature', and the human race is frequently identified as the rogue species which is uniquely responsible for upsetting this balance.

In the context of this book, it could be asked whether the growing move towards community care is an unconscious move on the part of society in an effort to restore equilibrium. If so, it is important for future health care planning that there is an understanding of the nature and function of a community. We need to develop a concept of community.

The assumption of the existence of the community as a cohesive agency, capable of thought, decisions, and action, appears to be implicit in legislation and reports related to community health care. Before implementing policies based on this assumption, we need to establish first whether this description may justifiably be applied to a community, and second, whether the community exists.

Definitions of the term 'community' all imply a group of people who share something in common. Examples of the common denominator may be neighbourhood, work, race, religion, or social activity. Minar & Greer (1969) suggest that:

> Communities are characterised by people's engagement in activities that demand inter-relationship of efforts, they give rise to shared culture, and they are often sited in a particular geographic locale.

The above statements immediately call into question the validity of the title of this book, *Community Health*! Community health care is usually understood to refer to care which takes place outside institutions. Within the nursing profession, for example, hospital care and community care are seen as alternatives. Yet those who work and those who are cared for within hospital walls share a common concern regarding disease and trauma. Nurses in particular share a common purpose in their nursing care. Surely these common factors accord the status of community to hospitals and to the professional body of nurses? Further, it appears that, within the hospital world, there are communities within the wider community. Perhaps the question of whether the person should be cared for in the community should be replaced by considering the type of community best suited to provide the care, given the person's present set of circumstances. It might be argued that the former question suggests lack of shared purpose and therfore an area of community breakdown within the body of those who profess to care.

Until this century the communities which have had the predominant influence on the lives of the vast majority of human individuals have been communities based on locality. In eighteenth century Kent '. . . most routes between village and town were poor, while those between one village and another were virtually non-existent or frequently lost beneath impassable mud' (West, 1973), so the community of work, race, religion, or social activity, was synonymous with the community of the locality: the village. Each person had his or her recognised place in that community, which, while it imposed great constraints on its members, also provided security, a sense of belonging, and sharing in adversity as well as in good times. The limitations of the village idiot may not have been fully understood, but it is possible that he had a greater sense of self-respect and personal identity in many eighteenth century villages than his counterpart has today in a mental subnormality hospital. Even today, nurses visiting in the more isolated rural communities are unlikely to find even the most unattractive members of those communities uncared for or unvisited. Sometimes hospital staff seem to have this kind of community hazily in mind when patients are discharged home without adequate preparation, yet such communities are becoming increasingly rare. At the other end of the scale, and becoming all too common, are localities where the characteristics of community seem sadly lacking. We are all familiar with newspaper headlines about neglected and forgotten old people. One 82-year-old widow, living alone, was trapped for 3½ days in her sea-front flat without food or water before help reached her. This incident took place, not in a deprived inner city area, but in the fairly affluent coastal resort of Bexhill, Sussex, where the Director of Social Services was quoted as saying that: 'It highlights the importance of neighbourly care in places like Bexhill where 47 per cent of the population are of retirement age.' (The Daily Telegraph, 1979).

This newspaper report seems to identify one of the factors which distinguish neighbourhoods which function as communities from those which do not, namely the age structure of the population. Also important is the length of time members of the population have lived in the locality. Resorts on the south coast with temperate climates like Bexhill and Worthing, are popular areas for retirement attracting people from all over the country. Some move from places where they had more roots than they realised and encounter greater difficulty in adjusting than they had expected. Loss of the familiar proves to be more traumatic than they had anticipated and so they exhibit behaviour patterns consistent with a kind of bereavement. For most people the ability to adapt to change apparently decreases with advancing years so that, in these circumstances, it takes proportionately longer for the elderly to build new relationships and to put down new roots. Some never succeed and this may become the point at which they withdraw into helpless isolation. By contrast, in a locality like Bermondsey, a working class borough of East London which lost its younger generation when the docks were closed, the elderly who remained and who had lived there all their lives retained a much greater measure of neighbourliness and self-help.

The age structure of the population and the time factor also appear to affect the quality of community in new town and housing estate developments. Where such developments are specifically intended to provide homes for workers in new industrial concerns, young workers and their families are brought together in a concentrated group which almost entirely lacks the older generation, and even the middle-aged.

One small new town development with which the author is acquanited, highlights a number of factors which appear to be related to the functioning of a community in a newly established neighbourhood with a young population. Despite the families being white and British almost without exception, regional origins were widely diverse and neighbours with different accents often seemed to regard each other with a degree of apprehension and uncertainty. A highly disproportionate number of families had a first or second child under one year old, and there were hardly any well-established families or older and more experienced individuals to whom young parents could turn for support, advice, and guidance. The incidence of marital breakdown was high, and couples whose relationship was under stress saw separation and divorce as the normal solution to their difficulties. All primary care facilities were hard pressed, and playgroup and child minding services were totally inadequate. It was a situation in which, in theory, self-help groups could have done a great deal to meet some of the needs, but the majority of couples resisted involvement. Apathy, depression, alcoholism, and a tendency to isolate themselves were disproportionately common features amongst the young mothers at home. Many expressed a sense of non-identity, of not belonging, and of being unimportant and insignificant. Many felt that the very architecture of the development heightened their sense of anonymity, saying that there was no point in going for a walk, since wherever they went looked the same as it did outside their own door. The limited community facilities provided, such as the youth/community hall, suffered repeated vandalism at the hands of the small teenage population, who felt that there was no scope for them to do what *they* wanted to and create something which belonged to *them*.

At this point it may be appropriate to pause and consider whether the new town described above merits the earlier description of a community as 'a cohesive agency capable of thought, decisions, and action'.

Inner-city areas are currently commonly referred to as deprived. Such areas are well represented in parts of the south-east, especially London. Primary health care workers find themselves continually involved in crisis intervention and, health visitors in particular, find it almost impossible to carry out the routine preventive work for which they are primarily trained. These are localities with a highly mobile, unsettled population, including immigrant and single parent families, desperate for whatever accommodation they can find. There is a disturbing incidence of child abuse and the streets generally are unsafe after dark. In many instances whose who live there do so because they have no alternative, and those able to choose have moved away. Such conditions are now common throughout the rest of the country, especially in the major cities. Social isolation is a feature of such a locality rather than social integration and community. If social isolation is the antithesis of community, it is sobering to reflect that: 'Social isolation is the common denominator of a number of factors correlated with a high suicide rate' (Stengel, 1964).

Professor Stengel went on to comment that

> The higher incidence of suicide in urban communities has been attributed to the greater risk of social isolation and the anonymity of life in the big cities . . . Investigations carried out . . . in London showed that the suicide rates were highest in those parts where the population was shifting.

Social isolation is not confined to the financially deprived, and Stengel points out that the highest suicide rates according to his evidence also occurred in the most prosperous sections of the city. My own brief experience of district nursing in Mayfair, an affluent area of London, brought home to me the possible social isolation of the wealthy. For example, I visited an elderly member of an internationally famous business family. She lacked no material comfort but, in her loneliness, she sought to give me some money because I smiled!

In his last chapter Stengel (1964) discusses prevention of suicide, and states that:

> . . . the fight against suicidal behaviour is only one of the aspects of a much bigger problem, which is the drastic reorientation of society to the social needs of its members . . . what is needed is a mobilisation of the latent resources for helping and healing in our society.

He then turns to a consideration of the concept of the 'therapeutic community' and suggests that society itself *could* become a truly therapeutic community. However, there are echoes of Toffler in one of his closing statments that:

> We are living in the age of a scientific revolution. At the same time, the incompetence of the human species in matters concerning the social well-being of communities is becoming more and more apparent.

Perhaps enough has been said to call into question the glib assumption that the community is a functioning social unit outside institutional walls, which may be depended upon to provide the continuing care a patient needs when he returns home.

It has earlier been mentioned that communities may exist independently of locality, and these need consideration. One such community for many will be the work community. The need for employment has, historically, exerted a considerable pressure contributing to the breakdown of existing local communities. With the advent of the industrial revolution, the growth of towns was inseparably linked with the search for work. Today, the road and rail network to the south and east of London is almost totally focused on providing access to London for workers of all descriptions.

Changes have taken place in the nature of the work community over the years, some of which parallel the changes in home communities. At the turn of the century work occupied the major proportion of the waking hours of the majority of the population. Workers expected to remain in one job for many years, if not for their working lives, in many instances. Many workers were part of an organisation small enough for them to identify with and have a sense of belonging. The relevance and importance of their particular contribution to the whole was more readily apparent. Today, concern is being expressed over the need to educate people for increased leisure and movement from one job to another is an almost universal expectation. Multinational corporations employ huge work-forces of people, many of whom perform apparently meaningless repetitive tasks, and who feel anonymous and lost in the vastness of it all. How much are factors such as the proliferation of strikes and demarcation disputes, the establishment of arbitration machinery, and pressure for closed shop legislation, symptoms of the breakdown of the work community paralleling the breakdown of communities at home? Further, is it evidence of Le Chatelier's principle operating in this area that the expression 'Small is beautiful' seems to be gaining in its appeal, and a measure of decentralisation is increasingly seen as desirable?

Even today, the work community provides the sense of belonging and identity for some, with opportunity for shared action towards a common purpose. This would seem to apply to members of the professions for whom job satisfaction is a real possibility, and who willingly engage in work-based activities out of hours for their professional development.

In the caring professions, for example, it may be asked whether there is another factor at work, related to the hall-marks of community, which encourages a willingness to go above and beyond the minimum required of their members. This is the element of vocation, which historically carried with it a commitment to involvement in the needs of others. According to Minar & Greer (1969): 'Community is then an aspect of the way men relate to one another . . . which goes far and away beyond the coerced and the necessary.'

In recent years the words 'vocation' and 'involvement' have begun to be seriously called into question, particularly by members of the nursing profession who find themselves at the sharp end of human need and suffering. At the same time, the National Health Service has followed the organisational pattern of industry, steadily distancing the deliverer of care further and further from those with power and authority. The number of tiers of management introduced with the 1974 Reorganisation of the National Health Service has come under heavy criticism. Although the present Government is at variance with the Royal Commission on the National Health Service (Department of Health & Social Security, 1979) over the appropriate changes to make, both are agreed on the need to reduce the total number of tiers. Within nursing there are many who feel that the distancing process was furthered by the change in nomenclature introduced with the Salmon Report, (Ministry of Health, 1966). The title 'Nursing Officer', they feel, is more impersonal and enhances anonymity. The effects of distancing on a community are commented on by Minar & Greer (1969):

> Beginning in the experiences of children in the family, (community) moves outward to include neighbourhood and peer group, congregation and collegium, the nation, and in some cases the human race. But it attenuates as we move further from the immediate; feeling and conception are replaced by principle and abstraction. There are limits to the possible inclusiveness of community.

Thus far the concept of community has been considered with respect to home and occupation. The increased speed and availability of world-wide transport has introduced new racial communities into Britain. In considering the significance of these within the wider community it is worthwhile considering the geographical locations from which the immigrants have come, and the life-styles to which they were formerly accustomed. Significant immigrant groups include Irish, West Indians, and Asians deriving very largely from North India. All of these groups largely come from extended family backgrounds. Indeed, from the Indian subcontinent, an immigrant family may come from a village setting where the entire village is a single social unit, consisting of several generations of the same family operating a joint economy with the father having absolute authority over his adult sons as long as he lives. Such a group has tremendous power over each individual member, and is characterised by a strong cultural uniformity. Whilst members conform they benefit greatly from the security provided by the group, with the unquestioned sharing by each with all, and by the powerful sense of belonging. At the same time the group exerts tremendous constraints and, of necessity, the cultural uniformity is consistent with a very parochial, narrow perspective on the part of the group. Thus, daughters who offend the taboos of, for example, the Sikh religion, may be punished by their families in a way which, while it is believed to be right by the Sikh community, is a criminal offence under British law. It is interesting to note how often teenagers of immigrant families which display social integration and are part of a local immigrant community prefer to support their parents' views on issues such as marriage and family, rather than those of the host community. Perhaps it is questionable whether in our legislation and our community health care policies towards immigrant groups in this country, we have taken enough account of the predictable characteristics of close-knit community groups such as many of our immigrant groups are.

Many immigrant groups are characterised by their religious affiliation, whilst statistics suggest that as a whole the British race has been progressively abandoning the traditional religion of the country, i.e. Christianity. (Frontier Youth Trust, 1976; Church Pastoral Aid Society, 1977). We are said to be living in a post-Christian era. Yet religions in themselves are a considerable force towards community, and generally require a high level of commitment from the members. The extent to which religions affect lives can be seen in a number of areas related to health care. The refusal of Jehovah's Witnesses to permit blood transfusion is familiar to any nurse. In meeting the dietary needs of sick people both food and cooking utensils have to be taken into account, with the need for kosher meat for the Jew and halal meat for the Muslim, for example. The religious necessity for the adult male Sikh to wear his turban conflicts with safety legislation requiring motor cyclists to wear crash helmets.

Like other strong communities, whilst religious communities provide benefits for the membership, they are inevitably exclusive as well as inclusive. Practically every major religion discourages marriage with partners of another faith, and in some religions the constraint is so severe that death is the penalty for the disobedient member.

It has been said that, with the growth of knowledge and scientific and technical progress, man no longer needs religion. However, it is a necessary consideration in a book on community health care on two counts. First, as has already been indicated, the individual committed to his religion is not concerned with the theoretical viewpoint of another that he does not need it, so it remains as a factor to be reckoned with. Second, far from dying out, in many parts of the world the major religions are increasing in membership.

The first type of community considered in this chapter was that of locality, as the community which historically has had the major influence on the lives of its members. The discussion at that point centred mainly on the breakdown of traditional local communities, and it was implied that the search for work and the meeting of material needs took precedence over the individual's social needs. However, there are exceptions to this pattern, and possibly even an alternative trend beginning. More and more groups seem to be experimenting with some form of communal living. Some groups have sought to abandon traditional family patterns and adopt the pattern of a commune, where a group of families live together and share their possessions and their responsibilities. There have been other modified forms of this kind of experiment. In some instances all the members of a particular community are also members of the same religious group. There are a number of communities in Britain, such as the Post Green Community in Dorset, which operate similarly to the joint family system in India. Under this system the life of the community comes first and, as far as possible, the needs of the individual are met by the community as a whole, which operates as a single economic unit. It is a caring community, which has a concern for the wider community in which it is placed. A number of local churches in Britain are beginning to follow the example of the Church of the Redeemer in Houston, Texas, where the choice of home and occupation for the members became part of their commitment to church membership. A family house would be chosen for its accessibility to the church rather than for its amenities. The church is committed to caring for local needs so that, for example, family homes expect to take in an extra member needing shelter or care during a crisis.

A different kind of move towards community has been attempted in what was a dying Welsh village. The villagers have turned themselves into a company, buying up houses so that young couples from the community have homes they can move into. They provide employment for 12 weavers and home knitters, and have set up a one man pottery in the doctor's garage. The resources for this achievement came from financial commitment within the community itself.

This chapter has sought to demonstrate the amorphous character of the community to which we all belong, and the intention has been to provoke thought and raise questions, rather than answering them. Do we have the right aims in relation to community health care? What level of participation in care should be expected or required from the community? What kind of national community should we be seeking to establish? Is it too late, and are we already helplessly in the grip of 'future shock', or is Le Chatelier's principle operating as increasing numbers of voluntarily formed communities begin to resist social disintegration? Your opinion is important, for in the words of John Donne (1571–1631):

> No man is an island, entire of itself... I am involved in mankind.

REFERENCES

Church Pastoral Aid Society 1977 The Nottingham Statement. The Second National Evangelical Anglican Congress
Daily Telegraph 1979 (27.8.79)
Department of Health and Social Security 1979 Report of the Royal Commission on the National Health Service. HMSO, London
Donne J 1571–1631 Devotions
Frontier Youth Trust 1976 Searching for values. Report of a study into youth and values
Minar D W, Greer S 1969 The concept of community. Butteworth, London
Ministry of Health 1966 Report of the Committee on Senior Nursing Staff Structure. (The Salmon Report). HMSO, London
Stengel E 1964 Suicide and attempted suicide. Penguin, Harmondsworth
Toffler A 1970 Future shock. Pan, London
West J 1973 The windmills of Kent. Skilton and Shaw, London

2

What is health?

Kate Robinson

It is usual to commence an essay of this type with an appeal to various dictionaries or thesauri for a 'correct' definition. Once we have consulted the appropriate tome, it is assumed, our definition will have substantive authority. Such an approach, however, mistakes the definition of the *word* for the analysis of the *concept*, and it is the concept that is important because it both reflects and shapes every aspect of health care, from the structure of the system to the daily interaction between health workers and clients. For anyone involved in designing, promoting or acting in a health care system the way in which the concept of health is understood will define the boundaries of her activity and set the goals of her policies.

Many different concepts of health have been proposed and practised, and perhaps the one statement that all participants in the debate would accept is that:

> health itself is not a precise or simple concept.
>
> Royal Commission on the National Health Service, 1979

The burgeoning 'what is health?' controversy has been nurtured by many different interests, including radical observers of the health scene and sociologists of health and illness. However, the participation of those actively involved in the provision of health care has emphasised one dimension of the debate, namely the implications of the practical application of any concept, They are concerned to use concepts to construct models of practice that can be used for the provision of health care. Much of this essentially practical, rather than theoretical, interest is generated by frustration at their apparent inability to affect significantly the health of particular groups of clients, primarily the chronic sick, the handicapped and the terminally ill.

For these professional workers seeking explanations for apparent failure and alternative programmes and policies, the adoption of new concepts of health around which to re-organise health care can seem very attractive, even seductive, particularly when the existing provision of health care is being eroded by government spending cuts. If we cannot progress along this road, it is argued, then let us choose a different destination. This is a much more radical approach than attempting a detour or using a different means of transport to reach the original destination. It involves abandoning that destination or goal as inadequate or irrelevant or impossible to achieve, and adopting a new goal and it is thus essentially an argument about ends and not about means.

Clearly it is important that the goals as well as the techniques and strategies of existing health care are open to continuous examination and evaluation, especially where the costs of that care are borne by the community as a whole. However, the consequences of re-aligning our entire health care system, especially in an era of zero growth, are profound and it would seem sensible, therefore, to examine very thoroughly any proposed model based on new concepts of health in order to discover its possible consequences, both intended and unintended. For the purposes of this discussion I will propose simply two opposing paradigms: a negative and a positive model of health. The negative model sees health as the absence of the constraint of illness. That is to say, you are healthy if you are not ill. For this model health and wellness are synonymous. The positive model sees health as the active management of life in a particular way. A specific pattern of living, if you like, that is equated with health. These two models may be seen as two successive stages, that is the removal of the constraint of illness may be necessary before the 'healthy' pattern of life is possible. But more usually, and more radically, it is claimed that the presence of a particular life pattern constitutes health *despite* the presence of disease or incapacity. This idea is particularly attractive to those who work, for instance, with the handicapped as it enables them to set health as the goal or achievable target despite the presence of an incurable handicapping condition.

Both these models have severe problems if one attempts to operationalise them in Britain today. Let us look first at the negative model.

It was widely assumed in 1948 when the National Health Service was established that 'health' was the opposite of illness, and illness was assumed to be synonymous with the presence of disease. The renewal of health in a diseased individual was the result of the removal of the disease, i.e. it can be expressed as the simple equation:

disease A + medical treatment a = health.

The problems involved were, therefore, firstly the correct diagnosis of disease A, and secondly the discovery or development of treatment a. These were difficult problems, certainly, but capable of solution by the 'holy' alliance of doctors and scientists. The major problem and the major area of controversy was considered to be achieving equality of access to treatment, and this was a financial and logistical problem.

Murcott (1979) reminds us that this was not the only available model around which to construct the National Health Service. It was inevitable, however, that such a model would be used, not only because the medical profession was based on such a model, but also because it fitted the whole character of the welfare state, which was not a revolutionary institution but rather a bureaucratic rationalisation of existing individualised services. The essential fabric of society was assumed to be satisfactory provided that protection could be extended to individuals against particular catstrophies. Thus sickness, like poverty or unemployment, was viewed as a potentially transient individual phenomena, and the scientific administration of services would conquer sickness as it would conquer poverty. This view owed much to the advances in medical science during the 19th and 20th centuries and the achievements in surgical technique and antibiotic therapy showed that such an approach could have spectacular results. However, the preventive personal and environmental services which had also produced very significant results received relatively little emphasis.

Thus the 'health' services of this country are primarily designed to cope with those who are ill.

Before mentioning the problems inherent in this model it is worth emphasising that for very many individuals this approach had been an unmitigated blessing: for the many people with cancers healed by surgery; for those with cataracts removed and sight restored; for those whose broken bones have been set and deformity avoided; all these and many more successes can provide a vigorous and justifiable defence of this 'negative' model. In viewing its deficiencies and judging it against other models we must not become blind to its achievements.

Not least of the problems of this model, however, is that the relationship between illness and disease is a complex one: doctors diagnose disease but people feel ill. Because people generally have to feel 'ill' before they refer themselves to a doctor many cases of disease are not seen by doctors, at least in the early stages, and consequently do not receive medical treatment, although they may be treated in other ways by other people. Similarly, many people feel 'ill' but the doctor may be unable to define their problem in terms of the disease states that he understands, and may therefore either offer no help or prescribe a placebo or treatments related to the separate symptoms.

Because of their increasing sophistication, scientific aids to diagnosis have rapidly reached the status of determinants of diagnosis rather than aids. Treatments are directed towards the scientifically defined symptom rather than towards the person as a whole. Thus, one is presented with the macabre spectacle of patients being discharged as 'cured' because their haemoglobin or blood pressure is now within 'normal' limits, despite the fact that they still complain of the feelings of illness that first took them to the doctor. Because of the mechanistic nature of this model of illness and because related expectations of cure have increased dramatically doctors find it hard to sustain interest in patients for whom a cure will not be possible. Either they refuse to admit the possibility of failure and turn to increasingly bizzarre remedies, or they attempt to pass the patient out of the system.

However, care as well as cure is a legitimate response to illness and can equally rest on the knowledge base of a 'sickness-oriented' training. Where care is required other than in relation to sickness, for instance for the mentally handicapped, the health service has traditionally provided assistance in the absence of any other source. However, this situation is changing with the increasing emphasis on care in the community and the Jay Report (1979) in particular, in advocating the removal of responsibility for the training of staff to care for the mentally handicapped from the General Nursing Council, emphasises the finite relationship between the provision of health care and sickness rather than welfare needs in general.

Thus, although the specific medical emphasis on the scientific definition of disease and on cure at all costs has distorted the current use of the illness/wellness model, it is not necessary to abandon all notions of treating illness in order to help those whom the National Health Service currently neglects. Those with chronic illness and degenerative disorders are sick and they can be aided provided that 'care' as well as 'cure' is admitted as legitimate treatment.

Similarly, the recent and timely emphasis on prevention of illness is not necessarily incompatible with this model, although financial competition sometimes encourages the view that it is. Advocates of prevention are divided into two camps: those concentrating on personal responsibilities and those concerned with wider environmental problems. The former school has been eagerly embraced by government policy makers (HMSO 1976) seeking relief from demands on the National Health Service in the transference of the consumer's role from victim to agent of his own misfortune. Although this argument has a certain libertarian attraction it ignores the obvious: that man lives inside a closely regulated framework and we are not free agents but have our choices largely circumscribed by the economic necessities of our society.

In any case we must note that such individualised preventive measures are based largely on preventing illness; which is a negative approach and not the giant step for mankind that some would have us believe. We must give up smoking to avoid cancer; butter to avoid coronaries; variety in sexual partners to avoid venereal disease.

Some of the environmentalists can be equally disease oriented. Lead pollution causes mental handicap, road traffic causes accidents; and this is the sole reason for their avoidance. Thus the link with sickness remains. However this relationship between disease and the environment has been developed into a more radical critique of the relationship between illness and modern industrial, and more specifically modern capitalist, society. Such a critique is not concerned merely with the connections between specific environmental factors and specific diseases but with the relevance to capitalism of a disease-free labour force, the supremacy of profit over health, and the relationship between health care and the private suppliers of plant, pharmaceuticals, etc.

This critique is a very telling and relevant one but clearly it points not to minor changes in orientation of the health care system, nor indeed to a major revision of the system, but to a reconstruction of society. Doyal (1979) concludes:

> 'any preventive medecine which was to be substantially effective, would need to interfere with the organisation of the productive process itself.'

Thus for health care workers seeking new orientations to practise it could lead not to less frustration but to more.

If we now examine other radical alternatives to the illness/wellness continuum we find that many reject any equation of health with the absence of disease and thus belong to the second of our opposing paradigms: positive health.

Probably the most widely known of such models is that of the World Health Organisation (1948), which defines health as:

> a state of complete physical, mental and social well-being and not merely the absence of disease or infirmity.

This definition explicitly states the assumptions of the whole group, who are in many ways a very diverse collection of propagandists, that to be healthy means something more or something different from just not being ill. The healthy individual is one who is in some undefined way fulfilled; who enjoys life; who ex- experiences wellbeing. Wilson (1975) has echoed this call to fulfilment with an emphasis on spiritual values, absent from the World Health Organistation definition.

These themes have also been pursued in government publications like the Court Report (DHSS, 1976) and publications by health care professionals like the 'Investigation into the Principles of Health Visiting' (Council for the Education and Training of Health Visitors, 1977). The former document rather tritely avoids the not inconsiderable question of what they consider child health to be by quoting from Katherine Mansfield:

> By health, I mean the power to live a full, adult breathing life in close contact with what I love — I want to be all that I am capable of becoming.

Unfortunately, this seems to have set a precedent, for the latter document, which devotes a whole chapter to considering health as a value, continues to discuss health in the context of practical health care as the achievement of full potential in all aspects of being, physical, emotional, social, intellectual and spiritual.

While no-one in this enlightened age would wish to deny fulfilment to any individual, we will see that such definitions only avoid the real problems of conflict between individual goals and community goals and of considering the nature of the contribution health services can offer. It may be inevitable that such definitions are expansive and ill-defined because their purpose is not to provide a working definition on which to base practice, but to define an area of life as 'belonging to' a professional group. Clearly one purpose of defining an area of life is to lay claim to it, to propose that one has special knowledge of its problems and therefore special rights to offer solutions. One can see this process operating between different branches of the medical profession and between the medical profession and other related occupational groups. For instance, the attempts to define childbirth as either a medical problem or a natural process can be seen as a dispute between rival claimants for power over a client group (Donnison, 1977).

However, the most forceful promoters of 'health imperialism', that is the expansion of health care practice into areas of life that were not previously defined as containing specifically *health* problems, seem not to be the doctors, the traditional targets of criticism on this score, but rather the nurses and other paramedical workers. Perhaps they have found that it is easier to expand into lay areas of expertise rather than challenge the doctors in the medical sphere. The health visitors' self-defined sphere of influence, for instance, seems to be rapidly expanding to encompass all of life; if health visitors have an interest in health and nothing falls outside the boundaries of health as they define it, then literally 'by definition' their work can be all encompassing.

Advocates of this positive view of health tend to concentrate on an idividualistic or an environmentalistic approach.

The environmentalistic approach relates closely to the radical critique of health in relation to modern society except that it emphasises that the sickness producing aspects of society relate not to any specific relationship between people and production but rather to any and every large-scale production. Thus advocates of this view cannot envisage any society in which technological progress can be harnessed for the benefit of people's health and must be detrimental; so any advanced industrial society is 'sick'.

Obviously there are degrees of radicalism within this viewpoint and certainly the rejection of any nuclear technology seems to be a growing trend. However, the logical consequences of this view involves a reversion to a pre-industrial society and the rejection of high technology. Mucking out cows becomes implicitly healthier than tuning a car engine. Presumably advocates of this 'green revolution' must accept a 'green medicine'* which not only rejects intensive care units and coronary care units but also large-scale production of antibiotics, anaesthetics, insulin, vitamins etc. and I wonder how many of us would care to get sick in such a society — and cows can cause nasty accidents! Some political commentators have seen this ecology lobby as the leading revolutionary influence of the 1980s but it is hard to see how the National Health Service could or should be leaders in the revolution.

However, this evangelical mission can also be practised on an individual basis, and is of particular interest because it is currently being debated and promoted by some community health workers. A striking example of this debate can be found in the 'Health Visitor', the official publication of the Health Visitor Association. Connolly, in her article 'Definition of health' (Connolly, 1978) discusses the problems of producing a workable definition of health to replace the medical mechanistic model. But Lesley Capel in her reply 'Yet Another Definition of Health' (Capel, 1979) goes further and offers a definition for consideration:

> a fundamental state of well-being periodically and fleetingly experienced during the dynamic process of environmental interaction and personal development.

By using this definition Capel agrees that she equates health with happiness, but as she dislikes the idea of being known as a 'happiness visitor' she will continue to be a 'health visitor'. Such implications of belonging to a profession dedicated to promoting happiness for all need to be examined closely before such a definition is taken up more widely. What would be the consequences of the adoption of this model for the profession, for the client and for the health service as a whole?

One of the major problems would seem to be how 'happiness' or 'fullness of life' is to be defined and by whom? Michael Wilson defines the health goal as 'what a people believes to be fullness of life' (Wilson, 1975). However, in Britain today, we are not 'a people', we are divided in many ways: by class, by culture and by ethnic group, and we probably have nearly as many concepts of fullness of life as there are individuals. One man's fulfilling life-style is not necessarily another's and indeed the state already intervenes to prevent the adoption of certain routes to fulfilment, for instance a drug enhanced route is illegal in many western countries.

A more profound problem, however, lies in the framework for individual activity laid down by the structure of capitalist society. If our current way of life demands that many people suffer unnecessary disease through accidents and stress, then the message of a health worker advocating a healthy lifestyle becomes either irrelevant or insulting. Indeed it could be argued that by urging the individual to

---

* I am indebted to Robert Dingwall for his help in preparing this paper, and particularly for this very evocative phrase.

adapt to prevailing conditions the health worker is reducing the likelihood of change in the level of disease-inducing factors in the environment. Thus the emphasis on 'positive' health will increase the necessity for 'negative' health care interventions.

A practical application of this positive model can be seen in an interesting booklet produced by John W. Travis (1977) of the Wellness Resource Centre. His *Wellness Inventory* contains a self-administered questionaire which readers can use to assess their wellness, and identifies the activities of life he equates with high level wellness. Many of the elements of the questionnaire relate to obvious ways of avoiding disease. One section, for example, relates to physical activity and you score points for agreeing that 'I climb stairs rather than ride elevators'. But the other sections are more contentious. To score really well you must also be able to claim that you vote regularly, have at least five friends and recycle papers, cans, glass, clothing, books and organic waste. These may well be good and useful things to do, but the implication behind their inclusion in any health questionnaire is that if don't do them, you are unhealthy and in our society if you are unhealthy you should seek the aid of health care personnel. Already health care workers are claiming expert knowledge and jurisdiction over areas of life previously held to be private. Health visitors and midwives would almost certainly consider it their business if you could not agree honestly with statement 99: 'I respect my child as an evolving, growing being' and many would be interested in your reply to statement 77: 'I like myself and look forward to the future.'

Although one might welcome in theory the sort of self-assessment being encouraged in this Wellness Inventory, the intervention of health service personnel in promoting such assessment or providing solutions to the problems discovered is a different matter. It represents an unwarranted expansion by the health services into essentially moral and political areas of life. Perhaps people do need help with these areas of life but many sources of help already exist, outwith the health services. In any case, expansion into morality and politics tends to lead to more problems, not less. As clients already expect cure for physical complaints they come to expect cure for these other 'ailments' and clearly such individual cures to essentially social problems do not exist. However, health workers trained in individualistic health care may seek solutions on individual psychology and individual weaknesses.

However, if such a radical model of health is to be widely promoted by existing health service personnel it is important to examine first how to train such personnel and how to avoid increased dependence on health service intervention by the clients.

The first problem is exactly that discovered by the Jay Committee (1979) when it was found that the sickness orientation of the nursing training could not be eradicated despite a verbal commitment to other models and goals. This could be circumvented by an entirely new training scheme to produce a positive health care worker though there is little evidence of a shortage of people to offer well-being to the populace.

The second problem must arise when clients are unable to make subtle distinctions between the health workers who are interested in their happiness and those more interested in their disease. The two would become inextricably entwined and clients would increasingly seek traditional health care solutions to emotional and social problems

It is easy to become enthusiastic about new models of health care based on different concepts of health which offer new challenges and new goals. However it is essential to examine the relationship between any proposed health care system and an historically discreet set of circumstances and relations between man and his environment. While the present system can be criticised for concentrating on the medical model and neglecting both the causes of disease and wider definitions of illness, it may not be possible for appropriate change to be generated by those working in the existing system without reference to wider economic and social issues.

The most attractive critiques relate health not to individual activity but to the way society is organised and this is clearly not amenable to change from inside the health care system. The danger is that, because the causes of ill-health are economic and social but the techniques and practices of health workers are individualistic, the results of attempts to change will be a kind of individualised environmentalism which inevitably puts the emphasis on micro-social and psychological factors in the absence of any ability on the part of the client or health worker to effect anything else.

REFERENCES

Capel L 1979 Yet another definition of health. Health Visitor 52: 3
Connolly P 1978 Definition of health. Health Visitor 51: 12
Council for the Education & Training of Health Visitors 1977 An investigation into the principles of health visiting. CETHV, London
Davis A G 1979 An equivocal change of policy: Prevention health and medical sociology. Social Science and Medicine 13A
Department of Health and Social Security 1976 Report of the Committee on Child Health Services. (The Court Report). HMSO, London
Department of Health and Social Security 1979 Report of the Royal Commission on the National Health Service. HMSO, London
Department of Health and Social Security 1979 Report of the Committee of Enquiry into Mental Handicap Nursing & Care. (The Jay Report) HMSO, London
Donnison J 1977 Midwives and medical men. Heinemann, London
Doyal L 1979 Political economy of health. Pluto Press, London
Murcott A 1979 Health as ideology. In: Atkinson, Dingwall, Murcott (eds) Prospects for the national health. Croom Helm, London
Strong P M, 1979 Sociological imperialism and the profession of medicine. Social Science and Medicine 13A
Travis J W 1977 Wellness inventory. Wellness Resource Centre, USA
Wilson M 1975 Health is for people. Darton, Longman & Todd, London
World Health Organisation 1948 The Constitution. World Health Organisation, Geneva

FURTHER READING

Atkinson, Dingwall, Murcott (eds) 1979 Prospects for the National Health. Croom Helm, London
Lesley Doyal 1979 The political economy of health. Pluto Press, London
Social Science Research Council 1977 Health and health policy. SSRC
David Tuckett (ed) 1976 An introduction to medical sociology. Tavistock, London

3

Concepts of prevention

Jenny Griffiths, John Dennis, Peter Draper and Jennie Popay

INTRODUCTION

In recent years the word 'prevention' has become much more prominent, not least in the vocabulary of those working in the health and social services. The need for greater investment in the prevention of illness has been stated in various government publications, for example 'Prevention and health: everybody's business' (DHSS, 1976a), and the White Paper, *Prevention and Health* (DHSS, 1977). The 1979 report of the Royal Commission on the National Health Service (NHS) regretted 'that more emphasis has not been placed in the past on the preventive role of the NHS. This must change if there are to be substantial improvements in health in the future' (Royal Commission, 1979).

This increased interest in prevention has been stimulated by growing doubts internationally whether the extensive and expensive provision of highly technological and specialised treatment services is the best means of achieving progress in health. The costs of such services are continually rising (for example, in the UK, since 1949 total expenditure on the NHS in real terms has more than doubled—Royal Commission, 1979), while at the same time there are diminishing returns in terms of decreased mortality and morbidity. Life expectancy has scarcely altered in economically developed countries over the last 30 years or so — the period which has seen the mushrooming of modern scientific medicine. This is not to argue that health services are unimportant. Furthermore, although the statistics quoted above may appear worrying, the NHS has avoided the worst excesses of health care provision in other countries. In particular, it has maintained a comparatively high commitment to caring (as opposed to treatment) services and, as we shall see, to preventive services.

Concern about the imbalance between resources devoted to the treatment of disease and to its prevention has also been supported by recent work demonstrating that the major improvements in health over the past century or so occurred before the advent of modern scientific medicine — with the lesson that public health measures, such as improved nutrition, housing and sanitation, were more efficacious (see McKeown, 1976). The great differences in health status between social groups also suggest that health services are not the sole determinants of health. In England and Wales, for example, the standardised mortality ratio of males aged 15–64 in 1970–72 for deaths from all causes ranged from 77 for social class I (professional) to 137 for social class V (unskilled) (Royal Commission,

1979). Such discrepancies have also been shown in other countries and are very relevant to preventive activity.

Finally, much of modern scientific medicine is tangential to the current health problems of developed countries. The major killers include cancer, for which, with a few exceptions, little effective treatment exists, heart disease and other chronic degenerative conditions. The rising incidence of chronic diseases is associated with the increasing number of elderly people (for example, those over 65 now comprise almost 15% of the UK population and occupy almost half of the non-psychiatric hospital beds in the NHS). Furthermore, much of this disease burden is preventable: much cancer is of environmental origin, and factors such as obesity, smoking and stress have been implicated in the causation of heart disease.

It can be argued that there are two markedly differing approaches to prevention: one tries to influence what might be termed 'personal health', while the other attempts to promote 'public health'. This chapter will attempt to demonstrate some common inadequacies in the 'personal health' approach and the need for complementary activities of a 'public health' kind.

THE 'PERSONAL HEALTH' CONCEPT OF PREVENTION

Preventive medicine is traditionally divided into three types: *primary prevention*, which takes measures to prevent accidents, disease or illness ever occurring; *secondary prevention*, which tries to diminish the effects of accidents or disease by early intervention; and *tertiary prevention*, which is concerned with minimising the disability arising out of existing disease or injury. This classification is often used by those who see the separation of curative from preventive medicine as artificial. From this perspective, almost any health care can be interpreted as preventive in some sense. For example, the treatment of haemophilia in specialist hospital units can be seen as preventing 'death; disability and handicap; educational problems, by minimising school absences; unemployment; and family breakdown' (Gray, 1979). In other words, such treatment is tertiary prevention for the patient, and primary prevention for relatives and friends. There is, of course, much justification in viewing prevention and treatment as a continuum. But the key word here is preventive *medicine* — prevention is seen as an adjunct of the clinical medical services directed at individuals.

This individualistic, or 'personal health' approach to prevention has underpinned the development this century of preventive health services and, more recently, health education. These will now be examined briefly in turn.

Personal health services

The NHS delivers a wide range of personal preventive health services. Their inception dates from concern about the appallingly high rates of infant and maternal mortality at the beginning of this century which led to the development of health visiting, of ante-natal and child welfare clinics, of school health services, and of vaccination and immunisation services. More recent developments include post-natal services, a birth control service, and screening programmes to enable the early diagnosis and treatment of disease.

These services span, in varying degrees, primary, secondary and tertiary prevention as defined above. The responsibility for their planning and evaluation lies with community physicians working in the NHS. The actual delivery of the services is carried out most obviously by clinical medical officers, birth control doctors and health visitors, and less visibly by general practitioners, district nurses and others. Preventive services have become part of the wide range of health services provided by the NHS, and thus tend to be seen as supportive to what is viewed as its major task — the treatment of existing disease and injury. In common with other 'neglected sectors' such as the elderly or the mentally ill or handicapped, preventive health services tend to lack finance and manpower. For example, the rate of increase in the number of health visitors has not been as great as that for hospital nursing staff. Preventive services require more resources, more research and greater consideration of how to tackle the very real problems of more effective delivery and increased accessibility for those in most need.

The importance of such services cannot be denied, though their contribution to improvements in health is difficult to measure. For example, preventive services were undoubtedly a factor in the decline in infant mortality from 142 per 1000 live births in 1900 to 59 per 1000 live births by 1940 (CSO, 1974). But much of this decline must be ascribed to wider changes in the social and economic environment.

One of the founding principles of the NHS was the aim of equalising the provision of services, and efforts at discrimination in favour of the socially deprived have continued ever since 1949 — though with varying vigour — the latest being action arising from the report of the Resource Allocation Working Party (DHSS, 1976b). However, such attempts at re-distribution of health services have not satisfied those who believe that services *per se* do not tackle the root causes of differences in health status — poverty, poor living and working conditions, amongst other factors. This subject will be returned to later.

Health education

As presently organised, health education is a comparatively recent innovation. The Health Education Council (HEC) for England, Wales and Northern Ireland, and the Scottish Health Education Unit (now the Scottish Health Education Group), were both set up in 1968. Their work consists of launching national initiatives, (for example, the HEC's 'Look after yourself' campaign), and of providing support for health educators in the field (including schools) particularly in the form of booklets, leaflets, posters and similar material. From the reorganisation of the NHS in 1974 to that in 1982, health education officers (HEOs) were appointed at Area and District levels. However, there is a shortage of suitable staff and six areas in England had no HEOs at all in 1978–9 (Royal Commission, 1979). What will happen following the April 1982 reorganisation is not yet certain. In addition to this formal structure, it is important to remember that health education has also been and still is carried out informally by a range of health workers, from general practitioners to health visitors.

Until recently, it was the unquestioned, underlying philosophy of health education that the individual bears the burden of responsibility for his or her own health. Statements such as the following are typical: 'to a large extent . . . it is clear that the weight of responsibility for his own state of health lies on the shoulders of the individual himself. The smoking related diseases, alcoholism and other drug dependencies, obesity and its consequences, and the sexually transmitted diseases are among the preventable problems of our time and in relation to all of these the individual must choose for himself' (DHSS, 1976a). In other words, the thesis is that much ill health results from individual and freely chosen patterns of behaviour and lifestyles. This philosophy tends to find its expression in a series of 'do's and don'ts' — don't smoke, don't drink and drive, do take more exercise, and so on. Such instructions are particularly directed at those in social classes IV and V who are seen as being less reponsible than those further up the social ladder.

The early pioneers of health education believed that simply giving people the facts, for example, about the damaging consequences of smoking, would be sufficient. However, it was gradually realised that exhortation and appeals to 'common sense' alone did not seem to work — at least, not quickly. Health education has therefore shifted its emphasis towards behavioural change through persuasion and propaganda. This is reflected in campaigns and publicity using the mass media which try to beat the purveyors of lethal goods such as cigarettes and alcohol at their own game, using the psychological techniques of commercial advertising agencies. But quite apart form reservations about 'social engineering', even for health reasons, it is the mouse trying to fight the mammoth: in 1976 about £½ million was spent on education about the dangers of alcohol in comparison with the £36 million spent on its promotion.

However, there is another cause for concern. Health education directed at individuals is being increasingly criticised, by health educators themselves as well as others, as being misplaced in its objectives, and for provoking unnecessary guilt and anxiety. At worst, it can be characterised as 'blaming the victim', at best, as 'preaching to the victim'. 'By focusing on behaviour itself, health educators do not deal with the social relations and structures that may underlie and contribute to the behaviour patterns they find objectionable and the disease they wish to prevent. The alienation of people from their bodies, stressful working conditions and inadequate nutrition due to insufficient income or inadequate food supply, are ignored' (Brown & Margo, 1978). Freudenberg (1978) expressed his reservations about behaviour shaping even more forcibly: 'to attempt to change individual behaviour without changing the forces that determine that behaviour is like treating symptoms while the patient dies'. No-one would deny that individually-determined behaviour contributes to health and disease. *Education* (in the sense of the provision of information rather than persuasion) about healthy and unhealthy habits, about body and mind, how they work and how to look after them, is obviously important. However, the approaches to prevention hitherto discussed do not go far enough. They typically ignore the social and economic processes and structures which damage health.

The word 'environment' has been mentioned several times in this chapter. A serious and committed policy of prevention must tackle the hazards to health in the wider environment — social, political and economic as well as physical. By ignoring the health-damaging nature of the wider environment, those working in prevention are effectively beating their heads against an insurmountable wall. Or, to change metaphors, they are doing what Zola (1974) has characterised as attempting to save an increasing number of people drowning in a river without refocusing upstream in an attempt to prevent them from falling (or being pushed) into the water in the first place (USHP, 1979). Much unhealthy behaviour is strongly shaped by influences external to the individual.

THE 'PUBLIC HEALTH' CONCEPT OF PREVENTION

Contemporary campaigners for prevention have a great deal to learn from the social history of public health — the 19th century public health movement. The pioneers of public health — Edwin Chadwick, Sir John Simon and others — were among the first to argue that environmental issues must be tackled. For a variety of reasons they fought long and hard against vested interests, both public and private, to secure the legislation — and the expenditure required to implement it — which has remained the bedrock of prevention. A crucial role in the public health movement was played by some of the Medical Officers of Health (MOsH) who were conceived of as the protectors and promoters of the health of the local authority population. Their work was by definition controversial, and it is important to note that their employment was protected so that dismissal would not be the reward for 'constructive trouble-making for health'. The MOH was, in a way, the 'guardian of the public health', and it is this type of watchdog and campaigning activity that is so lacking in prevention today. The absorption of the MOH at the time of the NHS reorganisation in 1974 can be regarded as having put the final nail in the coffin of public health.

This 'public health' concept of prevention focuses on the environment rather than individuals. 'In some respects our environment today is healthier than it has ever been' (DHSS, 1976a). Up to a point this is a valid statement. The concept of *prevention through legislation* to protect the individual from the worst excesses of the environment has a long and respectable history. From the mid-19th century onwards there has been a continuous stream of measures coming on to the statute book dealing with a whole range of health hazards: the prevention of infectious diseases; road safety; health and safety at work; standards for food, drugs and other consumer goods and so on. These laws are enforced by Environmental Health Officers working for local authorities (successors to the public health inspectors who used to work under the Medical Officer of Health), the police, trade union representatives and others. (A good summary of the role of law in prevention is given in Gray, 1979 Ch. 6.)

But the existence of such regulations to remove or reduce some of the health-damaging effects of the wider environment is too often taken as a justification for complacency today. In some respects the environment is *still* significantly unhealthy. An important point about contemporary hazards to health is that their causes often extend beyond the 'physical' environment (as usually defined) to the social, political and economic environment. Additionally, some of them (for example, asbestos) are more difficult to detect than hazards in the past. Some examples from agriculture, transport, employment and smoking will perhaps help to make the nature of such hazards clear.

Debates (and action) about agricultural and food policy tend to be dominated by questions of price, neglecting the nutritional implications of wider policies and practices (including those of the EEC) such as taxation and subsidies. For example, the 7% increase in butter consumption in the UK between 1973 and 1974 was at least partly related to the EEC retail subsidy introduced in 1973 which lowered the price of butter. Again, no-one really *knows* what the *long-term* effects will be of the 1500 chemical pesticides in use and the 7500 chemicals added to foodstuffs. Finally, attention is not paid to the availability of healthy foods — genuine wholemeal bread is often difficult to obtain — whilst checkout points in supermarkets (places of particular stress for parents) have prominent displays of confectionery.

To take another illustration, despite existing road safety legislation there are approximately one quarter of a million road accidents in Britain every year. These kill about 6500 people a year — on average, over 17 people a *day* — and seriously injure another 70–80 000 each year (CSO, 1977). More safety legislation, for example to make the use of seat belts compulsory, cannot remove all this carnage. This is not just a question of the relative use of safer and less energy-consuming modes of transport, such as buses, rail and waterways, there is much more transport overall than is necessary. The health costs of present transport policies should not, however, be measured in terms of accidents alone. For example, there has been a growing volume of evidence accumulating over many years showing impaired mental function in children exposed to lead levels below the present official 'safe' standard and relating this to atmospheric lead from petrol (see Needleman et al, 1979). Other countries have been sufficiently convinced of the dangers to strictly limit lead levels. Yet the UK government insisted until recently that the case was not strong enough to justify reducing the lead content of petrol. For these and other reasons, the ever-increasing transportation of goods and people by road does not make sense in health terms, any more than it does in terms of the prudent use of oil resources.

To turn to the area of work, involuntary *unemployment* is a serious and neglected threat to health (Draper et al, 1979). It has been shown that a 1% increase in the unemployment rate in America sustained over a period of six years 'has been associated . . . with increases of approximately 36 887 total deaths' from , for example, heart attacks, cirrhosis and suicide (Brenner, 1976). On the other side of the coin are the risks to health posed by some types of *employment*. British statistics suggest that 600–700 workers die each year as a result of industrial accidents (CSO, 1977). Less obvious, but equally important, is the impact of boring, stressful and alienating work on mental health, on the consumption of socially acceptable tranquillisers such as tobacco and alcohol, and thus indirectly on mortality from, for example, heart disease.

As a final example of pressures from the wider environment over which the individual has little control, the subject of smoking merits closer examination. Smoking is widely seen as a self-imposed risk, a personal addiction which it is the individual's responsibility to remove. Yet in the words of a recent report from the World Health Organization on smoking control (1979): 'It must be recognised that the tobacco industry has presented, and will continue to present, a formidable barrier to smoking control . . . no worthwhile progress can be achieved unless governments are prepared to put the interests of public health before those of private tobacco enterprise . . . The international tobacco industry's promotional campaigns are . . . direct causes of a substantial number of unnecessary deaths'. It is widely suspected that the relatively tough approach to the tobacco industry adopted by Sir George Young, the former Parliamentary Under-Secretary for Health, will not be sustained. In any case his successor will have to reckon with 'his cautious officials in the Department of Health and Social Security' (Lancet, 1979), whose present approach is based on 'education and persuasion of the individual and co-operation with the tobacco industry' (DHSS, 1977). Such 'co-operation' has extended to subsidising the establishment of tobacco factories to the level of no less than £30m between 1972 and 1979 (House of Lords, 1979).

Of course, the obstacles to a vigorous attack on tobacco consumption are considerable. Tobacco factories employ 30 000 people and many more are involved in one way or another in its promotion in the UK alone; the implications globally for the many countries producing tobacco are immense. Equally, the press is highly dependent on advertising revenue. (Dr David Owen, when Minister of Health, said that his major worry about banning cigarette advertising was the effect this might have had on some national newspapers because of the precarious financial state of the press. But these challenges must be faced and overcome. In this sense, prevention is *not* taken seriously, and a *Guardian* leader-writer was more than justified in commenting on the Report of the Royal Commission on the NHS: 'For not perceiving that even the DHSS has yet to become committed to preventive health, the Commission deserves some scorn. It has dug far too shallowly into departmental politics' (*Guardian*, 1979).

Prevention is not taken seriously because the health implications of other economic policies are neglected. The confused thinking of governments regarding smoking and the tobacco industry is but one illustration of this. Tobacco manufacturing contributes to 'jobs' and to the Gross National Product. As long as economic policy is obsessed by the desire to increase economic 'growth', 'policies designed to boost the total output of the economy may well mean greater production and consumption of health-damaging products — tobacco, alcohol, sugar and other refined carbohydrates and so on' (USHP, 1979).

There are perhaps even more compelling reasons why the current preoccupation with indiscriminate economic activity is in some respects lethal. Recent events have underlined the inevitability of serious and lasting oil shortages. But ecological issues in general, from dangerous pollution to the wiser use of finite resources, will have to be addressed if mankind is to survive — and survive with a reasonable quality of life. Marc Lalonde, as Canadian Minister of Health, challenged everyone working in health to consider what he saw as being:

> . . . the fundamental determinants of our health. I am thinking of the ecological, energy and resource limitations of this planet . . . I know this matter goes well beyond the normal terms of reference of the health professional . . . but as people who are manifestly concerned about the well-being of their fellow-men and women, I would urge you to extend your mandate to future generations and to support the analysis and action necessary to ensure their survival.
>
> Lalonde, 1977

PREVENTION, PUBLIC HEALTH AND SOCIAL CHANGE

The purpose of this chapter is to examine various approaches to prevention at the conceptual, rather than the practical, level. However, the issues raised in the previous section are wide-ranging and complex, and we would not wish to leave readers feeling overwhelmed and powerless in the face of the might of social, political and economic forces — apart from any other reason, they might take to smoking and excessive drinking! Though this chapter has argued that an effective policy of prevention must take account of environmental issues beyond the control of any *one* individual, individuals (and especially health workers acting together) *can* do much to contribute to the social changes necessary to make effective prevention a reality.

First, it is encouraging to note that changes in a health-promoting direction *are* taking place. For example, the Department of Energy's 'Save-It' campaign was based on the revolutionary idea that more consumption is *not* for the best. And other things being equal, less energy produced and consumed means less pollution. In the area of employment, workers at the Lucas Aerospace Factories when threatened with redundancy put forward a plan for alternative socially-useful work for the labour force (Elliott, 1977). In addition, in the last few years there has been a notable growth in the ecology movement, including the foundation of the Ecology Party, an umbrella group called the 'Green Alliance' and ecological groups in all three major political parties. (To some extent, 'human ecology' is simply another name for wise living in a sane environment — for 'public health'.)

So how can health workers interested in prevention contribute to what might be called the creation of a 'contemporary public health movement'? Perhaps the most important thing is not to fear opposition or initial failure. The 'great' Public Health Act of 1875, the Clean Air Act, or the birth control legislation would not have been enacted without persistence and dedication. Essentially, this implies a recognition that prevention is about social change and is therefore political — though not in the 'party political' sense. As the Council for the Education and Training of Health Visitors put it: 'If it is accepted that health is of value and worthy of achievement, then the health visiting profession has a responsibility to influence policies that affect health and in order to achieve this, health visitors will have to engage in political activity.' (CETHV, 1977). All health workers can contribute to creating a wider public awareness of issues of *health* policy. It is vital to destroy the myth that high-technology treatment *services* are the major determinants of health — a myth that is still daily propounded by the mass media.

At this point, interested readers may well be asking themselves what connection all this has with their day-to-day work visiting families, working in clinics or the GP's surgery. But this continual contact with people has great potential for 'grass-roots' preventive activity. Firstly, health workers can act as enablers and facilitators. As Brown & Margo (1978) argue, they could: 'provide the means for people to examine the social bases of their work and lives for unhealthful conditions *and* help them learn tools to change these conditions. This is a substantially different role than putting complete responsibility on the individual to change unhealthful behaviour . . . (The role of health staff should) be to help people challenge health-damaging conditions in their communities and workplaces and to work towards health-promoting conditions.'

Secondly, and this is also a means of achieving the objectives described above, there is a need for increased contact between people with a preventive outlook and commitment. The interest of some groups has already been mentioned, such as health visitors, health education officers and environmental health officers. But community nurses, community physicians, general practitioners, social workers, workers in community development, Community Health Councillors and many others are all involved at the interface between the health and other social problems of the individual and the wider environment. Increased communication and co-operation can only be beneficial to the local community and to such professionals themselves. Community initiatives for prevention, often lying dormant just beneath the surface of normal social intercourse, can also gain immensely from collaboration between health workers and local organisations, such as neighbourhood councils, law centres, tenants' associations or trade union branches. The possibilities are enormous — and it is important to realise that, whilst institutional changes are needed, much collaboration and communication does not necessarily require formalised structures*.

This chapter can only scratch the surface of a wide and complex subject. But concepts are ideas, and ideas should stimulate thought and action. It is positive thought and constructive action that are required if we are to make effective prevention a reality, to achieve a renaissance in public health.

REFERENCES

Brenner H 1976 Estimating the social costs of national economic policy. US Government Printing Office, Washington

Brown E R, Margo G E 1978 Health education: can the reformers be reformed? International Journal of Health Services 8(1): 3–26

Central Statistical Office 1974 Annual Abstract of Statistics. HMSO, London

Central Statistical Office 1977 Annual Abstract of Statistics. HMSO, London

Council for the Education & Training of Health Visitors 1977 An investigation into the principles of health visiting. CETHV, London

Department of Health and Social Security 1976a Prevention and health: everybody's business. HMSO, London

Department of Health and Social Security 1976b Sharing resources for health in England. Report of the Resource Allocation Working Party (RAWP). HMSO, London

Department of Health and Social Security 1977 Prevention and health. Cmnd 7047. HMSO, London

Draper P, Dennis J, Griffiths J, Partridge J, Popay J 1979 Micro-processors, macro-economic policy, and public health. Lancet 1: 373–374

Elliott D 1977 The Lucas Aerospace workers compaign. Fabian Tract, Fabian Society, London

Freudenberg N 1978 Shaping the future of health education: from behavior change to social change. Paper prepared for presentation at annual meeting of Society for Public Health Education, Los Angeles, California

Gray J A M 1979 Man against disease: preventive medicine. Oxford University Press, Oxford

Guardian 1979 Can the State give a nation health? July 19, p 14

House of Lords 1979 Hansard, 7th February. HMSO, London

Lalonde M 1977 Beyond a new perspective. American Journal of Public Health 67: 357–360

---

* The reader is referred to 'Rethinking Community Medicine: towards a renaissance in public health' (USHP, 1979) for a more detailed discussion of ideas for developing public health and preventive activity.

Lancet 1979 Unforeseen attack on tobacco industry. Lancet 1: 1415
McKeown T 1976 The role of medicine: dream, mirage or nemesis. The Rock Carling Lecture 1975, Nuffield Provincial Hospitals Trust, London
Needleman H L, Gunnoe C, Leviton A, Reed R, Peresie H, Maher C, Barrett P 1979 Deficits in psychologic and classroom performance of children with elevated dentine lead levels. New England Journal of Medicine 300(13): 689–695
Royal Commission on the National Health Service 1979 Report. (Chairman: Sir Alec Merrison). Cmnd 7615. HMSO. London
Unit for the Study of Health Policy 1979 Rethinking Community Medicine: towards a renaissance in public health? USHP, London
World Health Organization 1979 Controlling the smoking epidemic. Report of the WHO Expert Committee on Smoking Control. WHO Technical Report Series 636, Geneva
Zola I 1974 quoted in McKinlay J B 1974 A case for refocusing upstream: the political economy of illness. Behavioural Scienc Data Review, June

FURTHER READING

On the development of preventive services and health education
Gray J A M 1979 Man against disease: preventive medicine. Oxford University Press, Oxford
A critical look at health education
Brown E R, Margo G E 1978 Health education: can the reformers be reformed? International Journal of Health Services 8(1): 3–26
Tuckett D 1979 Choices for health education: a sociological view. In: Sutherland I (ed) Health education: perspectives and choices. Allen and Unwin, London
On lifestyle and environment — a seminal government document
Lalonde M 1974 A new perspective on the health of Canadians. The Government of Canada, Ottawa
On public health today, weakness and proposals
Unit for the Study of Health Policy 1979 Rethinking community medicine: towards a renaissance in public health? USHP, 8 Newcomen Street, London SEI IYR
An evaluation of modern scientific medicine and the importance of the wider environment
McKeown T 1976 The role of medicine: dream, mirage or nemesis. The Rock Carling Lecture 1975. Nuffield Provincial Hospitals Trust, London

4

Health education

Ann Burkitt

In 1954 the World Health Organisation described the aims of health education as follows:

1. To make health a valued community asset
2. To help individuals to become competent in and to carry out those activities they must undertake for themselves as individuals or in small groups, in order to realise fully the state of health defined in the constitution of the WHO
3. To promote the development and proper use of the health services.

This definition often rewritten in a different form but retaining the same basic meaning, is generally accepted as the working aims of health education. The problem with all generalised statements of intent is that they are open to numerous working interpretations and also, for reasons of simplicity, ignore other equally important but conflicting aims.

Aim one appears to be an aim no-one would quarrel with until you consider the frequently conflicting aim of economic growth and a healthy community. A free market politician would argue that you need to generate wealth in order to pay for a health service. A conservationist, however, may argue that the type of industry needed to create the wealth in itself creates illness which then requires a more sophisticated and expensive health service to provide treatment.

Aim two directly challenges the professional expertise of professionals. Part of the definition of a professional is to have knowledge and skills not possessed by others. Health education directly challenges that situation by offering 'medical' knowledge to the laity. The conflict in hospitals amongst medical and nursing staff over who should talk to the patient about diagnosis and treatment and how much patients should be told is just one aspect. If you are going to undergo surgery or be prescribed drugs it does not seem unreasonable that you should have as a right, information about the procedures, yet the evidence of surveys (Cartwright, 1967) shows this does not happen for all patients.

Once you are a patient you have entered into a sick role with rights and obligations, with the giving and receiving of informations as part of that role. But what about the public at large, what do they receive to achieve aim two?

Most receive haphazard information from parents, brothers, sisters, friends, school and the mass media. Some children leave school with excellent human and environmental biological knowledge, a few have information on child care, drugs, alcohol and V.D. but many more remain in ignorance.

Magazines directed at women have health pages but they are missing from magazines for men. Health items in newspapers are again usually on the woman's page. Radio and television do have a range of health programmes but there is no guarantee of continuity of message, nor can misunderstandings or uestions be dealt with, except in phone-in programmes and the advice columns and then only for a few.

In other words systematic health education which would ensure that individuals or groups could be competent in and carry out activities to make themselves healthy does not exist in our society.

Yet there are constant pronouncements from health professionals that people must look after their own health and that the ills of modern society are due to personal behaviour with smoking usually quoted as the main problem. This ignores the fact that British American Tobacco is one of the largest international companies in this country, that tobacco earns millions of pounds revenue for the government and that millions of jobs here and abroad are based on some aspect of the tobacco industry.

The third aim is based on a value judgment. It depends on which point of view you take as to what are 'proper' uses of the health services.

A constant complaint of general practitioners is that too many people consult them for trivial complaints, and yet most health advice leaflets end 'Consult your doctor.' How is the member of the public supposed to reconcile these two conflicting messages?

The truth of the matter is that most people make great use of self medication (Wadsworth et al, 1973). Why individuals do or do not consult doctors is the subject of much medical sociological research but what is important for the third aim of health education is that the development of and access to medical and health care facilities is a *political* one. Whether it is financed through tax with open access, combined tax and private insurance or a free market, the decision is political and the type of health service and subsequent health education will be a reflection of the prevailing political climate of the time. Therefore the interpretation of the aims of health education and how they are to be carried out will be based on the concepts and values system of a society or groups within that society.

In this chapter I intend to explore some of those concepts and values and how they lead to (a) a model of health and (b) an allied type of health education. Because Britain is a complex class and multi-ethnic society all these concepts and values will be found to varying and overlapping degrees.

EDUCATION

Most discussion about health education tends to stress health rather than education but it could be asked, and often is in educational (rather than health service) discussions about health education, why should education about health be seen as any different to education about English or geography.

Thousands of philosophers of education are employed in universities and colleges throughout the world debating the concept of education. O'Connor (1957) states that Education refers to:

(a) a set of techniques for imparting knowledge, skills and attitudes

(b) a set of theories which purport to explain or justify the use of these techniques

(c) a set of values or ideals embodied and expressed in the purposes for which knowledge, skills and attitudes are imparted and so directing the amounts and types of training that is given.'

Much debate is devoted in academic educational circles to what techniques are permissable. This of course depends on the values referred to in (c) and books on the Philosophy of Education debate the issues of whether training, instruction, propaganda and indoctrination are or are not a legitimate part of an educational process (Gribble, 1969, Ch. 2).

This debate is rarely heard in health service circles and health propaganda is seen as acceptable by some health professionals in a way that would be unacceptable in an educational institution, i.e. giving only one side of the story without explaining the underlying rationale.

The techniques widely advocated for health education are well described in the books given in further reading at the end of the chapter. To illustrate my point about the differences between health propaganda/indoctrination, health information and health education, I will use a common health slogan.

1. *Propaganda/Indoctrination*
   'Small Families are Healthy Families'
   No explanation is given with this statement.
   Compare this with:
2. *Health Information*
   'Research has shown that families with two children have a higher protein intake per person than families with six children. On average children from smaller families were taller and heavier than those children from large families.'
   This is a factual statement, if you accept the research, which leaves the reader to draw his own conclusions.
3. *Health Education* (directed at 12-year-old children)
   'What foods do we require to:
   1. Help us to grow and become strong?
   2. Protect us against disease?
      Consult the books on the *health* shelf of the school library).
   3. Plan a shopping list for food for one week for a family of two children and for a family of six children. You have £20 to spend on each family. Make sure you include in the right proportion all the foods you have found out are needed for growth and health.'

In the third example the children are asked to consider basic principles, i.e. what is a basic diet necessary for health and then to apply that knowledge. They may end up agreeing with statement one, but they will at least know why they agree.

Just as the concept of education covers a wide range of emphasis and interpretation so does the concept of health. Put these two together and as I hope to show, a wide variety of approaches to health education emerges.

MODELS OF HEALTH

Health is a concept like truth which cannot be defined. To define it is to kill it. Nor can it be possessed. It can only be shared. There is no health for me without my brother. There is no health for Britain without Bangladesh.

Wilson, 1975

In his influential book *Health is for People*, Michael Wilson, a doctor and theologian, presents a humanistic view of health based on the notion of Christian concern and justice. (A CIBA Foundation Symposium in 1973 had the theme Human Rights in Health). Although he does not attempt a definition of health such as the World Health Organisation's 'Health is not just the absence of disease but a positive state of physical, mental and social wellbeing', he does list 10 pages of important characteristics of what in his opinion constitutes health.

In contrast, Essex-Cater's *A Synopsis of Public Health and Social Medicine* (1967) 739 pages long, does not even discuss what health is although the aim of the book is to show procedures for its maintenance. This is a common occurence in all medical books written on a medical model of disease as opposed to health. Frazer Brockington in *The Health of the Community* (1965) defines public health as 'the application of hygiene, the science which seeks to preserve health, to the body corporate, the community.' In Chapter 8, entitled 'The Education of People for Health', he defines health as 'a state of feeling well in body, mind and spirit, together with a sense of reserve power, based on normal functioning of tissues, a practical understanding of the principles of healthy living, a harmonious adjustment to the environment (physical and psychological); it implies an acceptance of itself as a means of a richer life of service.' (p. 129).

The fact that this definition is rift with value judgments is not discussed. For example, what is normal functioning of the tissues? There is a medical dispute as to when blood pressure is high, i.e. abnormal as opposed to normal reuiring medication. At what point should an individual be recommended treatment and become 'a patient'? There is no universal agreement to this problem. What does Frazer Brockington mean by 'a richer life of service'? The lack of agreement between nutritionists over what constitutes a healthy diet can be seen from the continuing debate about cholesterol and its role in the development of heart disease.

Numerous books discussing the organisation of hospitals and community care discuss 'health care' when in reality they are concerned with the treatment and care of illness. As Illich (1976) says: 'Fifteen years ago it would have been impossible to get a hearing for the claim that medicine itself might be a danger to health.' As he and many writers, including Titmuss and Abel Smith, point out, Beveridge's calculation that the National Health Service costs would fall as therapy reduced the rate of illness was hopelessly wrong.

Instead, access to medical treatment raised people's expectation of what is possible but has also facilitated, as Illich points out, the medicalisation of everyday life. Natural events such as menstruation, birth and death have become the province of increasing medical specialisation and high technology.

The mounting costs of such services have so alarmed politicians and others that there is an increasing demand for personal responsibility for health which can be viewed in both a negative and positive manner. Negative in that illness is seen as personal failure on the part of an individual with possible punitive results, e.g. patients with lung cancer or injuries as the result of a road accident being made to pay for treatment. This of course is not new — the concept of illness as a result of sin is well established in most cultures.

Illich (1976) presents a positive view: 'Health designates a process by which each person is responsible, but only in part responsible to others. To be responsible may mean two things. A man is responsible for what he has done, and responsible to another person or group. Only when he feels subjectively responsible or answerable to another person will the conseuences of his failure be not criticism, censure or punishment but regret, remorse and true repentance. The conseuent states of grief and distress are marks of recovery and healing and are phenomenologically something entirely different from guilt feelings. Health is a task, and as such is not comparable to the physiological balance of beasts.'

Those with experience of self help groups such as smokers' clinics, weight watchers and Alcoholics Anonymous will recognise in this uote, elements of the process through which new members proceed. It bears a strong resemblance to religious revivalist meetings only instead of standing up and being saved for Christ, you jog, diet or give up drinking for health.

A totally different view of health is implicit in the 'Balint' school of therapy: 'Health is the crucial word. . . . I see it as indicating the patient's capacity to deal with his problems in a more realistic and productive manner coinciding with the loss or great diminuition of the symptoms which lead him to the doctor originally.' (Balint et al, 1973).

The patient centred therapy of the Balint school is closely allied to psychotherapy and its various traditions and modern humanistic psychology and the theories of A. Maslow and C. Rogers. Practitioners are found inside and outside the health service and private schools and therapy groups full of leaders with California accents abound in most urban areas. In health education programmes the main influence is on a personal relationship approach to health as opposed to a biological one. A growing influential view is that central to good health is positive self esteem. It is the underlying rationale of the Schools Council Health Education Projects, 5 to 13 and 13 to 18.

The growth of concern for the environment has given a new dimension to the traditional hygiene, environmental view of health and is best seen in the books of Rene Dubos:

> Man can function well only when his external environment is in tune with the needs he has inherited from his evolutionary, experiential and social past, and with his aspirations for the future. Because they are concerned with all the various aspects of man's humanness, the biomedical sciences in their highest form are potentially the richest expression of science.
>
> Dubos 1970, p 168

Ecology has become an important branch of biology and social biology an 'A' level subject.

In contrast to the above quoted authors who all operate in the context of Western scientific tradition there are those operating outside the legal sanction of the health service, except for homoeopathy (which is just tolerated) who have many followers. These are called traditional healers and range from faith healers, herbalists, forms of massage and manipulation, colour therapists, to vegetarians and whole food

Table 4.1

Model	Site of action	Agents & disciplines
Pathological (The Medical Model) 1, 2, 3. *Dominant models in the N.H.S.*	A part of a body Identifying pathogens, or abnormal functioning degeneration.	Doctors, Nurses, Paramedical, Medical Journalists. Teachers
		Medical sciences Epidemiology
Sociopsychological 1, 2, 3. Emphasis on sociological explanation	A human person A human group Stressful interpersonal interaction, attitudes, socialisation, group norms, culture, alienation, deviance.	Social Planners Public Health Drs & Nurses. Some G.P.s. Medical sociologists. Personnel staff Social workers Teachers
		Sociology & psycho-sociological research, Medical sociology and social policy Epidemiology
Psychosociological 1, 2, 3. Emphasis on psychological	A human person A human group Stressful interpersonal interaction, attitudes, socialisation, group norms, culture, alienation, deviance.	Health visitors, Balint Drs, Social workers, Teachers — especially those with pastoral responsibilities. Counsellors Psycho-theraphists — Gestalt, transactional analysis, self discovery groups. Alcoholics Anonymous
		Social Psychology Humanistic Psychology Management Theories
Ecological 1, 2.	Man in relation to his environment. Community action	Environmental engineering. Public Health Drs and Nurses. Environmental Health Services. Health and Safety Commission. Teachers Conservation pressure groups such as Friends of the Earth, population control advocates
		Ecology Occupational hygiene Demography Epidemiology

Therapy	Approach to health education
Drugs, surgery, diet, remedial exercises, screening tests, accident prevention.	*Topic based* e.g. smoking and lung cancer, overweight and heart disease. *Subject content*: Disease recognition, forms of treatment, acceptance of sufferers, use of services, anatomy and physiology, nutrition, physical education, *Techniques*: Personal advice, formal lectures, mass media campaigns, mass media information, shock techniques — *mainly directed at individuals.*
Social policy, e.g. type of housing, social support systems, social security, community development. Some occupational health services and personnal support in industry, e.g. Marks & Spencer. Occupational health service.	*Target group based* e.g. Epidemiological and community studies identifying at risk or socially deprived groups. Needs of the group determine subject content of health education. *Techniques*: Social planning and provision, campaigns to make the public aware of their rights and services available, group work, community development.
Raising self esteem and self awareness, teaching social skills, sensitivity training. Parentcraft Relaxation Self growth Family therapy	A. *Individual or small group based* Felt needs of individual or group. Content of health education based on those needs. Emphasis on emotional needs. *Techniques*: Counselling, individually or in groups, different types of groups, discussion, T.A. etc. Teaching relaxation *Face to face education individually or in groups*
Legislation, e.g. sewage, clean water, pollution control, factory acts, etc. Public awareness Campaigns — clean food, Intermediate technology	*Directed at* (A) *policy makers* e.g. Pressure groups to change or introduce laws. B. *At the general public or special groups* e.g. representatives. *Techniques*: Face to face or group advice and information. Mass media campaigns Enforcement of law Pressure groups to change public opinion, e.g. campaigns against factory farming.

Table 4.1 *(cont'd)*

Model	Site of action	Agents & disciplines
Traditional 1, 2, 3.	A human person	Traditional Healers, e.g. a. herbalists b. massage and manipulation c. faith d. diet
Traditional Chinese medicine Taoist 1, 2, 3.	A human person in relationship to their world. The balance of Chi. Yin and Yang	A Master of Taoist Medicine and his/her students, the patient, a barefoot doctor, health workers Taoism
Socialist 1, 2, 3.	Collective action of a class or group of humans to understand and change their conditions.	Politically aware groups, leaders, pressure groups. Socialist/Marxist Economics, Maoist China

enthusiasts. They are not mutually exclusive groups and patients frequently move between several alternative treatments and conventional medicine. Groups offering alternative medicine may have opposing theories of health and have only been put together because they are legally separate from services supplied by the N.H.S. and therefore judged by the medical profession to be outside their (the medical profession's) view of health and health maintenance, even though many doctors go to alternative practitioners for treatment themselves.

A totally different view of health of growing influence in this country is traditional Chinese medicine. Based on a concept alien to Western scientific medicine it is difficult for non Taoists to understand although there is increasing scientific evidence to explain some of its basic concepts such as Chi, the life force, the meridians, the pathways through which the Chi circulates and Yin and Yang, the balancing forces of life. To most Westerners, Chinese medicine is sticking needles into parts of the body but Taoist medicine is a system of health maintenance developed over three thousand years of experience, experiment and observation, based on diet, attitude of mind, exercise routines, of which the central system is

Therapy	Approach to health education
Correcting with 'natural' means imbalance in the body.	Information and acceptance of the therapy offered. Usually the client seeks out the service. e.g. Festival of Mind and Body.
Diet, Exercise, Stimulation or depression of Chi by a variety of methods including massage, accupunture, moxibustion, herbal treatments to maintain a balanced circulation of Chi and Ying and Yang	*Master to students* *Health worker to community* Establishment of personal discipline of diet, rest, meditation, exercise. Total life style.
Alteration in the social structure of society, positive discrimination for the disadvantaged, redistribution of resources according to need, collective action for health.	*Target groups*: Workers of all types. *Techniques*: Didatic and group discussion. Political education, recognition of the social and economic basis of ill health. Encouragement for group action to change conditions, e.g. trade union activity. War on Want's, work on international companies role in the Third World, e.g. baby food, drug testing, tobacco.

Tai Chi, and includes the martial arts, art, music and sex. The active participation of the patient, in treatment through education is central. In the West doctors were traditionally paid when you became ill and needed treatment. In traditional China the doctor was paid only when his patient or community were healthy. With such a tradition it is not surprising that China has the only health service in the world where the main emphasis is on prevention and simple technology with gratifying results. Some other countries such as Tanzania are experimenting with a Chinese type system. (Chagula Tarmino in Newell, 1975 and Horn in Ciba Foundation (1971).

The final model of health is a political interpretation. It is an epidemiological fact that there are distinct patterns of morbidity and mortality related to socio-economic groupings. The lower down the scale you are the worse your life chances. The advent of the Welfare State and the N.H.S. has not altered this pattern and although overall mortality rates have improved, the distance between social class 5 and social class 1 has widened.

In addition there are pronounced regional differences. The explanation provided for why this is will be dependent on which model of health you subscribe to, e.g. a psychosociological explanation would be that social class 5 does not have the social skills to use the system to its advantage and ecologists would point to greater pollution and substandard housing in the north-east compared with the south-east as an explanation as to why the north-east has a poorer record.

The political model which I will call socialist would point to the relationship between work and disease and work and income and argue that the roots of disease are social injustice, inequality and in the relationship of man to means of production Although the relationship between work and disease is well documented, occupational health is not part of the National Health Service. The introduction of the Health and Safety at Work Act 1974 and the subsequent training of safety representatives has now raised questions in the minds of many workers over means of production and the organisation of power in society, (Kinnersley, 1974) and its relationship to health.

To clarify the different models of health, their site of action, their agents, their therapy and health education approach, I have constructed Table 4.1.

The numbers in column Model represent whether the model operates in any one of the three stages of prevention, i.e. *primary*, before a problem begins (1); *secondary*, preventing an extension of the illness or injury and preventing further illness or injury to the individual or others (2); and *tertiary*, preventing the deterioration of a chronic condition and improving life within the limits of the condition (3).

These seven models are of course paradigms or aids to interpreting what you observe in the real world to help to understand how people behave and possible explanations for their action.

None of these models are mutually exclusive and many people, professional and lay, may operate on a combination of two or more.

For example, a chest surgeon tried telling patients to stop smoking with little result. He decided to try a psychosociological approach and start a smoking clinic with the help of a psychotherapist. Balint type doctors started with a medical training based on the pathological model and changed to the psychosociological one whereas doctors and nurses who choose to go into public health become very influenced by both the ecological and sociopsychological models which may lead them on to the socialist model.

Branches of the women's movement are found mainly in either the socialist or sociopsychological models but often with varying influences of the traditional and Taoist models. The interest in traditional Chinese medicine may come from a starting point of a political interest in China and the barefoot doctors.

Disagreements over health education policy, content and techniques become understandable when you realise that health educators and their allied professionals — teachers, doctors, nurses — may all be working on different models of health and priorities in health education and yet appear to be using the same words.

It is not the purpose of this chapter to advocate one particular model but to point out that these differences do exist and that to develop any health education programme it is essential that the people involved first establish their own beliefs and values and to decide if they are appropriate to (a) the needs of the client group or community and (b) the needs of the health service.

Ultimately the most successful health education will be that which most closely engages the values, needs and aspirations of the community it serves. Britain in the late 20th century is a multicultural society and therefore needs a multicultural approach to the health education provided.

REFERENCES

Reports

DHSS 1976 Prevention and health. HMSO, London
Radical Statistics Health Group 1977 In defence of the National Health Service. Radical Statistics Health Group Expert Committee
World Health Organisation 1969 Planning and evaluation of health education: T.R.S. No 409, 1969. World Health Organisation, Geneva
World Health Organisation 1974 Expert Committee on Health Education of the Public: T.R.S. No 87, 1974. World Health Organisation, Geneva

Books

Abel–Smith B 1976 Value for money in the health service. Heinemann, London
Argyle M 1976 Psychology of interpersonal behaviour. Penguin, Harmondsworth
Benjamin P 1955 Health, culture and community. Russell Sage
Cartwright A 1967 Patients and their doctors. Routledge, London
Ciba Foundation 1971 Teamwork for world health. Churchill, London, p 77–86
Ciba Foundation 1974 Human rights in health. Elsevier, London
Draper P 1976 Economic policy and health unit for the study of health policy. Guy's Medical School, London
Dubos R 1970 Man, medicine and environment. Pelican, Harmondsworth
Essex–Cater 1967 A synopsis of public health and social medicine, 2nd edn. John Wright, Bristol
Frazer Brockington 1965 The health of the community, 3rd edn. Churchill, London
Gribble J 1969 Introduction to philosophy of education. Allyn Bacon, Boston
Grundy F, Grundy P 1974 Community health and social services. H K Lewis, London
Illich I 1976 Limits to medicine. Marion Boyars, London, p 221, 273
Kinnersley P 1974 Hazards at work and how to fight them. Pluto Press, London
Maslow A H 1968 Towards a psychology of being. Van Nostrand
Newell K (ed) 1975 Health by the people. WHO, Geneva, p 145–168
O'Connor D J 1957 Introduction to philosophy of education. Routledge & Kegan Paul, London, p 5
Rogers C 1961 On becoming a person. Constable, London
Wadsworth M et al 1973 Health and sickness. Tavistock, London
Wilson M 1975 Health is for people. Darton Longman Todd, London, p 117
Young M 1971 Knowledge and control. Collier Macmillan, London

Background Reading Information

Dalzell Ward A J 1976 A textbook of health education. Tavistock, London
Official Chinese Paramedical 1977 A barefoot doctor's manual American Translation. Running Press, Philadelphia
Parker E 1975 Introduction to health education. Macmillan, London
Health Education Council, 78 New Oxford Street, London W.C.1. (has an excellent library and resources centre which will supply specialised bibliographies)
Information and courses on Traditional Chinese Medicine from: Liu Academy of Traditional Chinese Medicine, 13 Gunnersbury Avenue, London, W. 5

5

Handicap or special need?

Brian Hodges

Handicapped people are first and foremost people: people with the same basic human needs as the rest of humanity. Physiological needs of food, warmth, shelter, sex, and those needs that contribute to self-fulfilment; safety, security, love, a sense of belonging, self-esteem, social esteem, opportunity for new experiences, personal growth and creativity or mastery. As a result of such things as biological insult or the denial of a basic human need, love or stimulation for instance, handicapped people are disadvantaged compared with their fellows. Many caring strategies for the handicapped deny basic needs, ignore their essential personhood and overlook their special needs. What is required is a recognition of the ordinary and special needs of people who are handicapped and the implementation of policies to meet such needs as are identified.

Impairment affects different people differently, being related to personal life-philosophy, coping mechanisms, social motor and occupational skills, beliefs, value systems and attitudes to disability. For a low-key example take the retort of Gilbert Harding on the 1950 television panel game 'What's My Line?' : 'Of course I get indigestion — but I don't suffer from it.' Impairment is a very personal thing.

The variation and variability of individuals is most marked when handicapped people are considered. Not only does handicap vary both in nature and degree from one person to another; the fluctuations in an individual's handicap varies over time, idiosyncratically. The differences between individuals exceed expectations. Assumptions about future performance of any one person cannot be predicted with any degree of accuracy either by reference to personal history or the experiences of others. Although people with handicaps have common elements in their personal histories, to overlook their uniqueness as individuals is to do the handicapped a disservice.

Assessment, patterns of care, intervention strategies are dependent to a large extent on the philosophy, values attitudes, orientation and expectations that surround the notion of handicap. The philosophical framework, constructs, or model adopted will have a profound effect on the lives of people with handicapping conditions. This is reflected in the terminology used, those necessary lables used to order our world with all the disadvantages that such labels encompass. Labels have a nasty habit of becoming self-fulfilling prophecies. Terms present problems in having different meanings for different people, they become redundant and frequently carry little meaning at all. In this context there is the notion of compensatory education that failed to compensate for the cumulative and pervasive effects

Table 5.1

Harris, 1971	Wing, 1974
impairment lacking part or all of a limb, or having a defective limb, organ or mechanism of the body.	*impairment* defect or loss of a part of the body or malfunctioning of internal organs or other body mechanisms, whether or not it results in handicap
handicap the disadvantage or restriction of activity caused by disability	*handicap (or disability)* the disadvantage resulting from the loss or reduction of functional capacity
disablement the loss or reduction of functional ability	*disablement* the socially disabling effect of handicaps

of the childs environmental milieu. The Head Start programme in the United States commenced with much enthusiasm in 1965 failed to live up to its optimistic beginnings and by 1969 had been shown not to give the desired 'head start' to children disadvantaged by an environment hostile to personal development and thus resulting in under achievement. Similarly the various terms used for the handicapped may lead to confusion rather than elucidation.

The survey 'Handicapped and Impaired in Great Britain' (Harris, 1971) drew distinctions between impairment, handicap and disablement. In the paper presented to the Central Council for the Education and Training of Social Workers Working Party on Training for Social Work with Handicapped People Professor Wing used the same terms, defining them differently (Wing, 1974).

Peter Townsend outlines five concepts of disablement in *Poverty in the United Kingdom* (Townsend, 1979):

1. anatomical, physiological or psychological abnormality or loss
2. chronic clinical condition altering or interrupting physiological or psychological process
3. functional limitation of ordinary activity, whether that activity is carried on alone or with others
4. pattern of behaviour which has elements of a socially deviant kind
5. socially defined class and status.

> An individual who is 'disabled' is not just impaired, or limited, or different in his activities; he occupies a position in the social hierarchy determined by the kind of resource allowed to people like himself and a (usually) corresponding status which the disabled, when recognized as such, occupy in that particular society.

Handicap may thus be an attribute of the person, remaining with them whatever their circumstances, or may result from the situation in which they find themselves. A person may be disadvantaged as a result of physical, mental, emotional, educational or social handicap. A growing awareness of gender disadvantage is emerging — girls underachieving in science subjects for instance — and there is a wealth of literature on the disadvantage of race or social class, although the disadvantage of being middle-class is under-represented. These areas which may be of minimal interest to community health care workers show that handicap is not only multifactorial but has a wider connotation than might be expected on first encounter.

A distinction can be made between intrinsic and extrinsic handicaps, primary and secondary handicaps. An intrinsic handicap is one that remains with the person no matter what his circumstances — limited exercise tolerance, ataxia, sensory deficit, depression or disfigurement being examples. Extrinsic handicaps are situation dependent, existing independently of any intrinsic handicap. These arise as a result of social factors — poverty, under-stimulation, lack of opportunity to develop motor, social, or occupational skills are examples. Intrinsic handicaps have been classified by Agerholm (1975) into nine groups of handicapping factors: locomotor, visual, communication, visceral, intellectual, emotional, invisible, aversive and senescence handicap. Each handicap is subdivided into components, communication for instance contains impaired — hearing, talking, reading, writing. Each of these components could be further sub-divided, identifying specific handicapping conditions both qualitatively and quantitatively. For those people with multiple handicaps it should thus be possible to construct a profile of handicapping conditions on the basis of which appropriate intervention may be planned.

Whilst exception may be taken to 'aversive handicap', the classification gives momentum to the movement away from causation, so long the preoccupation of health care personel, towards a consideration of effect, functional deficit or special need. Attention to functional deficit, irrespective of causation, is potentially more productive. People with schizophrenia, perceptive deafness, mental retardation. dyslexia or autism, all have a communication disorder. Brain malfunction arising from cerebral vascular incident may also manifest as a disorder of communication. In each case the caring strategy adopted should give greater import to the particular effect rather than to the causation.

Primary handicaps equate with intrinsic handicaps. Secondary handicap arises as a direct result of the primary handicap discounting the belief in the single handicap, e.g.

Deafness. People with impaired hearing have difficulty: perceiving sound, in language development, perceiving symbols, initiating or maintaining conversation, and have a tendency to become socially isolated. Some of these characteristics persist after hearing has been restored.

Cerebral palsy. This non-progressive motor disorder gives rise to: characteristic dysfunction or deformities, susceptibility to pressure necrosis — respiratory or urinary infection, constipation, reduction of the opportunity to learn through exploration or manipulation and distortion of body image.

The person who remains a cardiac cripple some years after recovery from a coronary infarction and the psychological concomitants of facial disfiguration are further examples of secondary handicap.

Primary handicaps are by definition irreducible, it is possible however to reduce, if not to eliminate, the effect of secondary handicap, the extent to which the handicap is intrinsic or arises from other factors should be considered.

PREVALENCE

The difficulties inherent in establishing criteria for disability has as a consequence a certain vagueness about the number of people who can be described as disabled.

The Poverty Survey (Townsend, 1979) indicated that people who would not describe themselves as disabled would, on careful questioning, reveal difficulties in aspects of daily living that indicated disability. One conclusion to be drawn from published figures on disability is that they are unrepresentative. Townsend estimates $6\frac{1}{2}$ million people with some degree of disability from the results of the Poverty Survey where 12% said they had a disablement condition and that it prevented them doing things which were normal for people their age. In the case of handicapped children, if the experience of the Scottish Home and Health Department is a guide, then the numbers of handicapped children must be considerably in excess of 200 000.

There is potentially a large section of the populace who will require skilled intervention by a health care practitioner. The special needs of the client must be ascertained using an appropriate assessment schedule before an effective intervention strategy can be adopted.

DEVELOPMENTAL SCREENING

The identification of children at risk commences before conception by identifying mothers from disadvantaged groups known to be at risk. Such disadvantage may arise from social class, working with hazardous substances, known genetic or familial predisposition, or geographical location.

Whereas the screening for genetic and familial abnormalities such as Down's syndrome and spina bifida are well known if not well established, much less is known about the influence of social factors, locale, ignorance, poverty, industrial pollutants or occupational hazards. Exposure to lead is known to cause brain damage in children; working with lead is forbidden for the pregnant woman; it is some time however before the fact of pregnancy is known.

Published Government figures have shown alarming geographical differences in perinatal mortality rates: Dudley 24.1/1000, Oxford 9/1000. Improving the welfare services for the pregnant woman has been the concern of such organisations as the Spastics Society, with its 'Save a Baby' campaign, and the Trades Union Congress which sought to improve services for the working pregnant woman. The scheme that prompted the interest of the TUC was organized by Strathleven Bonded Warehouses in conjunction with the Argyll and Clyde Health Board. On confirmation of pregnancy women workers were given an identity card that allowed them time off to attend antenatal clinics, free milk in the works canteen and permission to finish five minutes before co-workers to avoid the onslaught of the homeward rush. A visit to the plant nurse was encouraged after each clinic appointment. This contrasts with previous practices of loss of wages incurred through leaving work to attend clinics and the preliminary concealment of pregnancy for fear of becoming unemployed. A charter for the working pregnant woman is long overdue.

Assessment from birth is necessary if early intervention is to be implemented. A schedule for a basic surveillance programme was outlined for children up to 5 years of age in the Report of the Committee on Child Health Services (DHSS, 1976). A wide range of complex child development schedules are available for the ascertainment of developmental delay whilst assessment techniques using simple equipment, a small piece of paper and ten bricks are useful to identify specific areas of dysfunction (Illingworth, 1972)

The health visitor is the person best placed to ascertain developmental delay or potential handicapping conditions using appropriate measures; this should be reflected in their training. Referral to the General Practitioner and through him to the District Handicap Team should take place automatically.

The low attendances at child health clinics — in 1973 73% of children under one year attended; of the children between two and four years of age 28% attended — makes the specialized role of the health visitor the more important. It is probable that as a result of non-attendance children whose handicap is either not obvious or who have developed strategies to cope, inappropriately with dysfunction may remain undetected.

Mia Kellmer Pringle, Director of the National Children's Bureau, has frequently advocated financial incentives for parents to encourage attendance at developmental clinics where potential impairments can be detected. Considering the paucity of information and the potential personal benefits a survey to determine the nature and extent of handicapping conditions in children is urgently required.

ASSESSMENT

Assessment is in vogue, and is in danger of being discredited. There are assessment wards, clinics, visits, (by community, social, and health workers) and assessment centres. Whilst some are competent highly efficient services the assessment criteria in others is deficient, in some cases it merely means the client attended or was attended. Assessment is in danger of becoming a euphemism for something else, admission for long-term care or to give the impression that something is being done.

Assessment is not an end in itself but a means to an end and should lead to action; as Miss Nightingale remarked: 'Reports are not self-executive.' Assessment is not a once-and-for-all occasion but a continuing process. The days of the one-off assessment forms, dutifully completed and stored in the client's file until the case conference, are hopefully over. There is little point in carrying out an assessment procedure unless there is some clear idea and intention to do something with the results. Assessment is not the prerogative of any one profession, each will develop a programme for a client from their own base criteria, hopefully in concert with other agencies involved. The other agencies and professionals involved will vary in response to the person being assessed; it should however be comprehensive and multidisciplinary identifying the special needs of the client. Comprehensive assessment may not always be possible or desirable and an extra burden is placed on a family if the back-up services are unavailable. A base line of behaviour may need to be established or sufficient information on which to base a decision may need to be gathered and it is preferable if this can be done on some other basis than inspired guesswork.

Diagnosis of a condition is necessary for treatment but has little to do with care or meeting the specific individual needs of the client.

A scheme should be devised to ascertain what the person can do, what he cannot do and what he could do with specific intervention. The emphasis should be on areas of dysfunction in which intervention would be advantageous; concentrating on the help required to complete a given task rather than on the inablity to do it.

A wide variety of assessment methods exist to ascertain dysfunction. Some are tightly controlled and specific to a limited area of human experience, tests of intelligence, neurological deficit, and lung compliance being examples. Others are more general concerning for instance health or social competence, and some include personal, social, educational, economic and geographical factors.

If the client is a schoolchild unable to discriminate between complex shapes, the presence or absence of a bath in the home is of little consequence. If, however, the client is an elderly arthritic lady living alone, not only the presence of a bath but its accessibility is of cardinal importance. To continue the bathing theme; a schedule for assessing the coping ability of a person with spastic diplegia at bathing would contain many items in order to determine the extent ard type of help required — ability to wash left foot, leg, thigh, arm, shoulder, similarly right and drying. Such detail would obviously be unimportant in people whose bathing behaviour required monitoring but whose impairment was different in nature.

The nine categories of Dr Agerholm can be used as a 'coarse sieve' to isolate intrinsic handicaps; this should not however detract from the secondary and socially imposed handicaps which have not been so clearly identified. Having determined the major handicapping factors that prevent the participation in activities of daily living commensurate with their age, more specific schedules or procedures should be utilized to indicate intervention strategies promoting optimum performance.

Assessment as a basis for care must take into account the prevailing value system. Care for the handicapped frequently involves the notion of independence; a frequently expressed aim is to make the client independent for dressing. To be dependent on another person for a short period each day may be preferable to undergoing a lengthy dressing programme; the time involved could be used to try something rather more exciting. The system of assessment should identify the shortfall in the basic and special needs of the individual and give an indication of areas of imbalance in the personal profile of competence to which attention could be given with profit.

COMMON GROUND

People who are handicapped, whether the handicap be one of mental retardation, psychiatric disorder or physical impairment, share a common ground in a world where to be handicapped is to be different.

It is a paradoxical topsy-turvy world; the young with their green spiky hair, outrageous if smart, clothes emphasize their individuality. People with an impairment, obviously different, would rather not be so regarded. The adolescent and the impaired both experience problems of identity. The adolescent identity crisis is a transient phenomenon experienced during the passage from relative dependence to relative independence, from childhood to adulthood; for the person with an impairment the situation is rather one of a spoiled identity, of stigmatization (Goffman, 1963). Consider then the problem of the handicapped adolescent. The young girl with the current outrageous fashion, purple nails, hair streaked red and orange, and garish clothes eventually becomes accepted, for what she is as a person. Consider personal reactions if the person dressed in that manner was confined to a wheelchair. A more dowdy appearance would be expected. It is as if the person with a disability should be super-normal, being deviant in one domain they are not allowed to be so in another.

People who are not handicapped have difficulty dealing with people who are; they experience discomfort and embarrassment. People either do not know where to look or they stare, are not sure whether to speak or maintain an uncomfortable silence. A young girl severely affected by 'polio' on seeing a disabled person said, 'See that lady! I didn't stare at that lady!' (Davis 1962) reflecting on her own experience. To use a possibly sexist example, a beautifully proportioned bikini — clad young lady running across the beach carrying two ice creams in her hands receives a large number of long looks. A congenital malformation having placed her hands close to her shoulders meant that in all probability it was not her curvaceous figure that was being admired; with an healthy interest in the female form and an awareness of the problems of the handicapped, to look or not to look that is the question.

The embarrassment experienced in conversing with a person who has a speech impediment is reduced by the device of avoidance. This resolves the predicament of the non-impaired at the expense of the impaired, whose social encounters may be limited as a consequence. Such an avoidance strategy is not atypical.

Stigma, one of the common grounds of people with impairment, although common has unequal application. The wearing of aids to vision is more acceptable than the wearing of aids to hearing. A person with age-induced impairment of both sight and hearing is more inclined to accept being seen wearing glasses than a hearing aid. This phenomenon is not restricted to the elderly. In *Passage Through Crisis* Davis reports how a boy affected with polio was pleased when his mother did not enlighten a taxi-driver who had assumed that his plaster-encased leg was the result of playing football (Davis, 1962).

Being different affects interpersonal relationships to the extent that both people involved are aware of the different nature of the interaction. When confronted by a person with a stigmatizing condition, the perceptions and expectations that govern everyday interactions are confounded. To ignore an obvious handicap, treating the person as though it did not exist as though the person were normal, is clearly inappropriate. Concessions related to the handicap will need to be made. The handicap should not be allowed to dominate the relationship or indeed the life of the person.

It is not uncommon for children with a handicap to be over indulged and for parents to become trapped in a pattern of indulgence that may later need to be broken. The gifts, excuses for misbehaviour and lax discipline arising from a compensatory mechanism are not in the best interest of the developing individual who will need to live in a world of competing demands. The child with a handicap amongst normal peers at school or club is so often selected for the special prize, the largest present or is the child selected to present the bouquet to the visiting dignitary. The adult in a wheelchair is granted unsolicited concessions, allowed to jump the queue to view the floral-art, although the problem of mobility has little relevance to this particular occasion and the person would rather be treated without special consideration.

The problems of relationship change affects the family with a member who is diagnosed mentally ill. This is particularly acute when the person returns home after a short period of hospitalisation. The person returning home presents problems not of relationship development but of relationship change. The changed behaviour of the individual causes a degree of uncertainty in the interpersonal relationships as the family interpret and respond to different cues. Confirmation of mental illness induces a change in the behaviour in the absence of any real change in the behaviour of the client.

An area in which the embarrassment is the more acutely felt is in the realm of sexual relationships, in short the people with handicaps should not have them, or so some would have us believe. The handicapped as people are entitled to all the ecstasy that derives from a loving relationship and equally entitled to all the pain that derives from the breakdown of a deep emotional involvement with another person. To make this a reality involves a radical change in attitudes towards people with handicaps, more help to families with a handicapped member to encourage appropriate socialization modifying the perception and expectations of disability.

A common effect of a handicapping condition is that people, with whom the affected person comes into contact make unwarranted assumptions. Invariably, the person affected by a 'stroke' who then experiences difficulty articulating speech is spoken to in the language and condescending manner of the nursery. (Not that such an attitude is any more appropriate there.) From the presence of a physical handicap a mental handicap is assumed; 'Does he take sugar?' is a typical remark, to which the appropriate answer from the handicapped person is 'Tell him yes.'

A boy caught pilfering from the corner shop will be excused if he is regarded as mentally retarded. The activity, which is not exactly abnormal for boys, is attributed to his handicap rather than his boyishness. A tumble from rollerskates or a fall from a horse is put down to disability rather than the stone under the wheel or poor horsemanship.

People with disability are first and foremost people, they exhibit all the fads and foibles, virtues and failings of being human. They have similar drives and similar needs. Overall it is preferable to regard them not so much as handicapped people or even people with handicaps but as people with special needs.

REFERENCES

Agerholm M 1975 Handicaps and the handicapped: a nomenclature and classification of intrinsic handicaps. Journal of the Royal Society of Health vol 1

Davis F 1963 Passage through crisis. The Bobbs-Merrill Company Inc., Indianapolis and New York

Department of Health and Social Security 1976 Department of Education and Science Report of the Committee on Child Health Services. (The Court Report). HMSO, London

Goffman E 1963 Stigma: notes on the management of a spoiled identity. Prentice Hall, New York

Harris A C 1971 Handicapped and impaired in Great Britain. HMSO, London

Illingworth 1972 Predictive value of developmental assessment in infancy. In: Douglas C P, Holt K S (eds) Mental retardation prenatal diagnosis and infant assessment. Butterworths, London

Townsend P 1979 Poverty in the United Kingdom. Penguin, Harmondsworth

Wing J K 1974 Suggested teaching on handicapping factors with special reference to schizophrenia in order to illustrate its application. In: People with handicaps need better trained workers. CCETSW Paper 5, Central Council for the Education and Training of Social Workers, London

FURTHER READING

Boswell D M, Wingrove J M 1974 The handicapped person in the community. Tavistock, London
Fox M They get this training but they don't really know how you feel. Horsham West Sussex, Action Research for the Crippled Child. National Fund for Research into crippling diseases
Miller E J, Gwynne G V 1974 A life apart. Tavistock, London
Thomas D 1978 Social psychology of childhood disability. Methuen, London
Tjossem T D 1976 Intervention strategies for high risk infants and young children. University Park Press, Baltimore
Younghusband E 1970 Living with handicap. National Bureau for Cooperation in Child Care, London

6

Mental health

Anthony Butterworth

To consider mental health within a health care system usually leads to a notion of a *restoration* of mental health following mental disorder, not the *maintenance* of mental health for the community at large. This narrow definition misses many important ideas that can be included within the mental health umbrella.

DEFINING THE BOUNDARIES

Viewed from its widest perspective, mental health is woven into a compound of associated elements such as biological, psychological, environmental and social influences. These influences all contribute towards a complex model of life of which mental health is one aspect. This model because of its complexity brings with it macroscopic ideas which affect the mental health of the individual and the community. Adequate housing, full employment and successful interpersonal relationships all affect mental health, but the means to affect all of them, and bring about suitable change to promote good mental health is beyond the scope of most individual health care practitioners. To assume that a given population will want major changes to its social fabric for the sake of mental health indicates a certain naivete. As Mechanic (1966) points out: 'The real question concerns the price we are willing to pay to promote the basic social conditions conducive to mental health and the price is more than an economic one'. This difficulty can be seen for example in the problem of alcoholism. To ban completely the consumption of alcohol would certainly curtail the problem of alcoholism. It can in no way be considered a reasonable act, and would infringe upon the rights of the individual and his need for individual decision making. The desire for mental health is not at the top of everyone's shopping list for a more satisfying and worthwhile life!

The mental health of a given community is important to its well being and there are limited means at our disposal to affect it through the vehicle of the health care services. Representations through various bodies which affect the wider ranging aspects of a community life style will possibly have some marginal effect upon its resources for providing a suitable milieu for mental health.

Greater interest has been given to the individual and his mental health. Some more realistic approaches can be considered which provide a means of considering mental health rather than illness at an individual level.

AN APPROACH THROUGH PRIMARY PREVENTION

Primary prevention in mental health seeks to identify those things which precipitate mental illness and halt their influence thereby maintaining the mental health of the individual. It has been demonstrated earlier that the difficulties of doing this at a societal level are sometimes prohibitive in terms of resource usage, acceptability, and the legitimacy of involvement by health care practitioners may be questionable. To grasp the concept of primary prevention in mental health, parallels can be drawn between general physical health and illness, and mental health and illness. It has long been recognised in general medicine that prevention is far easier than cure. The same assumption can be made in mental health/illness after considering the devastating effects upon the person and his family caused by acute mental disorder and its subsequent treatment. In the same way that certain individuals have resistance to physical ill-health because of their own immunities and strengths, the individual has varying degrees of strengths and resistances to mental ill-health. Certain factors can be altered and manipulated, others cannot. Those which cannot be altered, include such areas as sex, social grouping and age, all of which affect the individual's potential to suffer mental ill-health. The elderly, for example, are prone to a variety of mental ill-health provoking situations, but the aging process is unavoidable. Other 'coping' factors are fixed over a period of time — capacity to relate to others, levels of integrity, problem-solving ability are all developed from an early age, and while they are open to influence, changes in later life are more difficult to accomplish. For many people these 'coping' factors are often quite adequate in assisting them to 'manage' with life.

Certain writers, e.g. Caplan (1964) and Brandon (1970) would argue that there are periods of crisis where the coping strengths of the individual prove to be inadequate and do not survive these crisis periods. Theories have been developed around crisis periods throughout a life span and from these approaches can be taken the notion of 'at risk' populations. These populations at special risk have been variously described, and examples can be drawn from: (i) death of a spouse in the elderly dependent, (ii) retirement age groups, (iii) parental death in the case of children aged five to seven years old. These groups could be observed to be in receipt of a threat to the maintenance of their mental health. To identify these 'at risk' groups may be fairly easy, but to intervene and to assist is not. Accessibility presents one of the more particular problems when dealing with preventive strategies in mental health. A family with a physically ill person will possibly welcome intervention quite openly, as the ability to deal with that family member is often seen as being essentially a task outside the family's competance. To intervene in a family where one member is not mentally well does not meet with such a welcoming response. As the involvement of the family often extends into the causative factors which have precipitated the events, such hesitance is understandable. Not all people will fall at the crisis hurdles, and it is therefore necessary to be able to distinguish between the needy and not so needy groups which once again is not easy.

The major means promoting primary prevention for health care services probably lies in health education. As far as mental health is concerned, however, education programmes are made more difficult because problems are produced for the health educators in providing concrete and usable information which the lay person can understand. Efforts are being made in this direction as can be seen from Health Education Council information. Services already exist which aim towards the maintenance of mental health. General health checks on children, unemployment benefits, social services support systems and many others all aim indirectly at the maintenance of mental health.

AN APPROACH THROUGH SECONDARY PREVENTION

Where intervention can be more positive and services are more effective is in the area of secondary prevention. Secondary prevention programmes aim to lower the prevalence value of cases within the community. Caplan (1964) argues that there are two routes: (i) lowering the rate of new cases (which has been previously shown to be difficult) and (ii) the rate of old cases can be lowered by early diagnosis and effective treatment. To discover the very early signs of mental ill-health and deal with them positively means redirecting detection and treatment programmes.

For those people who are mentally unwell the traditional route to help is through a means of self-referral, or referral through family and friends. Arguably, when the individual has reached such a stage, some damage has already been done. Efforts should therefore be directed to the earlier detection and resolution of mental disorder as this will assist in: (i) reducing the effects of long-term mental disorder and (ii) lessen the repercussions that the 'ripple effect' of such a disorder will have upon family, friends and the work situation. The health care services are presented with some difficulty in approaching this area, as the best place for effective secondary prevention is general practice, but the Primary Health Care Team, is very often ill-equipped to deal with it. The prescribing habits and psychotherapeutic skills of practitioners in this area often leave something to be desired. Brave efforts are being made in some areas to counteract these deficiences. The Livingstone Project (Haines & Rae, 1973) provides an interesting example where physical and mental well-being is given equal weighting in general practice. Specific programmes and strategies are worked out to combat mental ill-health in much the same way as counteractive measures are presented to combat physical health. The primary health care team means just this, and team approaches are used to carry out the programmes of care.

Experimental work is going on in other areas to look at the possibilities of screening out those people with a potential mental disorder before it becomes advanced. Johnstone & Goldberg (1976) have developed what they claim is a usable experimental tool in this area.

To accomplish effective screening demands a 'captive' population who can be screened, tested, retraced and collated. This requires the co-operation of, and accessibility to, the captive population, and is therefore selective in the choice of targets. Not everyone can be persuaded to participate in pre-testing for potential mental disorder. The targets are therefore going to be groups such as General Practitioners' surgery attenders or industrial work forces. This will limit its usefulness if it cannot be applied to other 'at risk' groups mentioned previously.

The follow-up to early detection must be prompt and effective treatment. There are those who would argue that to identify large numbers of potentially mentally unhealthy individuals, would place an intolerable strain upon services which cannot cope easily with existing demands, and there is undeniable truth in this. The remedies to the problem are not total, nor without trauma. The psychiatric service in the United Kingdom is quite often based upon limited concepts and time consuming practice. Where the psychiatric/mental health team could be devoting its energies to early case detection and early treatment programmes, much time is spent in hospitals and psychiatric units so that the community has to seek the psychiatric service and not the other way round. If the psychiatric hospital is truly a community resource, then it should be more actively involved at a community level. There are services where such efforts have been made (Courigan 'Soni, 1977) and the experience for the practitioners, although initially unsettling can be ultimately more rewarding. Much of the work carried on in the large 'back' wards of psychiatric hospitals could be safely left in the hands of psychiatric nurses and psychologists, thus leaving the psychiatrists and mental health care team of psychiatric nurses, social workers and psychologists opportunity to find out where the early intervention strategies work best in the community at large.

AN APPROACH THROUGH TERTIARY PREVENTION

The discussion of 'treatments' and hospitals and psychiatric units leads to the final part of a tripartite approach in preventive programmes. Tertiary prevention seeks to reduce the residual effects of mental disorder, which often leaves the individual with a reduction in social, occupational and interpersonal functioning. There are a number of ways in which the tertiary aspects of preventive work can be implemented, and many of these have been given recognition in this country for some time. By making treatment available in the community or encouraging social contacts for the hospitalized, social isolation is reduced. This is a preventive strategy. Producing such iatrogenic disorders as institutionalization makes the treatment programme much longer as there will subsequently be a need to include lengthy resocialization as part of treatment. Maintaining social contacts helps to counter this. Treatment programmes, which provide (a) intensive care without institutionalization, (b) follow-up which is close and on a personal basis, (c) support services which are varied and accessible, are likely to succeed dramatically. One of the difficulties encountered in tertiary care is that services are provided in this country by two different sources. Firstly, the hospital psychiatric units, psychiatrists and psychiatric nurses are provided by the Department of Health and Social Services. Secondaly, follow-up facilities such as day centres, hostels and supporting social services are provided by local government and to levels which, although working to nationally recommended numbers, are rarely met and almost never exceeded. This dichotomy in service provision is counterproductive to those wishing to start an active tertiary care programme. Those who must have suitable time to rehabilitate are not always given the community support they need, as the facilities are non-existant thus affecting their chances of success. To bridge these gaps in the service, some personnel are moving full time into the community, most notably psychologists and psychiatric nurses. This at least can provide the essential continuity of care, and the close supervision which some people need to achieve some measure of success in living in the community once more.

THE SIZE OF THE PROBLEM

The estimate of mental ill-health has often been roughly measured in terms of patient populations in psychiatric hospitals and units but more realistically the problem is much greater than this. Haines & Rae (1973) suggest that the hospital consultant sees no more than 1 in 20 of patients recognised by the general practitioner to be mentally ill; of these diagnosed as neurotic, 7% will be referred by them and only 1 in 5 of these require hospital treatment. Added to this is the problem that such mental ill-health as there is, is often blurred and partly camouflaged by social and environmental hardships. This makes the task of the diagnostician and the intervention agents much more complicated. The workload of primary health care teams will be increased if the number of these people with mental ill-health is large. Evidence has shown, e.g. Shepherd et al (1966), that patients designated by doctors as 'psychiatric patients' consulted more often than others and there is a positive association between the risk of physical disease and psychiatric disorder. This depends not unnaturally upon the skills of the diagnostician. There must be some truth in the argument that psychiatric labels may be applied to those patients who have a high nuisance value, and repeatedly present with minor physical ailments at a G.P.s' surgery. The definitions of mental ill-health are as intangible and as variable as those which can be applied to mental health. This results inevitably in the provision of services based upon varied and inaccurate estimates of need. If new services are provided, then they will be used, and as with all health services the demand always exceeds the supply.

PROVIDING FACILITIES FOR MENTAL HEALTH CARE

To estimate at the 'ideal' level the services which are going to be essential to mental health care may appear an ivory tower exercise, but there are targets at which the services should aim. Eliminating the more grandiose schemes which would entail the involvement of mental health services in all aspects of life, certain important areas must be catered for if the mental health service is just that, and not a paper exercise to satisfy fashions of the day. It is possible to consider both community wide and more personal approaches to these facilities.

Health education programmes should be aiming towards a number of objectives: (i) Educating the general public as to the true effects of mental ill-health by highlighting predisposing factors which lead to it and an awareness of early recognition of the signs of any symptoms of mental ill-health. (ii) Advertising the available services and facilities which exist to help those people who have mental ill-health problems. (iii) Aiming at the reduction of the stigma and ignorance with which people view mental ill-health. Community services are at present provided by the Primary Health Care Team and voluntary organisations such as Alcoholics Anonymous and the Samaritans. There may be a case for an access point at, and through which, the general public can make use of more formal psychiatric services. Such a centre has been described by John Gleisner[8] and the potential for such self-referral, walk in centres is enormous. The previously hospital based services of psychology and psychiatric nursing have now begun to make themselves reachable by moving into the community. There are many examples of useful community psychiatric nursing services which have developed in recent years and have been described at length (see Hunter (1974) and Carr, et al (1980)).

The large psychiatric hospitals are begining to run down, although this run down is not pursued with equal vigour by all Area Health Authorities. As 'asylums' become less fashionable new psychiatric units are appearing which are attached to District General Hospitals. This has both advantages and disadvantages. The more extreme stigma of mental ill-health is reduced by placing it in a general hospital unit and the general public may find care and treatment within such a setting more palatable. This situation does tend to 'medicalize' mental health and illness to an even greater extent and the chance of asylum in its truest sense, i.e. peace and solitude away from the pressures of life, may be more difficult to find in such a unit, where the emphasis is on active treatment and rehabilitation programmes.

This is the era of 'team care' which should mean the widest possible coverage of all approaches to mental health and ill-health. The inclusion of the various parties who have an interest must mean a healthier approach to the encouragement of mental health promoting activities, and the early anticipation and correction of mental illness, and ill-health provoking situations. There are a number of strategies which must be employed to help make such tasks come a little nearer to fruition:

(i) Psychiatric services must continue to make themselves more accessible to the community — the current move towards the community by psychiatric services needs to be continued. This can only serve to make the general public more aware of, and possibly more at ease with, aspects of mental health and illness.

(ii) Ongoing research is essential into the areas of screening, and prevention programmes — while many people are in agreement that prevention is better than cure, there is no hard evidence to show that such early interventions are more effective, less costly or practically possible to undertake.

(iii) Education of existing health care personnel into aspects of prevention and mental health — the training of existing health care personnel is based very much around the 'treatment' aspects of illness and rarely examines the routes to prevention and mental health. This produces narrow concepts, and 'treatment' orientated services.

'Mental health' is a slippery concept to grasp. Depending upon the definitive stance adopted, and the eagerness or otherwise of health care services to be involved, there will be many different levels of interest and participation. Mental health, if nothing else, forces the practitioner to consider the other sides of a very complicated and currently 'loaded' dice.

REFERENCES

Brandon S 1970 Crisis theory and possibilities of therapeutic intervention. British Journal of Psychiatry 117 (541 December)
Caplan G 1964 Principles of preventive psychiatry. Tavistock, London

Carr P J, Butterworth C A, Hodges B E 1980 Community psychiatric nursing. Churchill Livingstone, Edinburgh
Corrigan J, Soni S D 1977 Community psychiatric nursing. An appraisal of its impact on community psychiatry in Manchester, England. Journal of Advanced Nursing Studies 2: 347–354
Gleisner J 1979 And experimental crisis centre. In: Meacher M (ed) New methods of mental health care. Pergammon Press, Oxford
Haines A J, Rae J B 1973 In: The Livingstone Project — the first five years (Scottish Health Service Studies No 29). Scottish Home and Health Department, Edinburgh
Hunter P 1974 Community psychiatric nursing in Great Britain, an historical review. International Journal of Nursing Studies 11: 223–233
Johnson A, Goldberg D V 1976 Psychiatric screening in general practice. The Lancet March 20: 605–608
Mechanic D 1966 Community psychiatry: some sociological perspectives and implications. In: Roberts L M, Halbeck S L, Loeb M D (eds) Community psychiatry. University of Wisconsin Press, Madison
Shepherd M, Cooper B, Brown A J, Kalton G W 1966 Psychiatric illness in general practice. Open University Press, London

FURTHER READING

Brandon S 1970 Crisis theory and possibilities of therapeutic intervention. British Journal of Psychiatry 117, 541 December
Butterworth C A, Skidmore D 1981 Caring for the mentally ill in the community. Croom Helm, London
Caplan G 1964 Principles of preventive psychiatry. Tavistock, London
Carr P J, Butterworth C A, Hodges B E 1980 Community psychiatric nursing. Churchill Livingstone, Edinburgh
Gleisner J 1979 An experimental crisis centre. In: Meacher M (ed) New methods of mental health care. Pergammon Press, Oxford
Goldberg D, Huxley P 1981 Mental illness in the community. Tavistock, London
Haines A J, Rae J B 1973 In: The Livingstone Project — the first five years (Scottish Health Service Studies No 29). Scottish Home and Health Department, Edinburgh

7

Spiritual care

Peter Coleman and Mary Coleman

Martin Luther, in nailing his 95 Theses to the church door at Wittenberg, began the Protestant Reformation with its upsurge of new thinking and understanding which spread into many areas of life. We are neither so energetic nor so ambitious! In offering five insights into the nature of care that are derived from, or emphasised by, a spiritual outlook on life, we hope we may perhaps stimulate some new thinking and understanding, and contribute to the reformation of community care that has been continuing for some time.

Spiritual care, we believe, can be viewed in the following five ways:

1. as an integral part of total care.
2. as concerned with health as with disease.
3. emphasis on the importance of individual conviction.
4. recognition of the social dimensions of health and disease.
5. underlining the role of the non-professional.

It is not suggested for one moment that these insights derive solely from a spiritual viewpoint, but rather that such a viewpoint underlies and reinforces this approach to community care.

1. An integral part of total care

Human personality can no longer be divided into the traditional categories of body, mind, and spirit. Our understanding of the interacting, interdependent nature of human personality has rendered obsolete this kind of artificial division of human life. The diagnosis of illness can no longer be contained under the heading of physical, mental, or even spiritual disorder. Increasingly the need to consider the total personality presents itself. Stafford-Clark (1975) writes of 'The ultimate impossibility of treating states of mind apart from states of body, and states of body apart from states of mind'. He goes on to say: 'in taking a history and conducting an examination of the patient, attention must be paid to the entire life situation of the person concerned, to his background and personal history, as well as to his presenting complaint'. Part of that entire life situation is what is often called a person's spiritual life, i.e. his sense of the purpose of life, his recognition or otherwise of the existence and presence of God, his striving after ethical and moral standards, his consciousness of guilt and failure, his belief in the efficacy of prayer and worship. This spiritual life is not separate from a person's state of health. Stafford-Clark gives an example of a patient suffering from ulcerative colitis, which at one point was strongly related to moral conflicts over military service. This under standing of illness is at least as old as the New Testament and the words of Jesus: 'Is it easier to say to this paralysed man "Your sins are forgiven", or to say, "Stand up, take your bed, and walk"?' (Mark 2,9) The recognition that both are the correct response is a recognition of the totality of human personality.

The corollary of this understanding that personality cannot be divided and that diagnosis has to take into account all aspects of a person's life, is that cure and care must likewise be concerned with the total person. The restoration of a person to health is a many faceted process in which different disciplines will play a part in caring, and where indeed there is a danger that a too narrow concept of care may impair recovery. There is, in addition, a warning here for the specialist:

> We pursue different disciplines and within even the same discipline each of us has his special interests and his special expertise. No one is able to comprehend everything and we are therefore betrayed by our desire for an answer into overlooking the importance of those things of which we know little or nothing, or even into denying that they can have any relevance . . . . . we regard as hostile to truth any other interpretation which is based on categories different from our own. What we defend is not truth but the security of our own convictions, or worse, of our vocations, our vested professional interests. (Lee, 1973)

The recognition that care has many facets will mean that the specialist, whether nurse, health visitor, doctor, social worker or clergyman, will exercise care in both specialist and non-specialist ways. Thus the nurse who spends time talking to a patient about belief in life after death as well as attending to a pressure sore, or the hospital chaplain who allays the fears of a patient regarding the nature of an operation, as well as praying with the patient, are both alike exercising care in a total sense. Faced with a bereaved widow, the best kind of care may be sitting talking, letting the anger, frustration, and sense of guilt and sadness come out, rather than prescribing tablets to give an enforced tranquility and sleep. But what kind of care is this, and who is best able to give it?

2. Concern with health as with disease

Wilson (1975) begins his book *Health is for People* with these words: 'In his novel *Nineteen Eighty-four*, George Orwell describes four ministries through which The Party holds power: A Ministry of Peace concerned with war. A Ministry of Love for law and order. A Ministry of Plenty to deal with scarcities. A Ministry of Truth where a vast system of brainwashing is planned and executed. He did not need to describe a Ministry of Health which deals with disease: we already have one.' We support the view that so often caring has been too narrowly concerned with disease rather than health. Such a concern stems from a negative standpoint which tends to define health as the absence of illness and suffering. It is a Biblical and spiritual concept which sees health in the positive terms of wholeness and wellbeing, and which can countenance, indeed create, a healthy attitude to disease and death.

The Peckham Health Centre of the 1940s which Wilson also describes with its cafeteria, large hall, swimming bath, gymnasium and theatre, and its practice of family membership enshrines a very different concept of health than does its modern counterpart with its cluster of treatment rooms, consulting rooms and clinics. The former is concerned, as the name suggests with health, the latter with disease. A Church with its variety of organisations for young, middle-aged, and older people, which meet some of the recreational and leisure needs of a community, and its provision of voluntary day centres, luncheon clubs, street warden schemes, regular visiting of the elderly and housebound, telephone dialling services for the lonely and depressed, parties and holidays for the mentally or physically disabled, or for the elderly, is concerned with a concept of health which includes disease, and a concept of community care which provides for the fit and the able, as well as for the sick and the needy.

The overseas work of the Church makes the same point. From the early days of Christian missions, the emphasis has been on the provision of health in its broadest sense, so churches, schools, and hospitals stood side by side as they still do in many developing countries. Preaching, teaching and healing were considered part and parcel of the same concern, to which today has been added care for the hungry and the poor, with resultant work amongst refugees and the teaching and demonstrating of agricultural techniques to improve nutritional standards. This is not just a concern for illness, disease or deficiency, but a care for health, wholeness, indeed for life.

In a different way the growth of Hospices for the Dying which have been pioneered by the Church in recent years illustrates the same positive spiritual insight. The whole thrust of the philosophy that lies behind the creation of a hospice and the nature of its care, is that it is possible and indeed right to have a healthy attitude to illness and dying.

3. Emphasis on importance of individual conviction

Part of the Christian heritage that is enjoyed in the Western hemisphere is an understanding of human nature that is based on the Biblical concept of man being made in the image of God and therefore with a dignity and importance that gives to the individual human life a particular significance. This is not to suggest that such an understanding of human nature is not to be found in other great world religions, or indeed in non-religious philosophical world views, but to show that, whatever its origin, such a concept is a spiritual one. This view of man very clearly influences the attitude we have to those in need. In pre-Christian times human life was held cheaply, e.g. unwanted babies especially female ones were left to die of exposure, the ill were left to die uncared for, gladiators could fight to the death in the arena for the entertainment of others. Today, though sometimes denied by events, to which Belsen and Sharpeville bear witness, human life is in the main held as sacred, or at least lip-service is paid to the ideal. The continuing debate on the ethics of abortion and euthanasia only serve to show the strength of this belief about human life.

Along with respect for human life itself has gone respect for the beliefs and convictions of human individuals. Religious people at their worst have often been guilty, and still can be as the continuing tragedy of Northern Ireland shows, of intolerance towards those of other persuasions. However, it is worth remembering that the first full plea for religious toleration printed in the English language was written by a Christian as long ago as 1612, (Thomas Helwys, 1612), and it was a toleration which included the non-Christian religious believer and the atheist.

This belief in the sacredness of human life and a tolerance for the beliefs of others has a special place in caring, and should show in attitudes towards the convictions of those being cared for. Saunders (1973) has stated: 'We should never impose our own beliefs and our own feeling of meaning on to another person, but I am quite sure we can help to produce a climate in which patients can find their own meaning.' The patient who is helped by a prayer said by a minister, or by the sacrament of Holy Communion, or by annointing with oil, or by particular dietary observances, and to whom these things are important, has a right to expect that the carer will make possible such religious observances even if, to them, they have no meaning or significance. True spiritual care will also respect the beliefs, convictions and assumptions that individuals have about the meaning of life and death, the importance of worship, the existence of God, even if the person exercising care does not share such beliefs.

This is not to say that there will not be areas of religious conviction where the carers will find themselves in a dilemma. The rejection of blood transfusions on religious grounds is one such area. So also are the differing attitudes to birth control and abortion, made more difficult by the sincerely held religious views on both sides of the question. Caring is not a mechanical, robot-like activity, it is essentially the response of one human being to another, so inevitably tension and difficulty will arise on occasion. This same response will also give rise to compassionate sympathy and understanding which are part of the human components of care, often arising from a person's spiritual awareness and sense of commitment.

4. Recognition of the social dimensions of health and disease

If the last section has been concerned to show that people have a right to be treated as people who matter, with beliefs and convictions, rather than as interesting cases or diseases, this section is concerned to show that people cannot be considered in isolation but must be seen as members of a community. Much of Christianity, as much of the teaching of other world religions, is concerned with how man is to live in community and the nature of his relationship with his fellow man. The Church has taught that mankind is to be seen as a family with mutual dependence and mutual responsibilities. One of these responsibilities is to share in the creation of a healthy society. Brian Wren in a leaflet for Christian Aid quoted by Kane (1975) tells the parable of a factory employing thousands of workers on modern production lines turning out a high volume of machines every day, but with a high accident rate because of human error. Men came out of the factory with crushed fingers, broken limbs, and there were the occasional accidental deaths. An enterprising Christian minister organised a first aid tent outside the factory gates. As concern grew the Council of Churches sponsored a properly built clinic. With the interest and support of the Town Council, the Chamber of Trade and the Rotary Club, the clinic became a small hospital. Then the factory management, seeing the good that was being done, and wishing to be thought enlightened, gave unrestricted access to the factory for hospital personel, a small annual grant, and an ambulance to speed serious cases from workshop to hospital. But year by year as production rose, despite the work of the hospital, so did the accident rate and the number of deaths. Only then did people begin to ask if it was enough to treat people's injuries while leaving untouched the machinery that caused them.

Caring for health has a social, even a political dimension. What is true of accidents in the parable has been shown to be true of alcoholism, tooth decay, lung cancer, and the whole range of illnesses that are partly caused by a style of life and a social acceptance of that life-style which is harmful to human health. Too often we battle with the symptoms whilst ignoring the causes. Community care is not just caring in the community, it is care for the community in its widest sense, and a moulding of that community's life-style by values which are in the last resort, spiritual.

A second responsibility that arises from the recognition that man is mutually dependent, is the responsibility to create or encourage the kind of small group within which care can be exercised. In hospitals this kind of group can be seen most clearly in the group therapy unit which is an essential part of psychiatric treatment. In the community it can be seen in the work of groups like Alcoholics Anonymous, societies for the mentally or physically handicapped, day centres for the elderly and lonely, Cruse Clubs for those recently widowed, Cancer Anonymous and many others, whose basis is a sharing of experience and the recognition of a common humanity. It is significant that many, though not all of these caring groups are organised and staffed on a voluntary basis, and have their origins in a quite explicit religious concern.

5. Underlining the role of the non-professional

We ended the section on the concept of total care with a question: What kind of care is this, and who is best able to give it? Whilst not for one moment belittling the professional skills of doctor, nurse, social worker or clergyman, enough has been written to show that within the total care of a person there is a place for the non-professional — the close relative, the concerned neighbour, the old established friend, the fellow member of a Church or club, or the anonymous volunteer who gives valuable spare time to the work of Samaritans or marriage guidance. The value of such non-professional caring has been demonstrated by Bagley's study of Samaritans (1968), showing a correlation between the introduction of Samaritan services and a reduction in the suicide rate, making the U.K. at that time the only country in Western Europe with a declining suicide rate. Caplan (1961) underlines the importance of police, midwives, teachers, barmen, bus conductors, the man or woman who runs the corner shop or the bingo hall, the granny in a street, the mother of a family, who are the key people who listen to, advise and help their neighbours and who are to be found in every community. Nye Bevan in one of his speeches at the inauguration of the National Health Service said 'There is no substitute for the good neighbour.'

Such non-professional voluntary caring often, though by no means always, has behind it a religious motivation. It is seen by the volunteer as one of the ways in which the command to love God and one's neighbour is fulfilled. A volunteer or good neighbour is encouraged by the Church to see such service in terms of a stewarding of the God given gifts of time or energy or ability. Thus what is essentially a spiritual understanding is worked out in very practical and physical ways. Archbishop William Temple's comment that Christianity is the most materialist of all faiths would appear to ring true in this context. Even in those instances where an explicit sense of religious commitment is absent or denied, there is an inevitable dependence on the ethos of Christian culture which, with other influences, has permeated our society over the preceeding centuries, and which has left its mark particularly in attitudes to voluntary service. This is perhaps best illustrated by the existence of a number of voluntary agencies, which, though not specifically Christian or religious in the narrow sense, have their origin in Christian concern. Oxfam, Help the Aged, the Samaritans, and Cruse Clubs all demonstrate this, the last two betraying by their biblically derived names the close relationship with a Christian-caring philosophy.

These same two factors, the religious motivation of the volunteer and the religious origin of many voluntary caring organisations, are of course to be found in the professional side of caring. There are those who see their profession in terms of a religious vocation, and the origin of hospitals and care for the sick in the Christian Church has been charted in other places. To the extent that this common tradition still exists between the professional and non-professional, it is a factor contributing to the close working partnership between the two and the acceptance of a clear role for both.

As well as these five insights spiritual care makes an all-important general contribution to community care by widening the definition of caring — caring is not just technology, it is technology plus love. Dr Cicely Saunders (1973) Medical Director of St Christopher's Hospice, and previously trained as both a nurse and a social worker, when talking quite simply of a person having a cup of tea on the last day of their life says: 'this cup of tea comes best of all from someone who has compassion, understanding and practicality, someone who adds heart to skill and has a sense of meaning and the assurance of another dimension of life.' Love is a spiritual quality and, as the quotation demonstrates, derives from a person's understanding of, or attitude to, life including for some a belief in God. It is to be found in the professional and the non-professional, but it cannot be taught in the way that technology can. It can be deepened and broadened by a clearer knowledge and understanding of the total needs of a person. It is here perhaps that a wider role than is sometimes envisaged for the professional can be seen. The educational or teaching side of the work of a district nurse, health visitor, social worker, or doctor in enabling the non-professional to care more effectively is a side that may well expand of necessity in the face of increasingly stringent cutbacks in the professional caring services. We believe that it should expand regardless of such a possibility, and that the situation described by Sheila Hancock (1973) when wanting to care for her dying mother should never arise:

> I found a strange resistance in some nurses to teach me; they seemed to think I was invading their professional privacy in some way . . . . there was this curious attitude, as with a lot of specialists, that it was not my business.

That attitude as she was quick to point out, was a generalisation and certainly does not apply to all professionals. But where it does, it is technology without love, or sensitivity, or that spiritual dimension which is the vital and essential ingredient in caring.

REFERENCES

Bagley C 1968 The evaluation of suicide prevention scheme by an ecological method. Social Science and Medicine vol 2
Caplan G 1961 An approach to community mental health. Tavistock, London
Helwys T 1612 The Mistery of Iniquity. Facsimile published in 1935 for Baptist Historical Society. Kingsgate Press, London
Kane M 1975 Theology in an industrial society. S.C.M., London
Lee R S 1973 In: Melinsky M A H (ed) Religion and medicine, 2. S.C.M., London
Saunders C 1973 In: Care of the dying. Report of a National Symposium. HMSO, London
Stafford-Clark D, Smith Andrew C 1978 Psychiatry for students. Allen & Unwin, London
Wilson M 1975 Health is for people. Darton Longman & Todd, London

FURTHER READING

DHSS 1973 Care of the dying. Report of a National Symposium. HMSO, London
Melinsky M A H (ed) 1973 Religion and medicine, 2. S.C.M., London
Millard D W (ed) 1976 Religion and medicine, 3. S.C. M., London
Stafford-Clark D 1972 Five questions in search of an answer. Fontana, London
Wilson M 1975 Health is for people. Darton Longman & Todd, London
Wilson M 1966 The church is healing. S.C.M., London

SECTION TWO

Contexts

From time immemorial it has been recognised that there is a link between an individual's wellbeing and the environment in which he lives. In the 5th century BC, in a treatise entitled 'Airs, Waters, Places' the Greek physician Hippocrates exhorted doctors to study these subjects, for 'A physician who understands them well, or at least as well as he can, could not fail to observe what diseases are important in a given locality as well as the nature of the inhabitants in general, when he first comes into a district which was unfamiliar to him. Thus he would not be at a loss to treat the diseases to which the inhabitants are liable nor would be make mistakes as he would certainly do had he not thought about these things beforehand.' More than a thousand years later Florence Nightingale, in promoting 'sanitary nursing' made much the same point. The power of this knowledge for the prevention of illness was also recognised, and was especially important during times before the development of medical science made the cure of diseases a realistic alternative. The failure to use this knowledge, which is evidenced by the emphasis in the U.K. and most other developed countries on curative medicine and the direction of intervention to the individual rather than the environment, is as paradoxical as it is tragic. Part of the explanation may lie in the power system which determines decisions about health care provision — an issue which is directly addressed in the final chapter in this section. Part may lie in the deep-seated fatalism of ordinary people and in the awe inspired in most cultures by the interventionist 'medicine man'. Part of the explanation, however, must lie in the basic preparation of doctors and nurses in which the 'patient in the bed' is accepted without challenge as an unalterable 'given' — and it is towards countering this attitude that this section is mainly devoted.

The term 'environment' includes far more than Hippocrates' 'Airs, waters, and Places'; indeed, the treatise lists among the factors to be considered, alongside the seasons, the winds, the water supply, and the soil, 'the life of the inhabitants themselves.' The 'life' of people is not limited to, nor determined only by, physiological manifestations; the social, cultural, political, and economic environments within which people live, exert an influence on their health at least as great as that exerted by the physical environment. The health care system itself consistutes an environment which influences the givers and the receivers of care and, therefore, also the nature of the care given.

All these perspectives are included in this section, and it is for this reason that we have preferred the word 'Contexts' to 'Environment' for the title of the section.

Jeremy Cobb writes from the perspective of a community physician, whose unique function is said to be that of 'change agent' which has in turn been defined by Lakin as 'a paragon who had awareness of the need for change, was able to diagnose the problems involved, who could plan for change, implement his plans, and evaluate the results.'The ability to implement change, let alone to evaluate the results, is for community physicians and others more problematic because it is limited by constraints touched on within Dr Cobb's own contribution and expanded later by Jane Salvage. Caroline Cox discusses why these factors are important, and Alix Henley shows what happens when we fail to take account of them. Jennifer Barnard's chapter reminds us that since people spend approximately a third of each day for approximately half of their lives at work, both the fact of work and the environment within which it happens are important — as important for those who do not have work as for those who have. Jean Gaffin describes the field of social welfare, of which the NHS is only one part, and shows how what happens in one sector inevitably affects what happens in another. Finally, Jane Salvage analyses the political and economic environment, which perhaps more than anything else determines what kinds of health care will be provided, by whom and for whom.

The contributions contained in this section are as different from one another as are their contributors, and each was written quite independently of the others. Yet there are certain common strands. In this section one can detect, perhaps more clearly than in any other, a challenge to the appropriateness of modern curative medicine to society's needs. In several of the essays, but perhaps especially in those of Alix Henley and Jane Salvage, one can sense the anger provoked by our apparent inability to make the change which all (that is, all the contributors to this book) agree to be necessary.

One further issue, which is implied by several of the contributors and touched upon by Jane Salvage in her closing paragraphs, is commended for consideration. This is the dilemma for all health workers produced by knowing that environmental factors and social conditions are affecting a patient's health or recovery from illness and being unable to change those conditions. Social work has moved much further than either medicine or nursing in facing this dilemma and in taking action to resolve it. Nurses are only just beginning to consider a role as the patient's advocate in attempting to improve his situation. Yet caring for people, whether they are defined as patients, clients or consumers, must include measures to improve in whatever way is possible the conditions which are affecting their health, as well as providing the support which may be necessary to maintain health at the optimum level in whatever conditions they find themselves.

8

A healthy environment

Jeremy Cobb

In a society which has taken so enthusiastically to the curative idea of modern medicine, it is difficult to emphasise the environment as the crucial factor in health that it is. Many of its concepts are put forward in vague and over-academic terms so that environmental concerns fail to achieve the same status as the images so readily available to curative medicine. Can the sewers really be as important as 'intensive care'? Safety in the home does not appear to get the same attention as the event of an injured child admitted to a casualty department — and yet it must claim more if prevention is to mean anything.

The images that are projected by the communications which we all use are affected very powerfully by the need to capture attention by being dramatic. This concentration on the easily-made drama which is so encouraged in the health professions, has allowed curative medicine to become a dominant concern of society; the organisation and development of curative medicine is accorded a priority which is really false. The development of curative medicine has turned the health concern of the communnity away from the environment and focused it on the curative institutions — and yet the environment that *is* the community itself, is often ignored as the generator of ill-health.

Perhaps one of the most devastating analyses of the reasons why modern attitudes to health are so concerned with technology and cure, was made by Illich (1976). In the second chapter of his book *Limits to Medicine* he discusses the 'medicalization of life' and shows how the concern to find cures for all disease and discomfort has become accepted by Western society. It seems we are caught in a style of thinking that can only generate more and more technology and increasing numbers of professionals to 'fight disease'.

Such emphasis on cure has unfortunately detracted from the notion that change in the environment designed to prevent health problems could be carried much further than at present. The need now is to divert our attention from the restless search for cures, to look more closely at the environment in all its many aspects, and to consider how it is responsible for causing ill-health. The society and community which we inhabit is a piece of that environment.

Does the 'environment' really cause harm? Can examples be identified? The answer to both questions is unfortunately yes: examples can easily be identified:

(a) 68 010 people were killed or seriously injured by motor vehicles in 1978.
(b) Accidents in the home killed 6063 people and injured many more.

(c) In the same year 21 334 pedestrians — people just crossing the road or walking on pavements — were killed or seriously injured.

Such statistics can be compared with those relating to disease processes that are not so clearly connected with the environment. If all the accidental and violent deaths of people between the ages of 5 and 35 are added together, they cause many more deaths than any intrinsic disease process. Certainly the environment exerts a profound effect on life.

Amongst the causes of accidents in the home it is often possible to trace a clear link with poor environmental circumstances, which makes it easier to suggest means of improvement. However, links with the environment for some other diseases are not so clear, but the suspicion that the environment has some kind of effect on *all* health remains. Examination of all causes of mortality in the United Kingdom was made by Howe (1976). It is apparent that certain geographic areas are healthier than others — in general terms, the south-east seems the healthiest. The trouble is that the exact connection between the environment and disease is not clear-cut. There are some pointers: the dramatic reduction of respiratory diseases following the introduction of smoke-free zones in 1956 made it quite clear that smog was a very real hazard. Where such connections are clear it is possible to bring about improvements in respect of pollutants. Even when there is sufficient evidence that a pollutant is harmful, however, it is not easy to exert sufficient influence on the necessary bureaucracies to bring about effective control. Getting legislation passed and implemented can be a long and difficult process. Lead pollution is clearly too high in this country, and yet until very recently it was impossible to convince the government that action should be taken. How these problems can be tackled will be examined under different headings, but it is almost certain that there are other pollutants waiting to be identified in the environment which affect health. In these circumstances, community workers must know and follow the patterns of legislation that have been developed to cope with known dangerous substances. An exercise which any community worker might undertake is to trace the reports and published opinions about a particular pollutant into the legislation process, and on into the implementation of that legislation. Such an exercise on asbestos, for example, would give considerable insight into why most organisations take so long to respond.

The community worker must also be aware of newer pollutions, e.g. the extraordinary rise in noise levels throughout society, as well as in industry. The accepted levels of noise in some discotheques and dance halls will be as damaging to the ear as any factory clamour.

Environmental conditions can affect early life, and the deaths from accidents and violence reflect that important fact. After the early part of life, certain disease processes become more evident as a cause of death and disability. During the ages from 30 to 65 years of age, ischaemic heart disease and strokes make their impact. Ischaemic heart disease is the leading cause of death in men for this age group, whilst strokes are a very important cause of death and disability in both sexes. Lung cancer is also a leading cause of death in men and will also probably increase as a cause of death in women.

How does the environment affect these diseases? In terms of our personal environment, tobacco smoke causes lung cancer and it seems very probable that a polluted space containing tobacco smoke will affect even non-smokers. There also appear to be clear links between the lower exercise levels of individuals who suffer heart attacks when compared with those who do not. Any environment which makes it difficult for an individual to take regular exercise must be seen as contributing to the toll of death from heart attacks.

Dietary factors also play an important part in ischaemic heart disease. The dietary habits of a community are a reflection of a cultural pattern and environment. This cultural environment significantly affects life-style and can be understood as the immediate personal environment of family and friends together with the other everyday influences of the work place and recreation. In health terms there is much wrong with these environments where certain foods and alcohol have become so harmful and yet retain a status out of proportion to their real value. Between 1970 and 1977, admissions of patients under the age of 25 years with a primary diagnosis of alcoholism or alcoholic psychosis showed an increase in men of 139% and for women, no less than 375%! How much of this harm to health comes from the environment created by advertising or of social pressure is a matter for conjecture, but the dangers of excessive consumption seem to be poorly understood and the methods of teaching individuals to adopt healthy habits largely ignored.

In the nineteenth century, a major influence on personal environment came when sewers and clean water supplies were established. Cholera and typhoid were prevented by such measures but public opinion and medical opinion were hostile to such major capital investment. Yet these engineering efforts did more for health than all the medical practitioners together. Perhaps there is a parallel now — the environment, in a broad sense, has been forgotten because public opinion is too concerned with cure — those dramatic images of cure on which so much money is spent, with so little benefit.

The picture of the environment as a whole includes many physical factors which are seen at their most destructive in the decaying urban centres common to many of our cities. Overcrowding and pollution are the obvious effects of underlying social problems which are linked with economic and occupational factors. These factors are a fundamental part of the environment and are identified in the Black Report on Inequalities in Health (DHSS, 1980). In this Report, many clues can be found which point the way for future action to change services in urban communities.

Social class differences in health are marked. In 1970–1972, the infant mortality rate in Social Class I was more than 30% below the rate for all classes — whilst the rate in Social Class V was over 70% higher (OHE, 1979). Mortality from most causes is significantly worse in lower socio-economic groups (DHSS, 1980), and it is just these groups who generally find themselves in the worst environmental conditions.

In the discussion of the environment so far, it has been necessary to paint a jumbled picture. The problem confronting any worker in the community is how to understand the environment in all its complexity, so that such a worker can put energy into making improvement and without feeling that environmental matters are too complex or too big to change. Some kind of analysis is needed which, at the very least, gives some direction for positive action.

In approaching this problem, the distinction between *macro* and *micro* is useful because this is more readily understood within the framework of personal experience and individual perception of the community. The word *macro* is intended to imply all those environmental concerns which are affected by structured, well-defined authorities and established bodies who determine broad policy. These policies are the *macro* framework within which individuals must operate. Other *macro* environmental factors include climate and geography, widespread pollutants and large scale occupations that are harmful, as well as the large scale problems of poverty and deprivation.

Within the large scale environments exist a rich variety of activities closely related to human behaviour — the interaction between people. This is the *micro* environment, which includes personal habits as well as accommodation and housing, local community facilities and transport. Such a *micro* environment can be analysed in terms of human behaviour — the seeking of prestige and power, the deals done between individuals, the reward of others for favours granted. Also included in the *micro* environment is the local management structure and systems which affect operational community workers.

The importance of distinguishing between *macro* and *micro* elements of the environment lies in observing the links between the two. Clearly, little effect on the climate can be made by the activities in the micro environment (unless one believes in witchcraft!); but in terms of the policies that develop from the major bureaucracies, the micro environmental systems can have an effect — indeed it is the face-to-face relations, discussions and bargaining which are gradually turned into the more anonymous written reports and orders which are built up into the macro systems which direct environmental policy. This does not mean that such policies are good for the environment but it does mean that some kind of interaction exists which can be used to change policy.

The establishment of many health policies affects the micro environment of the individual. The community worker and activist have a responsibility to be aware of the issues involved, seeking wherever possible to influence policy in the positive direction of health improvement for all, even where this means emphasising the needs of a particular group of people. The evidence that the wearing of seat belts would improve the accident injuries and fatalities was clear for many years before the macro system (in this case Parliament) was sufficiently convinced to alter the law to enforce them to be worn, despite the fact that such prevention would help not just the injured individual, but all the members of family and work who depend on such an individual. If the current road death figures were caused by some famous infection like 'Legionnaires' disease', laws would soon find their way to the statute books.

Everyday interaction between individuals is the essence of the micro environment and is the vehicle of influence which the community worker must use. The basic aim is to supply knowledge about the health impact of the personal environment to individuals. Such information given must find room for all the possibilities that the individual can create to influence his own environment. The range should be wide; it must include not only hygiene and communicable disease information, but must be positive about the control of smoking and the need for exercise on a regular basis. The risks of travelling without seat belts must be clearly presented and it must be made clear that health rests for the most part with the individual and *not* with the medical profession. The individual must be encouraged to take action on his own behalf.

Anyone working in the community — that is anyone working outside a formal institution — has to learn to avoid a patronising approach to information giving. All too often professional education bestows an exaggerated sense of self-importance and regard. The clear objective of the health educator must be to raise the individual's awareness of advantages to be gained by reorganising the personal environment. To achieve this professional workers have to sacrifice their own prestige in order to raise the level of self-confidence in the people they serve.

Perhaps more crucial than any other task, a community worker needs to try to change his own and his clients' view of curative medicine and in particular the idea that there is a pill or operation for all troubles when the personal environment itself is the cause. The professional traditions that pervade the education of doctors, nurses and related professions can be seen as disabling to individuals struggling to manage their own environments (McKnight, 1977).

Analysing the case of a particular patient in the community is not an opportunity to atomise someone's environmental need into the divided specialty conditions of modern technological medicine; rather it is to create an awareness of the potential for healthy living by seeeing the individual's whole behaviour in relationship to the local environment and strengthening any desire to alter that environment to gain the advantages of health.

The hospitals and other institutions that have developed in a local community do *not* merit the priority that is often claimed — the priority should be given to asbence of pollution, stress and deprivation, to the space in architectural and urban terms to live healthily, and to the knowledge and desire to change to healthy living habits on the part of the population.

Reference has already been made to the link between the micro environment, consisting of the social interactions and geography of the local community, and the macro environment consisting of the formalised institutions and climates that make up the macro environment. The readily identifiable bridge between the two is the concept of organisations. A useful introduction to the concept of modern organisation is given by Etzioni (1964) and an evaluation of organisational theory by Silverman (1970).

Understanding organisations is basic to using them as a tool to improve the environment. Frequently, community workers are obliged to behave towards their clients in a way which reflects the macro policy of an organisation, instead of offering a genuine choice. What is on offer is something that the organisation is comfortable about, rather than a support for the individual's independent action.

Workers caught in this conflict will often find themselves declaring that they have 'no interest in management' or are only 'interested in people' or, more commonly, 'my reward comes from my patients/clients'. The unpopularity of organisations — the so called 'management' — serves only to reinforce those professional attitudes which insist that some cure or solution can only come from them or from the professionally trained person. This invasion of professionalism has occurred in health organisations to the extent that the original objectives of the organisation have been changed to meet the expectations of the professionals involved. A good example is the continuing debate about heart transplantation, performed for a handful of patients at great cost whilst the prevention of death from environmental causes is ignored. There have been some changes — attention has been drawn to the terrible waste of life on the roads, and the environmental encouragement which increases alcoholism.

The National Health Service itself was established during the post-war period as an organisation whose specific purpose was to make its services equally available to all when there was need. Yet inequality in health has still persisted (DHSS, 1980) despite the enormous social impact that the Health Service made particularly during its early years. Regrettably, the original objectives of the National Health Service have become supplanted by professional objectives which are characterised by a desperate search for professional prestige through technology.

Thus there is a clear need for those individuals involved in community work to re-enter the organisational framework to take the operational problems of the environment right into its formal structure. Policy *can* be influenced by people who are prepared to accept management responsibilities and to learn the organisation structure and behaviour patterns. However, this cannot be done without explicit and detailed study of how such organisations work. The community worker at the operational level must know how the policy forming machinery works *in all its detail*. The superficial outline of organisational theory which is sometimes included in conferences and courses is not sufficient.

To generate the energy which is necessary to influence policy the environmental worker needs to be able to recognise opportunities and to be aware of the issues that can be affected. This means being well informed and developing an ability to think politically. A useful guide to thinking in political terms has been written by Blondel (1978). Political activity is often held in the same poor esteem by professionals as the management and administration of organisations. Unfortunately, this tends to reduce the opportunities to make change since it involves rejection of the machinery that can achieve change. Thinking in political terms may not come easily to professionals but is essential if the proper links between the environment problems and means of solving them, are to be improved.

Greater recognition needs to be given by all community workers to the importance of the environment. Professional education must change, to reduce the inappropriate emphasis on curative medicine, to increase understanding of organisational behaviour at both the macro and the micro level, and to generate interest in political and managerial mechanisms for the improvement of health.

REFERENCES

Blondel J 1978 Thinking politically. Pelican Books, London
British Medical Journal 1981 282: 1177
Compendium of Health Statistics 1979 3rd edn. Office of Health Economics, London
DHSS 1976 Prevention and health, everybody's business. HMSO, London
DHSS 1980 Inequalities in health. Report of a research working group. DHSS, London
Etzioni A 1964 Modern organisations. Prentice-Hall, London
Howe G Melvyn 1976 Man, environment and disease in Britain. Pelican Books, London
Illich I 1976 Limits to medicine. Pelican Books, London
McKnight J 1977 Professionalized service and disabling help. In: Boyars M (ed) Disabling professions.
Morris J N 1964 Uses of epidemiology. 2nd edn. E & S Livingstone, Edinburgh
Silverman D 1970 The theory of organisations. Heinemann, London
Social Trends 1980 edition. HMSO, London

9

Class, culture and community

Caroline Cox

'Class' is not just a piece of sociological jargon. It is a word which refers to deep human experiences and relationships. It includes the diversities of wealth and poverty; of social snobbery and social deference; of inequalities in access to, and benefit from, various educational, health and welfare services. It may also be reflected in the avoidable death of a child and the tragedy of an impoverished, undernourished elderly person dying alone in a cold room from hypothermia.

Similarly, the word 'culture' is not a mere abstract concept, but a word used to describe the richness and variety of the world of human ideas. It refers to the realms of knowledge, beliefs, values, attitudes and prejudice; it comprises ways in which people in different societies or groups understand the world and interpret experience, and it is handed down from one generation to the next by the process of 'socialization'. A culture may be very stable and last for centuries — as in the case of traditional Indian caste society; or elements may change quite rapidly: for example, we in Britain in the late 20th century think and behave in ways which would have shocked our Victorian forbears. Moreover, one society may contain a variety of different cultures or sub-cultures and so class and culture often overlap.

Classes vary in life styles, standards of living, attitudes, beliefs and values. There are the famous accounts of family life in the traditional working class communities of London's East End (Young & Willmott, 1957) and others which describe middle class families (Bell, 1968). Other studies have highlighted the effects of occupation on the surrounding community and family life; graphic portraits of the life of deep sea fishermen (Tunstall, 1969) or of coal miners (Dennis et al, 1956) contrast vividly with those of people in the professions (Rapoport & Rapoport, 1971). Their life-styles will be different again from those of families who earn their living from the land — and among these, the lives of those who are engaged in capital intensive agriculture will be different from those in sheep farming in remote mountains and moorlands. So, even within the confines of our small islands we need to take account of a great diversity of class, culture and types of community and to consider their implications for health care.

Moreover, during the last 100 years and especially since the Second World War, Britain has become home for many people from other parts of the world. We are now a multiracial society and many of those who have settled here have come from countries with very diverse cultures, including those of Asia, Africa and other parts of Europe. We will need to look at some of the implications for health of these cultures and the ways of life associated with them.

The chapter gives a brief overview of those aspects of *social class* which have a bearing on health care with particular reference to:

1. the *incidence of mortality and morbidity*
2. the *provision of health care*
3. the *uptake of health care*.

and then turns to a consideration of the relationship between *culture* and health with particular reference to:

(i) cultural variations in the perception of, and response to, pain and illness
(ii) communication between people of different cultures or sub-cultures
(iii) health problems associated with particular cultures — especially those of some ethnic minority groups.

Finally the effect of class and culture on the provision of health care is considered.

SOCIAL CLASS

The concept 'class' has been discussed by social scientists for over 100 years, and is still the centre of much debate. However, in this chapter a practical working definition will be used — the Registrar General's classification based on income and occupational status — as this is most frequently used in health care studies.

Social class variations in mortality and morbidity

There are significant and persisting differences in the patterns of disease and death between social classes in our society. Sir John Brotherston reviewed the situation in the Galton Lecture in 1975 (Brotherston, 1976) and it has been usefully discussed by Blaxter (1976). A more recent account is provided by Morris in his paper 'Social inequalities undiminished' and recently all the evidence has been brought together and reviewed by the working party under the chairmanship of Sir Douglas Black. (DHSS, 1980). These reviews reveal differences in perinatal mortality, and show that inequalities in ill health increase in childhood and that overall mortality and morbidity rates also increase as one moves from Social Class I to Social Class V. However, before looking at these inequalities in some detail, it must be stressed that they should be seen in the context of many changes and improvements in the general state of health of our society as a whole. The virtual eradication or control of many of the killer disease of earlier decades such as tuberculosis, and of epidemic diseases such as cholera, has meant that the overall state of health for all sections of the population has improved greatly. So discussion of the worrying persistence of continuing inequalities, must take account of dramatic improvements in general health resulting from rising standards of living, and advances in public health, medical science and health care.

There is only space here for a few illustrative examples of social class differences in disease and death. I have chosen perinatal mortality; mortality of adult males of working age; and sickness — acute and chronic.

Perinatal mortality

This table shows rates for perinatal mortality increasing consistently and persis-

Table 9.1 Perinatal mortality rates in England and Wales: social class (legitimate single births only) per 1000 live and still births. (Source: Population Trends 4, 1976)

Social class	1950	1973	Percentage decrease 1950–73
I Professional	25.4	13.9	45
II Managerial	30.4	15.6	49
III Skilled	33.6	19.2	43
non-manual		17.3	
manual		19.7	
IV Semi-skilled	36.9	21.8	41
V Unskilled	40.4	26.8	34
All social classes (including armed forces, students, etc)	34.9*	18.9	46

* Estimated

tently from Social Class I to V. It also illustrates the point made a little earlier: that there has been an overall improvement and that the rate for Social Class V in 1973 had almost dropped to that of Social Class I two decades earlier. But there is no room for complacency. Lambert (1976) emphasized that our perinatal mortality rate is still well above that of other countries (e.g. Sweden's 14.3). He pointed to some of the main factors influencing this and suggested: 'Substantial progress towards lower levels of perinatal mortality might be made if a greater proportion of all births were to be clustered at the optimal maternal ages (20–29 years), if fewer mothers had more than two children and if the rates experienced in Social Classes I and II could be extended to all babies.' More recently the Short Report on perinatal mortality has confirmed this view.

Adult mortality

Table 9.2 shows the variation in death rates for men of working age (i.e. 15–64) by social class.

Table 9.2 Mortality of men* by social class, ages 15–64, 1970–72. (Morris, 1979)

Social class	Standardised mortality ratios (*Refers to all men in England and Wales 100)
I	77
II	81
III (non-manual)	99
III (manual)	106
IV	114
V	137

Morbidity

When we turn from death to disease, we must remember it does not follow automatically that variations in mortality rates are precise reflections of rates of morbidity. Many illnesses and disabilities are not lethal. Many factors may influence a person's decision when, or whether, to seek medical treatment for particular ailments. Much illness may go unreported for many reasons — some of them linked with social class. For example, a person in a professional occupation, or

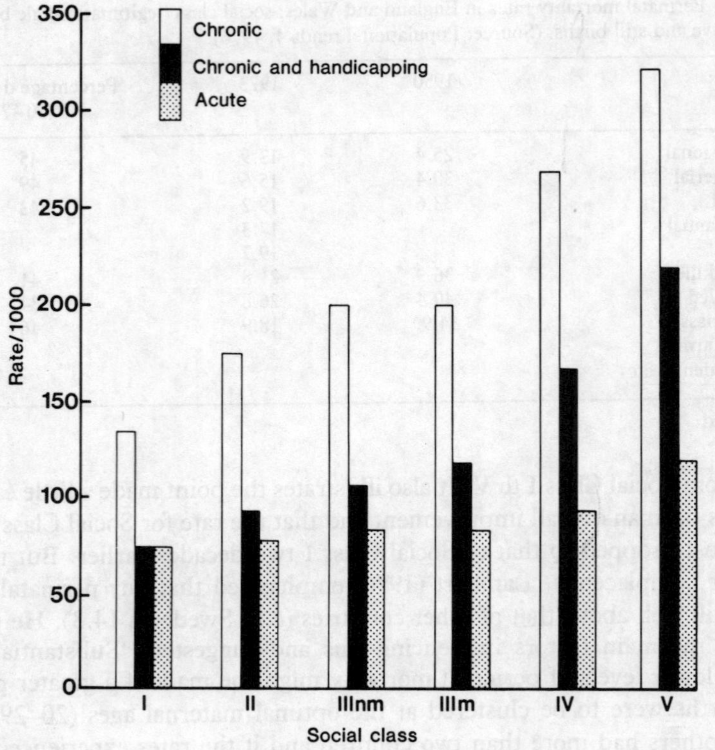

Fig. 9.1 Rates of self-reported illness by social class, per 1000 people, men and women, all ages, Great Britain (General Household Survey, 1972).

who is self- employed, may not need a 'certificate' for a short-term incapacitating illness, whereas a manual worker may need to see his doctor to obtain one: he is thus more likely to appear in the GP's surgery and so to feature in the statistics. In contrast, a working class mother with small children, and dependent on public transport, may find it harder to visit the doctor for consultation than her middle class counterpart with a car; she will, therefore, be less likely to figure in the statistics and to receive treatment for a comparable condition. Consequently, statistics of morbidity may not be a very accurate indicator of the actual amount of illness in the community. However, they obviously do indicate the presence of ill health and they also show correlations with social class (Fig. 9.1)

Commenting on the statistics from the General Household Survey, Blaxter (1976) wrote: 'Even if examination is confined to the more stringent and objective condition of handicapping chronic illness, prevalence rates in Social Class V, at over 200 per 1000 people, are well over twice the rate of 75 reported in Class I.' (p. 117)

The provision of health care

Class variations occur in literally 'concrete' terms (such as buildings), in staffing and in the professional-patient relationship.

The general situation has been described by Tudor Hart (1971) as an 'inverse care law': that the quality of health care tends to be lower in deprived neighbourhoods, although it is here that one finds a greater concentration of people with the highest mortality and morbidity rates and who could therefore be deemed to need better quality health care. There is also a tendency for lock-up surgeries to be found in deprived inner city areas with all the problems this creates for patients who need medical help 'after hours'. These problems are most severe for patients with no telephone, who have difficulty in communicating by telephone and who live in areas where vandalism may have put telephones out of action.

Even when a patient comes into contact with health care professionals, social class may influence the duration of the consultation, together with the quality of communication. Buchan & Richardson (1971) in Aberdeen found a social class gradient in the length of time that GPs spent with their patients, with upper class patients receiving longer consultations, and Cartwright & O'Brien (1976) showed that GPs tended to know more about their middle class than their working class patients.

A crucial aspect of communication is language. The extent to which the health care professional and the patient 'speak the same language' will therefore affect the degree of their mutual understanding and rapport. Sociological work on class differences in the use of language, most notably by Bernstein (1961), shows that middle class people may use a more complex or elaborate form of language than the more restricted form characteristic of some working class cultures. If professional and patient are using different forms of language, this might affect vital transactions including the presentation and interpretation of case histories, the discussion of diagnosis and prognosis and details concerning treatment. A salutary study undertaken by Boyle (1970) showed that many patients, especially working class patients, had gross misconceptions about basic anatomy and about key terms such as 'palpitation' or 'diarrhoea'. They could thus be talking at cross purposes with their doctor. (I, myself, remember being somewhat nonplussed by a patient who presented with pain in his 'sweetbreads'!)

The uptake of health care

This is a complex field and many studies have demonstrated different aspects of

Table 9.3 Need and service utilization: percentage of seven-year old children assessed in National Child Development Survey, 1965.

Need/Service	Social class I	II	IIInm	IIIm	IV	V
Had poor dental health (10 or more DMF teeth)	6.5	8.8	10.0	9.7	11.4	9.6
Had ever attended dental clinic, dentist or orthodontist	83.3	79.9	80.9	76.2	72.5	67.6
Had not fully intelligible speech	5.5	8.4	9.5	14.9	18.3	22.1
Had ever attended for speech therapy	2.8	2.0	2.1	2.4	2.8	3.0
Had signs of past or present otitis media	6.8	5.8	7.7	7.4	6.8	9.6
Had ever attended a hearing or audiology clinic	8.6	7.0	7.9	7.7	7.6	7.1

class differences. We give one example, relating to children. Blaxter summarises some of the findings arising from the National Child Development Survey (1972). Table 9.3 shows that among seven-year-old children, those with greater clinically-defined needs for specialist services (needs which may have profound implications for their future) tended to use the relevant specialist services less than others.

In summary, this brief and selective overview shows that despite 35 years of the National Health Service and of generally rising standards of living, inequalities between social classes persist, not only in health, illness and death rates, but also in the provision and use of health care.

CULTURE

Cultural variations in the perception of, and response to, pain and illness

There is an abundance of fascinating anthropological and sociological studies which describe variations in ways in which people from different cultures perceive and respond to illness. Two examples will illustrate the importance of such differences. The first is an account of attempts to provide contraceptive devices for a number of West Indian women living in Britain and the problems which emerged. Some of the women were very reluctant to accept contraceptives as they believed that there is a passage leading directly from the vagina to the mouth; consequently, they feared that they might choke if they inserted anything into the vagina or uterus. An understanding of their 'body fantasies' was clearly essential in appreciating their apprehensiveness with regard to various methods of birth control (Kitzinger 1972). This example illustrates relationships between culture and health behaviour — although it must be stressed that not all members of a social group will necessarily have the same beliefs. The second example takes us into the realm of 'folk medicine'. Many people hesitate before seeking professional medical help, preferring lay advice and the traditional remedies of their subculture. I remember an elderly patient who had been suffering from acute follicular tonsillitis for a whole week; when asked why she had not sought treatment earlier, she replied; 'Well, I've been taking the usual treatment.' This involved 'gargling with vaseline and jam'. It was only after this 'treatment' had manifestly failed to cure the really severe infection that she came to orthodox medicine, as a last resort.

Communication between people of different cultures

Another example illustrates how people from different cultures may respond to illness and pain in different ways. It is an American study, but it is relevant to all concerned with providing health care to people from different cultures. Zborowski (1952) described how members of three different ethnic groups (Jews, Italians and 'Old Americans') responded to pain associated with identical pathological conditions. On the surface, the Jews and Italians reacted similarly: they behaved emotionally, tended to be relatively uninhibited and were highly sensitive. But, underlying the similarities there were profound differences in their anxieties about the meaning of the pain and the illness causing it. The Italians were predominantly concerned with immediate pain relief, while the Jews were more worried about the long-term implications of their illness for their families and their jobs. In contrast, the 'Old Americans' were less overtly emotional, tending to keep a 'stiff upper lip' although beneath this, they were deeply anxious about concerns similar to those worrying the Jews. As far as British health care professionals are concerned, a traditional British 'stiff upper lip' and 'no fuss' behaviour, with stoical inhibition in the face of pain, anxiety and grief may be more compatible with our cultural images of what constitutes 'good patient behaviour' than the more noisy, demanding and imperious behaviour which may characterise patients from other cultures. Some understanding of their cultural background may facilitate our sympathy and promote a more sensitive rapport, thus enhancing our ability to respond to their spoken and unspoken needs.

Health problems associated with different cultures — especially ethnic minority groups

We have seen that there are variations in patterns of health and in health behaviour between social classes and groups amongst our native population. We have also seen that there may be problems of communication and of rapport between people who apparently speak the same language. We should, therefore, expect much more variation in patterns of health and many more problems of communication when we consider those people who have come to settle in Britain from different parts of the world, with very different cultures. Therefore, consideration of the health problems of some of the ethnic minority groups is important, especially for health care workers in the community.

It is very hard to obtain accurate population statistics, but figures cited by Lomas (1973) indicated that there were then about 650 000 immigrants from India and Pakistan, 446 000 West Indians and 168 000 Africans. There are also considerable numbers of white immigrants: an estimated $1\frac{1}{2}$ million, including about 615 000 Irish and 265 000 Mediterranean Europeans. The reasons for their coming have been a combination of what sociologists call 'pull' and 'push' factors. Among the former was Britain's need for labour in the post-war period, and it must be remembered that active recruitment campaigns were initiated by British firms and other organisations such as London Transport to encourage people from places such as Barbados to come here to work. Among the 'push' factors have been wars, persecution, political conflict and unemployment in the immigrants' countries of origin. On arrival here, immigrants have tended to settle in certain areas, with the big cities attracting the largest numbers to work in factories and public services such as transport and hospitals. Certain parts of London have attracted West Indians (e.g. Paddington, Notting Hill and Lambeth) while the Asians tend to have settled in other areas of London, such as Southall, or in other towns such as Bradford, Leeds, Luton and Leicester. Their life-styles and associated health behaviour are as diverse as the cultures of the countries they have left and it is only possible to mention a few significant examples here.

Birth rates and infant care

The number of children of immigrant families tends to be larger than that of English families, although the differentials appear to be diminishing. Reasons for the high birth rates include cultural-religious beliefs and the agricultural economies in the societies they have left which encourage the birth of children as a source of cheap labour. Moreover, some of the ethnic groups place great value on the birth of sons and so the birth of a daughter, particularly if she is the first baby, may be seen as a disappointment. This may result in problems in encouraging the mother to relate warmly and affectionately to the baby girl and thus to establish a good bonding relationship; it may also mean that she will be under considerable pressure to conceive again as soon as possible in order to give birth to a son. Other factors which may be conducive to high birth rates in newly arrived immigrant groups are lack of sexual instruction and knowledge about contraception, and the pressures for large families in their own lands where high infant mortality rates generate a need for replacements. For example, in Bangladesh, a woman has an average of 12 pregnancies, resulting in two miscarriages, three deaths in infancy and seven children who survive to adulthood. It is not surprising if it takes a little while for patterns of family life to adjust to a very different social context, and here health education may be very helpful on matters such as contraception.

Feeding of babies

The way in which some immigrant mothers feed their babies is a cause for concern. In Asia and Africa, they would traditionally be breast-fed. However, recently, particularly in West Africa, tinned powdered cows' milk has become available and has been advertised in ways which make it appear superior to breast milk. Moreover, when immigrant mothers arrive here, they see the majority of British mothers bottle-feeding their babies. It is not surprising then if they are led to believe that 'bottle is best'. But there are problems associated with feeding babies on cows' milk, which are particularly acute for a mother who may be illiterate, unable to speak or understand English and who has poor knowledge of hygiene. She may not follow the instructions correctly and may mix the feed too strong or too weak. If she makes it too strong, the baby may become too fat and liable to hypernatremia; if too weak, the baby lacks adequate caloric intake, does not thrive and may be susceptible to infection. This may be especially significant as the risk of gastroenteritis is much higher with bottle fed babies, and poor standards of hygiene may increase this risk. Lobo (1978) suggests that there are important implications here for health education, especially in the ante-natal period, and that immigrant Asian mothers in particular should be encouraged to breast feed. He argues that 'audio-visual propaganda in the two major languages — Punjabi and Hindustani — would be the most effective form of encouragement and should be made available for the Asian television and radio programmes, as well as for selected hospital ante-natal clinics and Asian organisations.'

Common diseases of children in immigrant families

Two examples are highlighted: anaemias and rickets.

Anaemias. The child of Asian parents is often fed on milk for a prolonged period; when weaning does occur, foods tend to consist of rice, potatoes, milk puddings and fruit; eggs, meat and fish do not feature. Consequently, the diet may be deficient in iron, and may result in anaemia which becomes most pronounced by the age of three. A survey in 1975 (cited by Lobo) of children born in Luton to Asian mothers, found that 24% were anaemic (less than 70% Hb); none of the children in the control group of English and West Indian families had anaemia. There would seem to be a clear case here for the education of Asian mothers in infant welfare clinics to help them to give balanced diets to their toddlers, and also for screening tests to discover anaemic children and to facilitate treatment with oral iron preparations. Other anaemias are inherited, such as sickle cell and thalassemia major. The genes for both of these conditions are recessive and may be carried by parents who are themselves free of symptoms. But if two carriers marry, their children have a one in four risk of inheriting the disease. According to Lobo, thalassemia trait is seen in about 5% of Southern Italians, 10% Sicilians, 15–20% Cypriots, Greeks and Turks, and in some other ethnic groups. In Britain, in 1977, there were 300 children known to be affected, of whom 60% were Greek-Cypriot, 30% Northern Indian and 10% of Italian or Chinese origin. Sickle cell trait is found in 10% of West Indian Negroes, 20% West Africans, 40% East Africans and in some Arabs — the world distribution resembling that of malaria, for which sickle cell trait gives some protection. The implications for health care lie in the fields of detection, diagnosis and treatment. Issues concerning prevention may also be discussed, recognising that the ethical and personal problems are profound. Lobo suggests that all children of affected groups could be screened before leaving school and carriers could then be identified; they, and their families, could then be aware of the situation and of the risks involved in marrying another carrier.

Rickets. This disease used to be found amongst the poorer classes in Britain, and although it had been virtually eliminated, it began to recur in some very deprived urban areas such as Glasgow in the 1960s. However, in the last decade, it has reappeared in new sections of the population, most notably among children of Asian immigrants, where it features most prominently in pre-school age youngsters, in adolescents and in young women. A survey by Goel et al (1976) of vitamin D levels in children in Glasgow and Bradford showed a relatively higher incidence of both florid and of sub-clinical rickets among Asian children (10 and 15 respectively, out of 200), than in a mixed group of 300 African, Chinese and Scottish children. Lobo suggests that the factors which make Asian children particularly prone are the type of flour used for making chapattis, the high vegetable fibre content of their diet and the lack of exposure to sunshine. Dunnigan et al (1972) make a case for the routine fortification of the wholewheat unrefined flour used by the Asian community with calcium and vitamin D, and Lobo claims: 'In my opinion, the fortification of chapatti flour is an effective, cheap, safe and sensible way to prevent rickets, and the sooner the DHSS approves its use, the better.' Alternatively or additionally, the use of vitamin drops containing vitamins A, D and C would help to prevent rickets and promote the growth of healthy bones in children.

Diseases acquired abroad

Many immigrants have a great desire to return to their homeland for holidays, and to take their families with them. Such trips may entail various health hazards, especially for the children, and health care workers in the community should be alert to these in order to encourage preventive or remedial action where necessary. The hazards arise from exposing children to infectious diseases to which they may have developed no resistance, as they now live in the relatively hygienic conditions of Britain. The main risks are the water-borne infections (such as amoebic dysentery and typhoid); malaria; droplet or contact infections (such as tuberculosis) and worm infestation (e.g. by hookworm, roundworm or whipworm). Adequate preventive measures should be taken for all conditions where these are available, for example, with typhoid and paratyphoid, malaria and tuberculosis. Lobo reports that in Luton it is policy to vaccinate routinely, with BCG vaccine, all newborn babies whose mothers were born in the New Commonwealth countries, and in Pakistan and China, and advocates the adoption of this policy on a national basis. With regard to infestation by worms, various debilitating effects can ensue and treatment should be given as soon as possible.

In conclusion, in this very brief account of some aspects of the interrelationships between culture, life-style, health and disease, I have tried to show the importance of understanding the significance of cultural differences for the provision of health care. Some policy implications have already been mentioned; others will now be considered, together with those arising from the earlier discussion on social class.

GENERAL POLICY IMPLICATIONS

Our brief overview has shown that, despite the establishment of the National Health Service, serious inequalities persist in the health of different social classes and subcultures in our society. What can we do? The following suggestions are not comprehensive, but indicate some possibilities.

The basic philosophy of the National Health Service is that of a self-help service: free treatment at the point of demand. But this assumes that people will come forward for treatment as and when appropriate. We have seen, however, that the assumption that if services are available people will use them, does not always hold. Brotherston (1976) argues that if:

> these assumptions are not warranted we must be prepared to re-examine the assumptions and draw appropriate conclusions in relation to the groups and services for whom the self-help system does not operate effectively. We require policies of positive discrimination in the direction of greatest need. And since such positive discrimination runs counter to the normal flow of our efforts, it is essential to monitor to ensure that the desired deployment in fact takes place.

Developing his theme, he draws a distinction between 'self-help' and 'outreach' — the latter policy being designed to identify people most in need of health care and to take care to them. This clearly raises the question of identification and here studies such as those by Davie (1972) on child development or Lobo (1978) on immigrants are relevant. They indicate some of the groups most at risk and highlight strategies for helping them. Both emphasise the importance of health education, especially in antenatal care.

Blaxter (1976) also supports positive discrimination and extends the discussion by considering a possible redeployment of health service resources and personnel away from some of the exciting and expensive developments towards consolidation at a more mundane level — especially given current financial stringency. She asks whether we need 'not more doctors but more health visitors, district nurses, medical and psychiatric and social workers, and with more responsibility.' This seems a pertinent question. For it is well known that there have been significant shifts in the nature and proportions of health problems over recent decades, with growing numbers of elderly people, the chronic sick and the disabled. Medicine has little to offer to many of these people by way of a cure; what they need is care

(Cox, 1979). And there is a notorious shortage of personnel available to provide that care in both hospitals and in the community. Moving further along the treatment-prevention continuum: some of the examples cited above have shown the need for 'outreach' in both prophylaxis and education. As we have seen, some of the class and ethnic variations in health are associated with ignorance of health behaviour, or reluctance to use health facilities. Here, health education may play a crucial role. We have emphasised its importance in antenatal care. Perhaps another positive measure would be the extension of the role of the school nurse as a health educator — with all the opportunities she could have for influencing young people.

Perhaps all we can do at present is to try to correct the most glaring anomalies which now exist, to create the conditions for as healthy a population as possible, given our current state of knowledge and of resources, and to remove those obstacles which prevent any class or group within our society from having access to the positive freedoms and opportunities for well-being enjoyed by others. These are challenges which will require all our intelligent concern, energy and commitment. Beyond this we may not go. For: 'Man is not and never will be the master of his fate: his very reason always progresses by leading him into the unknown and unforeseen where he learns new things.' (Hayek, 1978).

REFERENCES

Bell C 1968 Middle class families: Social & geographical mobility. Routledge & Kegan Paul, London

Bernstein B 1961 Social class & linguistic development: A theory of social learning. In: Halsey A, Floud J, Anderson C (eds) Education, economy & society. Collier-Macmillan, London

Blaxter M 1976 Social class and health inequalities. In: Carter C O, Peel J (eds) Equalities and inequalities in health. Academic Press, London

Boyle C M 1970 Differences between patients' and doctors' interpretations of some common medical terms. British Medical Journal (2 May 1970). Reprinted in Cox C, Mead A 1975 A sociology of medical practice. Collier Macmillan, London

Brotherston J 1976 Inequality: Is it inevitable? In: Carter C O, Peel J (eds) Equalities and inequalities in health. Academic Press, London

Buchan I C, Richardson I M 1971 Time study of consultations in general practice. Scottish Health Service Studies Number 27, Scottish Home & Health Department, Edinburgh

Carter C O, Peel J (eds) 1976 Equalities and inequalities in health. Academic Press, London

Cartwright A, O'Brien M 1976 Social class variations in the nature of general practitioner consultations. In: Stacey M (ed) 1976 The sociology of the National Health Service. Sociological Review Monograph No 22, University of Keele, Staffordshire

Cox C 1979 Who cares? Nursing and sociology: The development of a symbiotic relationship. Journal of Advanced Nursing 4: 237–252

Cox C, Mead A 1975 A sociology of medical practice. Collier Macmillan, London

Davie R 1972 From birth to seven: The second report of the National Child Development Survey (1958 Cohort), Longman and The National Children's Bureau, London

Dennis N, Henriques F & Slaughter C 1956 Coal is our life. Tavistock Publications, London

Dunnigan M G 1972 Biochemical response of late rickets and osteomalacia to a chapatti-free diet. British Medical Journal 2: 446

Goel K M 1976 Florid and subclinical rickets among immigrant children in Glasgow. Lancet 1: 1141

Hart J T 1971 The inverse care law. Lancet 1: 1179–1190. Reprinted in Cox C, Mead A 1975 A sociology of medical practice. Collier Macmillan, London

Hayek F A 1978 The three sources of human values. The London School of Economics & Political Science, London. Also in Hayek F A 1979 Law, legislation & liberty, Vol III: The political order of a free people. Routledge & Kegan Paul, London

Kitzinger S 1972 Body fantasies. New Society 21: 510
Lambert P 1976 Perinatal mortality: Social and environmental factors. In: Population Trends 4, Office of Population Censuses and Surveys, HMSO, London
Lobo E de H 1978 Children of immigrants to Britain: Their health & social problems. Hodder & Stoughton, London
Lomas G B G 1973 Census 1971: The coloured population of Great Britain, Preliminary Report, The Runnymede Trust
Morris J N 1979 Social inequalities undiminished. Lancet 1: 87 (Jan 13)
Office of Population Censuses & Surveys 1976 Population Trends. HMSO, London
Rapoport R, Rapoport R 1971 Dual career families. Penguin, Harmondsworth
Tunstall J 1969 The fishermen. MacGibbon & Kee, London
Young M Willmott P 1957 Family and Kinship in East London. Routledge & Kegan Paul, London
Zborowski M 1952 Cultural components in response to pain. Journal of Social Issues 8

FURTHER READING

Carter C O, Peel J 1976 Equalities and inequalities in health. Academic Press, London (especially chapters by Brotherston and Blaxter)
Cartwright A 1967 Patients and their doctors: A study of general practice. Routledge & Kegan Paul, London
Cox C, Mead A 1975 A sociology of medical practice. Collier Macmillan, London (especially chapters by Boyle, Hart, Milio and Zola)
Lobo E de H 1978 Children of immigrants to Britain: Their health and social problems
Morris J N 1979 Social inequalities undiminished. Lancet 1: 87–90 (Jan 13)
Wandswroth Council for Community Relations 1977 The Health Service and The Asian Community

10

Monocultural health services in a multicultural society

Alix Henley

The NHS was designed in 1948 to provide for the health needs of the British people; its provision naturally grew up around British social and family patterns, religious and cultural beliefs, and around the expectations and health needs of the indigenous population at that time.

More than thirty years later we have a very different kind of society in Britain. It contains people of a great diversity of cultures, pulled into Britain (as into the rest of Western Europe) by the tremendous industrial and economic expansion of the 1950s and '60s.

Inevitably, many of the people now living in Britain have different social and family patterns, different religious and cultural beliefs, and different expectations and health needs from those of the indigenous population. Much of the health care provision that we offer is therefore inappropriate for them: we may provide it in a way that is unacceptable; the kind of health worker-patient relationship that we offer them may be off-putting and unhelpful; the advice we give them may not help them; the way that we think they should handle illness, family crises, and hospitalisation may make no sense to them at all.

In other words, traditional monocultural health care provision will not reach many of the people in our present multicultural society. Worse, it will not reach many of those who are most at risk in terms of health. Most members of ethnic minority groups find themselves at the bottom of our economic pile, doing the less desirable jobs and living in less desirable housing in areas with poorer facilities. If they are new to this country they are also usually coping with major changes in climate, environment and pace of life, and are cut off from many of their normal and vital sources of support and help. Low wages, long hours, poor housing, living in deprived areas, continual experience of racism and discrimination, isolation, and language problems, all increase physical and mental stress and therefore increase the risk of ill health. For this reason members of ethnic minorities are in fact likely to need more in terms of health care than the rest of the population.

This is well known, and yet the evidence shows that, even after more than twenty five years, the Health Service is failing to provide for the real health care needs of these vulnerable groups.

Why is it failing? The most important single reason is the general belief that it is the responsibility of the minority groups to change and to make themselves accessible to our provision. We do not feel that it is our responsibility to learn about them and to adapt ourselves *and our services* to their needs and way of life.

In maternity units in most areas, for example, Asian women are expected to accept examination by male doctors, newborn babies are removed to sleep in separate nurseries, staff insist on certain positions for delivery, jewellery and clothing with religious significance are summarily removed. In hospitals and in the community the values and assumptions of an individualistic Western culture are applied to people from cultures where an individual is primarily a member of a much larger family group, and where decisions and actions have a very different basis. We seem to believe that culture and values are like clothes, and that when people migrate they can and should cast off one set, and put on and live by another. Do we really think that it is the moral duty of all cultural minorities to change their ways as fast as possible?

Most of us do. And we firmly believe that if we were to migrate we too should change completely to fit in with our new country, though the evidence indicates that the British have always been slow to change their values and beliefs and social patterns when living overseas. It is, after all, a very difficult thing to do, and can be destructive. We all need a group identity, and a migrant who gives up his own culture and roots is usually left without any group at all; he is neither part of his old group nor accepted by the new.

But let us look more closely at the belief that ethnic minority groups should abandon their own identity and take on ours. Is this really just naivety and inexperience on our part? Have we just not thought fully about what it means? Or is it something nastier? Is it that we look down both on them and on the culture and values they bring with them? Is it that our attitudes are, at bottom, racist? That we do not place any worth on, and so will not try to understand, the social and family systems, and religious and cultural beliefs of any group but our own? Have we not yet grown out of the self-centred and destructive belief that if people are different from us they are wrong? And that our ways and beliefs are always better?

Why do we resent minority groups and refuse to consider co-operating when they try to maintain parts of their own lifestyle? To bring up their children according to their own values? To continue to follow their own religious observances, cook and eat their own food, preserve their own standards of dress, and to pattern their lives in their own way? Is it because we respect neither them nor their values? Because we consider them essentially inferior? So that they can only become respectable, only have the right to equal treatment from the Health Service or any other institution, if they become more British and less themselves? Does it, in the end, all come down to racism?

In my work in developing training materials for health workers. I have spent some time going round hospitals and training schools asking medical and nursing students in all disciplines to write down for me the kind of differences they have found when working with ethnic monority patients, particularly Asians.

Their replies were disturbing. They were almost always negative, though I had specifically and carefully asked about differences not problems. A selection of not untypical replies (unamended) is given here. They indicate vividly the students' ideas about 'correct' behaviour, and the values through which they see the world and which often prevent them respecting or valuing other people.

Asian patients

They eat with fingers.
Sit up cross-legged on bed.
Ignore simple instructions.
Rub skin with horrible smelling oil.
Habits: toilet problems; linen problems.
They have too large families.
Want private room to pray.
Very demanding and reluctant. Do not want to exercise.
Will not undress for doctors.
Too much sugar in tea.
Will not eat hospital food. Want food brought by relatives.
Old ladies all pick up and handle new babies.
When children are admitted, nurses have difficulty in co-operating with child because of relatives.
Seek attention all the time.
Wash their private area with water using their hands.
Parents want to stay with children all the time.
Hygiene problems.
Do not put on open-backed gowns. Will only wear own clothes.
Reluctant to take baths.
Always fear what's going on.
Too many visitors.
Use fingers to eat — will not use knives and forks.
No common sense.
No outside interests: life taken up with own family.

The attitudes implicit in these comments are that the way British people eat, sit, care for their skin, wash, care for children, run their families, dress, and organise their lives is the only acceptable way. Other ways are deviant, inferior, unacceptable, and a problem for responsible people.

The discussions that occurred with the students during these sessions confirmed my impressions. The students were, almost without exception, critical and antagonistic towards ethnic minority patients particularly when they exhibited different behaviour or characteristics from those expected from indigenous British patients. They showed none of the idealism and liking for people that leads people into the caring profession. They seemed to have little idea that there are other values, other cultures, other equally valid ways of living and behaving and seeing the world; and that in providing health care we must recognise and respect other values, other ways of doing things and people who are different. Had they been told that judging everything in terms of one's own norms is completely inappropriate when those norms are not shared by the people one is judging, and that we need to learn about and respect other people's norms in order to work effectively with them? That in a multicultural society we need consciously to become multicultural health workers?

This refusal to respect other ways, to accept people's right to choose their own ways and values wherever they live is surely the greatest barrier between the Health Service and the minority groups. This is the barrier that stops us considering ways of adapting our provision to make it more acceptable and useful to them. We still plan and cater and train for a monocultural world, but on the wards, in the waiting rooms and clinics, in patients' homes, we work in a multicultural world and we need to be prepared to adapt to it in all kinds of ways, or face the increasing anger of people who receive inferior health care because they belong to a minority culture.

The issue for the National Health Service seems clear therefore: if we will not accept the right of ethnic minorities to choose how they wish to lead their lives, and to choose the values they wish to live by (a right which we grant to ourselves), we cannot provide effective health care for all the members of our multicultural society.

And if we do not accept that ethnic minorities have the right to choose, even in Britain, we are in effect offering them a stark choice: 'Behave like us, think like us, conform to our ways and standards, or deal with your health care yourselves'. In other words, we are saying that we are only prepared to offer a White Majority Health Service — something which most health workers would surely dispute violently.

But let us look at some of the evidence: There is in Britain at present what many experts would consider to be an epidemic of rickets among the Asian communities. Rickets used to be known in Europe as the British disease but was wiped out among the indigenous population in the 1940s largely by the fortification of certain popular foods. It has now reappeared, almost entirely among the Asian population who do not eat any of these foods, both because of religious dietary restrictions, and because they are unfamiliar to them. In 1979 it was estimated that one Glasgow Asian child in seventeen, and one Bradford Asian child in forty-two, could expect admission to hospital with severe rickets before he/she is sixteen years old. What would be the reaction to an epidemic of these proportions among the white population? What policy decisions would result? What urgent measures would be taken? Rickets is a preventable disease, but it is not being prevented among the Asian population.

Another problem which affects only the racial minorities in Britain is sickle cell anaemia and thalassemia. There is no adequate screening and counselling service for these two serious hereditary diseases. Doctors and nurses are rarely trained to recognise or cope with them, or to counsel, support, or educate families affected by them.

Among the Pakistani community in Britain the infant mortality rate is 23.5 (per thousand live births); among the total population it is 14.4. Why does the antenatal service not attract and meet the needs of Asian women in Britain? It is because too often, services are offered as if this were a monocultural, monolingual society. Because they fail to take into account the different needs and cultural and religious values of the ethnic majority groups, because they make Asian women feel unwelcome, humiliated and despised. Because they provide an arrogantly uniform service in a plural society. Despite the efforts of many health workers, most of our services *are* still generally organised as if we were a monocultural monolingual society. And there is too often a real unwillingness to alter or extend provision so that it reaches minority groups. 'Their ways are inferior, the sooner they become like us the better'.

But it is not only provision. As individual health workers too, we may fail to reach people, partly because we lack the information we need to be really effective, and partly because as mentioned, most of us have not been prepared for the extra and difficult demands of working in such a diverse society. What kind of preparation do health workers need? As a beginning, extra information. Much of our work revolves round practical matters such as diet, weaning, physical care, keeping records, giving advice on the care of babies and children, helping people cope with the physical aspects of pregnancy.

With our indigenous clients we are familiar with most of the habits and practices that are likely to occur. On diet for example: we know, within a broad spectrum, what people are likely to eat, how they are likely to prepare it, what they are likely to think is suitable for weaning their children, the probable routines into which they organise their days, what may trouble them and what advice might help them.

With our ethnic minority clients most of us do not know these things. We are suddenly no longer competent in all sorts of areas that we normally take for granted, and where we normally have confidence in our ability to be useful and to meet people's needs. We no longer have a basis on which we can discuss people's dietary preferences and needs.

Let us concentrate further on the subject of dietary advice. Looking at it in very practical terms, what kind of additional information do we need to be sure that we can give useful dietary advice to ethnic minority clients?

1. General information

General information about the *minority group* to which a family belongs. e.g. What the normal diet is in their country of origin. Staples, protein, vegetables, fruit, sources of essential vitamins etc. Which methods of cooking they are likely to be most familiar with. Whether there are any religious restrictions regarding food that they might follow.

Whether there are any additional cultural factors that might affect their diet at special times, e.g. during pregnancy, illness, hot or cold weather.

These are the facts we need to be armed with before we begin. If we can come prepared, and have an informed discussion, our clients are more likely to have confidence in us, and in our genuine desire to accept them as they are and help them, rather than change them.

Collecting this kind of information is not the mammoth task it might appear. In most areas one or two minority groups predominate, so it is not necessary for health workers to find out about twenty or thirty different diets. More and more information is being produced on the diets of different groups. If a health worker is in contact with a local group on which there seems to be no information, he or she must press for some. Health workers cannot work effectively with clients if they are not given the information that is an essential tool of their trade.

2. Particular information

Particular information about the *family*: e.g. How long they have been in Britain (if they are immigrants).

Who decides what the family eats.
Who does the shopping and who does the cooking.
What shops they use.

The basic principles on which we give advice are the same for any family, but different family dynamics, different authority patterns, and the different ways that people perceive our role as visiting health workers may affect the way that the principles are worked out in practice.

Here are some guidelines:

(i) Aim, as usual, to give advice as far as possible on the basis of your client's existing diet and preferences.

(ii) Find out, as usual, about anything particular the client does not eat, either out of individual preference or for religious or cultural reasons. But bear in mind that most ethnic minority families have experienced racist attitudes. They are likely to feel that British people will laugh at or despise their customs. They may tell you what they think you would like to hear rather than risk exposing themselves to ridicule. Expect most people to follow religious and cultural restrictions on food, and accept without question (particularly at the beginning of your relationship) the restrictions that they do follow. It is almost always possible to give nutritional advice that does not clash with people's beliefs and practices.

It is important to tread a fine line in this respect and not to assume that every client follows traditional customs and practices regarding food completely. Discuss this with clients. Some clients may wish to adopt more local foods and should be given help in doing so.

(iii) Work with whoever is responsible for decisions about food, but note that it may not be the person you would expect. In most English families a young mother is responsible for decisions about what she cooks for her family and what she eats. In an Asian family, for example, there may be several people responsible for such decisions. It may not be the young mother alone who needs to be involved, but her mother-in-law, or her husband, or her older sisters-in-law. Their support is crucial and their opposition, should they decide to exercise it, unbeatable. Work within the authority structure of the particular family to avoid embarrassing them and frustrating yourself. Insist that you are given an interpreter if the people in authority in the family do not speak English.

(iv) Look critically at any major dietary changes (in the client's terms) you might advise and decide whether they are really crucial to the client's health. What is standard and easy-to-follow advice to people on a British diet may require major decisions and changes in, for example, a normal Vietnamese diet. Require as little major change as possible. Leave out all but the most important advice if it is going to be difficult to follow.

(v) Try recommending some new foods that are easily available and fairly cheap here. Tell people the names of suitable foods that you think they might be able to use in their cooking. Many people who are new to this country would like to use cheaper local foods but are as baffled by them as we would be by most foreign foodstuffs. If possible, demonstrate how to prepare them. (Peel, or scrape, wash, length of cooking time needed etc.) The foods most likely to be accepted are those which can be cooked according to traditional methods. Many Asians, for example, find boiled vegetables unpalatable.

(vi) Indicate your respect for and understanding of your client's dietary choices. Build up a relationship of mutual trust and respect. Members of minority groups are only too aware that many British people believe they should change completely now that they are in Britain and should even give up their own food habits and adopt an entirely British diet, and, for example, British weaning patterns. They are likely to be extremely sensitive to any implications of disapproval on a health worker's part. None of us willingly accepts advice from people who we feel look down on us or whom we do not trust.

Implicit in the guidelines above is our acceptance of differences and of people's right to choose their own ways and standards. Without this acceptance, all the information in the world will not help us or our clients.

Acceptance too, may be an area in which we need preparation. The answers listed on page 85 above do not indicate acceptance of, or respect for, other groups. Students who go out into the world with the attitudes reflected there are unlikely to be able to build relationships of mutual trust and respect with patients and clients from minority groups. They are therefore unlikely to be effective health workers.

What is the process that helps us to develop acceptance and understanding and a respect for other groups? Part of it is the examination of our *own* cultural attitudes and beliefs. It is very difficult to be truly sensitive to other people's values and beliefs unless one understands a lot about one's own values and beliefs and how important they are to one. As long as we talk about culture as though it was something other people had but not us, it all seems strange and alien. But the cultural barrier is a two-way barrier. Our culture also forms a barrier to access to health care for minority groups and we need to understand it. Until we understand, for example, the influence of British ideas about the family in the way we offer our health care, we cannot assess how our preconceptions and assumptions may be forming a barrier between us and our ethnic minority patients.

We need, therefore, to articulate and learn about our own culture and values, and understand them in terms of our own history and development. We need to recognise how our culture and values affect all our actions and attitudes. They act as a lens through which, almost inevitably, we view the world and make all our judgements about other people. We must learn to stand back from our own values and accept them as just one possible set of lenses among the many that exist in the world. We need to acknowledge and accept other people's sets of lenses as equally real, equally valuable, and equally worthy of respect. We need to examine our own attitudes to people of different cultures and races. To be truly multicultural we need to develop the ability to look through different sets of lenses at different times, to make judgements that are appropriate to the particular family or individual we are with, and to see the issues and priorities as they see them. Without the understanding that this gives us, we, as individuals, cannot offer them the kind of service appropriate to a multicultural society.

REFERENCES

Davies Isobel Macdonald 1980 Perinatal and infant deaths: social and biological factors. Spring. Population Trends OPCS, HMSO, London
Glasgow Health Education programme 1979

11

Social welfare

Jean Gaffin

INTRODUCTION

The health services are a major part of the social welfare provisions in modern Britain. The National Health Service spends less than the social security scheme, but employs more people than any other public service and is used by virtually the whole population at one time or another. Why look at *other* social welfare provisions in a book focussing on health?

The needs for medical care that the health services meet are rarely self contained. A general practitioner prescribing an antibiotic for tonsillitis or a surgeon removing an appendix show the health services meeting purely health needs. But most needs, translated into demands by patients and accepted as valid demands by the doctors acting as 'doorkeepers' to the medical care system, are more complex. The old lady blocking a hospital bed because of shortage of places in a residential home; the child with a chest condition aggravated by damp, inadequate housing; the woman admitted to psychiatric hospital with depression related to her husband's unemployment and her family's poverty — all these problems have more than just a health aspect. Problems do not come neatly wrapped up, tied with string, labelled 'health' or 'social', correctly delivered to the provider of the most appropriate services. Providers need to know about a range of social provisions if these are to be mobilized for that patient or client. It is as important to realize that social conditions such as bad housing and poverty generate health problems as it is to see how health problems generate a need for social support. This need for social support can be for tangible services (e.g. home help) or intangible ones (e.g. help in adjusting to a life of dependency).

It is also important to recognise that the major improvements in the health of the British population are due more to improved economic and social circumstances than to improved health services (McKeowen, 1977). This chapter therefore outlines the scope of the major social service provisions in modern Britain and attempts to pinpoint some of their implications for community health care.

SOCIAL WELFARE: ONLY THE SOCIAL SERVICES?

This approach can be criticized as too narrow. Social welfare is usually seen in terms of activities (mainly stemming from central and local government action but also initiated and implemented by voluntary agencies) which meet the needs of the population. These needs include minimum income, health care, education, housing and help and support with a range of needs arising from dependency. Social provisions are linked with the political system by Robson (1976) who argues:

> what is not open to serious question is that a welfare state must be democratic. By that I mean the government must have been freely chosen by the citizens . . . public criticism of the government must be unrestricted and freely tolerated . . . But political and social freedom are in my opinion essential ingredients of the welfare state; and this excludes totalitarian regimes or dictatorships from being welfare states.

Equally critical of an examination of social welfare in isolation from other aspects of society is Titmuss (1974) who argues that the social services are the 'observable part of the welfare phenomena'. He goes on to argue that the operation of the tax system (fiscal welfare) is relevant to a study of the social services, explaining how allowances and tax relief provide similar benefits to the benefits received under the social security system but are *not* treated as social service expenditure. Titmuss is not concerned only with the relationship between social welfare and fiscal welfare: he sees occupational welfare as relevant too. Occupational welfare means the benefits provided by employers, such as occupational pensions, free private medical care, meal vouchers and motor cars.

Titmuss says that they are:

> in effect if not in administrative method 'social services', duplicating and overlapping social and fiscal welfare benefits. The rapidity of their growth in recent years has increasingly diminished the value and relevance of salary, wage and income statistics.

SOCIAL PROVISION AND PUBLIC EXPENDITURE

In stressing the other ways, distinct from the social welfare system, in which social needs are met, Titmuss is concerned that we see the provision and use of the social services as part of the rights of citizenship, rather than as a system selecting special groups for special treatment leading to the users of the social services feeling stigmatized and the general public seeing recipients of help as a 'burden'.

The advocates of reduced public services and increasing private provisions rarely consider the likely effect on the quality of provisions and the feelings of its users as the public sector declines. The debate between the advocates of increased public spending as a way of achieving social justice and those seeking more use of the private market as the mechanism for meeting need is a fascinating one.

Leaving aside those who criticise the isolation of social welfare from other aspects of society, and also the debate on just how much of the nation's wealth could or should be devoted to social provision, it is important next to examine the current social provisions in Britain. Looked at in terms of the legislation on the statute book, the provisions appear comprehensive. Looked at from the perspective of someone with a need about to be translated into demand, the provisions look rather less comprehensive! This is due to administrative factors: the way the legislation is in fact put into practice by a wide range of national and local government agencies, and by the individuals staffing these agencies. Local authorities vary in their capacity to raise funds and the services to which they give priority — so meals on wheels may be available once a week in one local authority but daily in another.

In addition, it is important to remember that the biggest provider of social provision to those in need is in fact the members of the individual's own family.

This gap between what legislation proposes and the State disposes is due to a range of political and economic factors. Public expectations about the quality of social provisions are rising, and with an increasing elderly population, needs are growing along with demands. But the changes made when the public expenditure cuts begun with the 1979 budget turned into the reality of postponed new buildings, staff reductions and a halt to new developments have serious implications for the community health services whose already stretched resources may well be stretched more thinly still.

We now look at some specific areas of social welfare provision.

Social security

The social security system is designed to maintain income when it is interrupted (e.g. of sickness) or stops (e.g. due to retirement). There are two major kinds of benefit. National Insurance Benefits include maternity grant, sickness benefit, widows' benefits and retirement pensions, and depend on the claimant having contributed to the scheme. Contributions are made whilst working but are credited in times of sickness, unemployment and since 1978, for women at home looking after children or a disabled adult. The other major kind of benefit is the non-contributory Supplementary Benefit Scheme which helps those who have insufficiently contributed to the scheme, have been unemployed for over a year or who cannot manage on their National Insurance Benefits. Benefit under this scheme depends on a means test — looking at income, expenditure and savings — either at the claimant's home or in the social security office. Apart from a regular allowance, special payments may be made such as help with rent or heating.

In July 1978 (Social Assistance, DHSS 1978) just over a fifth of all the retired, about half the unemployed and lone parents, and about a fifth of sick people were in receipt of supplementary benefit. In addition it was estimated that about 600 000 retirement pensioners were not claiming supplementary benefit to which they were entitled, due perhaps to fear of means tests or ignorance of eligibility.

The Supplementary Benefits scheme is currently under review — in February 1979 3 000 000 were dependent on it which meant, including dependants of claimants, 9% of the population. As demands on the scheme have grown it has become ever more complex with more rules and increased discretion by officials over the interpretation of these rules. For the community health worker anxious to advise a patient this complexity makes the giving of advice more essential and yet more difficult. A useful booklet called Family Benefits and Pensions (FB1) is available free from social security offices to members of the helping professions in contact with the public. It is revised regularly.

Other social security benefits include the Child Benefit which is slightly higher for the children of the one parent family, and Family Income Supplement for the low wage earner with one child or more working 24 hours per week. Benefits for the disabled include the Attendance Allowance, Mobility Allowance and Housewives Non-Contributory Invalidity Allowance.

In addition, there are many means-tested benefits outside the scope of the social security system. These include relief from paying prescription or school meal charges, whilst Council tenants may be entitled to rent rebates, private tenants to rent allowances and everyone to a rates rebate.

Attitudes to social security vary. Some are most concerned with abuse of the system, others with the inadequacy of existing benefits compared to the average national wage. New Society (16.11.1978, p. 395) estimated that £3 250 000 was fraudulently claimed in the *year* 1976/7 out of the £36 000 000 paid out *daily*.

In the years following the introduction of the social security scheme it was thought poverty in Britain would disappear. Research from the mid-'50s onwards has shown that is not so. Low wages, rising unemployment, the growth of one parent families and low social security benefits are all relevant. In addition, our concept of poverty is changing. It is no longer seen as low income alone, but also in terms of a wide range of inequalities which include poor housing and the higher mortality and morbidity figures associated with the lower socio-economic groups.

Housing

There is a link between poverty and bad housing — also between bad housing and poor health. Anyone able to afford a mortgage for the purchase of a house will have relatively little housing problem, but houses tend to be cheapest in areas of high unemployment.

Not only is family housing in short supply. So too are community facilities for the mentally ill, sheltered housing for the elderly and purpose built accommodation for the disabled.

Since the war the number of dwellings owned or being purchased has risen, and now accounts for over half the total. Local authority housing accounts for about one-third. The rest are rented by private landlords, a shrinking part of the housing market, with rents often high and conditions often poor. Local authorities have responsibility, under the Homeless Persons Act, 1977, towards families with children, the elderly, the handicapped, the vulnerable and victims of family violence. Otherwise the extent to which local authorities build housing for rent depends on the political and economic circumstances of each authority.

Those purchasing houses are greatly helped by tax relief on mortgage interest, which means that much of the public money available to help with housing costs goes to the better off. For the vulnerable — the low wage earner, the unemployed, the family new to an area, the large family — only public housing can solve their housing need. The sale of council housing, whilst satisfying the legitimate aspirations of existing council tenants, will reduce the total stock of housing available to rent, and can hardly help those on the waiting list or those waiting to be rehoused from unsatisfactory accommodation.

Rising expectations mean that tenants of run down estates are anxious to transfer and prospective council tenants refuse to accept dwelling on estates with poor reputations — accelerating their decay. This seeming paradox of increasing numbers of homeless and increasing numbers of empty low quality local authority dwellings is not easily solved. Solutions include tenant control, renovation and more money for repairs and maintenance. Public expenditure cuts makes this kind of expenditure more difficult, and some inner city local authorities are becoming slum landlords on a massive scale. The health service will no doubt be approached for medical aid to patch up the minds and bodies harmed and disturbed by poor housing.

The personal social services

The social services that have developed since 1945 were initially organized in three separate departments supplying services to defined groups in the population, at local government level. The Welfare Departments had responsibility for the elderly, physically handicapped and homeless, under Part III of the National Assistance Act 1948. The Children's Department was responsible for children deprived of a normal home life, (for reasons including death or desertion of parents or the child being in need of care, protection and control), under the Children's Act, 1948. Under the National Health Services Act 1946 the local authorities were responsible for services to the mentally ill and mentally handicapped, for day nurseries and child minding and a wide range of other provisions.

The major trend in social service provision since the 1950s has been towards community care, although this does not mean the end of institutions which heal, shelter, confine, teach or protect groups in society, as Jones (1975) reminds us. Community care suggest groups or individuals receiving care in the community rather than in institutions. For some groups, such as the elderly, community care means domiciliary services in their existing home or a sheltered flatlet, rather than a bed in a local authority residential home. But for other groups, a bed in a local authority hostel is community care when compared to a bed in a large psychiatric hospital or hospital for the mentally subnormal.

It is also important to remember that relatively few of, for example, the elderly are in institutional care at all, as the Table 11.1 reminds us (Central Statistical Office 1979). It is usually cheaper to keep people out of residential care. Fostering a child is cheaper than a place in a residential children's home. However, in an attempt to determine the real costs of domiciliary care for the elderly, Opit (1977) suggested that for the bedfast the average cost of domiciliary care was £25.60p in Birmingham in 1974–75, when the average cost per week in a residential home was £34 and in geriatric hospital about £45 per week. Opit pointed out that it is possible to keep many seriously disabled persons at home but suggests that the quality of life for some of these patients may be

> far from compatible with any civilized humanitarian standards . . . If the present policy of passively transferring the elderly chronic sick from hospital to home continues by limiting the various types of accommodation available for them, a substantial additional financial allocation for domiciliary care will be needed. If this does not occur then domiciliary care for the elderly will be increasingly "economic" simply because the level of care provided becomes increasingly inadequate.

The trend towards community care is not uniform throughout Great Britain but depends on the policy and resources of each local authority as well as local opinion. It is one thing to support community care for the mentally handicapped but seemingly another to agree that such a hostel should be opened in *our* road.

This trend towards community care, together with demographic changes such as increasing numbers of elderly in the community, dominate the history of social service provision since 1945 but equally relevant are changes in family structure including the changing role of women and the rapid growth of the single parent

Table 11.1 Elderly people: by type of household or institution, 1971 and 1977

Great Britain	Men				Women			Percentages
	65–74	75–84	85+	All 65+	65–74	75–84	85+	All 65+
Living in private households 1977 General Household Survey (percentages)								
With wife/husband:								
and others	13	11	5	12	6	4	1	5
no others	66	54	36	63	41	18	6	31
Without wife/husband:								
but with others	9	13	32	11	16	25	44	21
of which: living with child(ren)	34	47	52	40	41	49	49	45
living with siblings	33	10	10	24	31	21	17	25
Living alone	12	22	27	14	37	53	49	43
Total in private households	100	100	100	100	100	100	100	100
Sample size (numbers)	1344	436	66	1846	1720	904	177	2801
Resident in institutions: 1971 Census[1] (percentages)	**1971 Census**[1] (percentages)							
Old people's homes	1	3	9	1	1	4	12	2
Hospitals	1	1	3	1	1	2	6	2
Other institutions	–	–	1	1	–	–	1	–
Total percentages of elderly people resident in institutions	2	4	13	3	2	6	19	5
Numbers (thousands)	34	29	14	77	49	81	62	192

[1] England and Wales.
Source: General Household Survey, 1977; 1971 Census; *Department of Health and Social Security*; *Welsh Office; Scottish Education Department, Social Work Services Group*

family. These changes are linked to the administrative changes which led to the creation of the Social Service Departments in 1971, replacing the Welfare and Children's Departments and taking on much of the work of the Local Health Authority.

This new Department arose from the recommendations of the Committee on Local Authority and Allied Personal Social Services (Seebohm Committee) which was set up in 1965 and reported 1968 (HMSO, 1968) It reviewed the organization and responsibilities of local authority social services in England and Wales and was asked to consider changes desirable to secure an effective family service. One member of the Committee, Roy Parker (1970) defined personal social services as:

> usually considered to be those lying outside the general fields of health and education, which are adjusted in some special way to the particular social needs of families or groups and which require personal contact between provider and recipient. The skill involved is often labelled social work.

The Committee was concerned at the lack of resources for social care, finding inadequacy of provision, inequalities of service, poor coordination between services and poor cooperation between the staff of the various services examined. One recommendation quickly implemented was that mentally subnormal children should no longer be seen as totally ineducable, and junior training centres became Schools for the Educationally Subnormal (Severe) within each Local Authority's Education Department.

The most important recommendation was that a new department was needed, geared to the needs of the population served, forming a large powerful local authority department. The Chief Officer would have status, and be backed by a Committee of councillors able to argue on equal terms with other important committees such as education or housing. More training for social work staff was stressed as was accessibility: the department was to be organized into area offices, several to each local authority area. The Social Services Act, 1970, brought the new departments into being in 1971, with the Department of Health and Social Security as the directing central government Department.

When formed, the new departments provided a large number of senior posts which meant that experienced social workers were promoted to management jobs, leaving the inexperienced, often unqualified staff, at field level. This dilemma is equally familiar to those involved in the health service.

The problems not resolved by the proposals of the Seebohm Report remain unresolved. One such problem is what kind of family relationship the State should support. One social service department, Kent, is experimenting with making fairly high financial payments to relatives who stop work to care for dependent relatives. One observer, (Moroney, 1976), argues that the social welfare system in Britain *substitutes* when the family cannot or will not care, but does little to *support* the family that does want to care.

Some social workers feel that much of their work arises because of poverty and bad housing, and they may resent being used to help people to adjust to adverse situations created by the society in which we live.

Rising expectations of social service departments by the community, shortage of trained staff, and current economic policies, make it harder than ever for social service departments to function at the level society expects. Social workers feel that when other professionals find a problem insoluble, they tend to ask the social services to cope. The mentally disturbed adult discharged from the mental hospital on the grounds that nothing more can be done is left to the social worker in the community. When the social worker fails, it is usually the police who are involved, and the even more inappropriate prison may become home to the inadequate former psychiatric hospital patient.

Since local government reorganization in 1974, social service departments have been the responsibility of London Boroughs, non-Metropolitan Counties and Metropolitan Districts. In the early 1970s the new departments had many new demands made upon them, fully explored in Sainsbury's study (1977), but briefly mentioned here.

The 1963 Children's Act had been concerned that preventive work be undertaken to reduce the need for children to be received into care. The Children's and Young Persons' Act, 1969, involved social service departments in offering social work support and a wide range of residential and community provisions to children brought before the courts. In fact, the growing workload makes crisis work rather than preventive work the norm. In 1977 101 000 children were in care, compared with 87 000 in 1971. There is a tendency for children to stay longer in care although most are in care for short term reasons such as temporary illness of parent.

From the point of view of public opinion as expressed through the media the major problem of the social service departments in relation to children is child abuse, which involves health and social service personnel, teachers, police and educational welfare workers. Studies show how complex the causal factors in child abuse are, and thus how difficult is effective prevention. (Kempe, 1978; Freeman, 1979). Much valuable work is undertaken by a voluntary body, the National Society for the Prevention of Cruelty to Children, whose annual reports make useful reading. Work with children at risk of abuse is seen as primarily a social worker role but during the social worker strikes in 1978/9 it was the health visitor who often played the major role, whilst the general practitioner and the hospital are often the first agency to recognize the 'battered child'.

The Chronically Sick and Disabled Act, 1970, imposed new duties on the newly created social service departments as did the 1971 decision to implement Section 45 of the Public Health and Services Act, 1968, giving local authorities permission to promote the welfare of the elderly. There is an overlap between the elderly and the physically handicapped: arthritis is the major of the handicapping diseases, but the needs of the young disabled are perhaps the most urgent. It is also important not to generalize about the elderly, as Hunt reminds us in her study of the elderly at home (Hunt, 1978) Ninety percent of the elderly can go out without help but this falls to less than half if we isolate the over 85s.

Despite these two Acts, there are great variations in the help the elderly and disabled receive, whether one looks at special housing, meals on wheels, home helps, day centre places, provision of aids and gadgets or adaptations to the home. There are also variations between those taking advantage of the rehabilitation programmes available in some hospitals and followed through into the community, and those equally disabled who do not go through the hospitals. Even such a basic service as chiropody is in desperately short supply, with its obvious implications for the mobility of the elderly and disabled.

As the population ages and domiciliary care improves, the population of the residential homes run by local authorities become older and more infirm, with the decision about residential home or geriatric bed becoming more a question of supply than sensitive assessment of needs. Geriatric patients may be accepted only if a rehabilitated elderly patient is accepted by the local authority, for one of its residential homes. The senile demented patient is in an even worse situation: not physically ill enough for a geriatric bed, not capable of help in a psychiatric bed; too difficult for many local authority residential homes. Often they remain in the community, perhaps a danger to themselves, certainly creating stress for any family with whom they live. It is important to relate these dilemmas to shortage of resources — rationing by waiting list or deflection is inevitable in conditions of scarcity.

The problem of the senile demented patient shows clearly the link between the client of the social service department and the patient of the health services, with the role of the family doctor in trying to find a satisfactory solution crucial. This is equally true of the mentally disordered (covering the mentally ill and mentally handicapped), the other major group helped by the social service department.

Provision for the mentally disordered is at present governed by the Mental Health Act, 1959, which was concerned to move more rapidly from compulsory to voluntary admission, and to promote community care facilities. With the drug revolution that followed the Second World War, the closed door of the psychiatric hospital became a revolving door, with day care and hostel facilities supposedly available for those unable to cope unaided in the community. Of low priority in most local authorities — and within the National Health Service — community facilities remain inadequate.

The 1959 Act is under review, (DHSS 1976, 1978) and whilst some critics argue for reform on 'civil liberties' grounds, (Gostin, 1978), other commentators, (Jones 1977) are more concerned that adequate resources be made available to the existing services.

There have been a series of adverse reports on the large mental subnormality hospitals, ranging from the Report on Ely Hospital (DHSS 1969) to the one on Normansfield, (DHSS 1979). These reports are unlikely to be the last, despite the Health Service Commissioner and the work of the Health Advisery Service and the Mental Handicap Development Group. The movement towards more community care for the mentally handicapped is very slow. It means not just support for parents, but residential provision to relieve the parent, to cater for the profoundly handicapped child that cannot be cared for at home and to ensure that parents are not *forced* to cope at home by the absence of alternative facilities.

This brief survey of social welfare provisions has shown their complexity although variations in provision from one part of the country to another have been insufficiently stressed. To illustrate the complexity as it affects one client group, and to show the need for coordination of service and cooperation of health and social service staff if the client is to be effectively helped, an outline of services for the disabled is given in Table 11.2.

Coordination at field level can only come with understanding of, and respect for, the role of other professional groups within the caring professions. Perhaps this is most crucial in the field of child abuse (Freeman, 1979). For the consumer it is delivery that matters. Not just quantity and quality of service but the way in which it is offered. Coordination at the level of provision of service is important too and the 1974 NHS reorganization recognized this when it insisted that local authorities and the NHS consult and inform each other through the medium of the Joint Consultative Committees. Health care planning teams can involve non-NHS personnel in focussing on the needs of patient groups in their District. But the most hopeful development is joint financing.

Joint financing between the NHS and local authorities was introduced in 1977. On capital and revenue projects the Area Health Authority can make a 60% contribution to the total cost of a scheme if it will be in the interests of the NHS as well as the local authority, and can make a better contribution in terms of total care than if applied to health services directly. Area Health Authorities and local authorities are expected to choose schemes that relate to the DHSS national priorities. In 1979/80 schemes made possible because of this injection of NHS money into the squeezed local authority sector included adult training centres, residential homes for the elderly and the mentally infirm and day centres for the young physically handicapped. When the projects are revenue, the NHS contribution is reduced to nil over a period of 7 years, when the local authority is fully responsible. Revenue schemes included additional meals on wheels or home helps, but also more innovative schemes such as using private nursing homes to give families a break from an elderly relative, or night sitters for patients with terminal illness.

Table 11.2 Services for disabled people

Access/Mobility
Provision in this area cannot be the responsibility of one single service giver. Significant factors range from the availability of aids like wheelchairs to the provision of ramps in public and private buildings, the removal of high kerb stones, the appropriate design of public transport vehicles like buses and the judicious placing of 'street furniture'. The 'mobility allowance' provides significant financial support for around 200 000 very severely disabled younger people. It has risen relatively rapidly in value in the last few years, in line with the high costs of motoring reflected in the 'motor-bility' scheme for disabled drivers. But many less disabled persons capable of walking only short distances, or who happen to be over retirement age, receive no special assistance.

Education
Officially some 2 % of Britain's school age population (a little under 200 000 individuals) are classified as handicapped, although perhaps 15–20% are in need of some form of special educational help. Over 80 % of the former group are in segregated schools. Following the Warnock report government has moved towards recognising the need to 'integrate' more fully the education of many such children with that of their able bodied peers, both on academic and social grounds. However, some commentators (see, for example, Low 1981) fear that lack of economic resources and confused philosophies of support mean that little real progress is likely to be made in the foreseeable future.

Employment
Of the half a million plus individuals on the MSC register of disabled people over 15% are unemployed, about twice the national average figure. At present the quota scheme established by the 1944 Disabled Persons (Employment) Act is under review, as has been the future of the Disablement Resettlement Officer Service and that of certain Employment Rehabilitation Centres. Yet it seems unlikely that any radically new pattern will emerge. A key point is that government policy generally has concentrated on 'lubricating' the existing employment market rather than attempting to create significant numbers of jobs 'tailor made' for groups like mildly mentally handicapped people. A case can be made for a considerably more interventionist policy, especially in periods of lower overall employment levels. However, this may involve regarding 'jobs' as commodities in themselves, rather than merely a means to producing valued goods.

Housing
In the period 1970–75 only one purpose built dwelling was completed for every 400 disabled individuals defined by the OPCS as in need of rehousing. Since then, with economic recession, the rate of provision of either new homes or even of adaptations may have dropped. For instance, *Shelter* recently noted that in 1980 the number of 'starts' on disabled housing units was down by about a third on the previous year. In the case of home adaptations the recent imposition of charges by a number of authorities may have discouraged some clients from proceeding with requests for such assistance.

Income
Financial support for disabled persons and their families increased through the 1970s, although groups such as the Disability Alliance and the Disablement Income Group still stress the need for a comprehensive disability income designed to cover the special expenses that disability imposes as well as lost earning capacity. Estimates of the additional costs of such a scheme vary between £1500 million and £3000 million. Its advantages would include the possible elimination of inequities relating to assessment for benefits like housewives non-contributory invalidity pension (married women are at present subject to particularly stringent criteria) and the poverty trap suffered by partially disabled people of working age. A government study of this area has recently been re-initiated, and should eventually lead to a green paper.

Source: Disability in Britain – The Processes of Transition. OHE Briefing. Office of Health Economics. London. July 1981.

If allowed to grow the importance of such developments for community health staff is obvious but the money spent so far is a very small proportion of the NHS budget and the future of the scheme is not clear.

CONCLUSIONS

However inadequate the social welfare provisions may be, they have lifted the fears of unemployment, motherhood and illness that dominated working class lives before the Second World War. It could be argued that these changes have had a cost in terms of the strength of community feelings and changes of values within communities. This theme is explored by Seabrook (1978), who raises issues of importance to those concerned with community health in its widest sense.

In my view the social welfare provisions are nevertheless inadequate when looked at in terms of the average standards of the average family — even more so if we look at the distribution of wealth in this country. (Field, 1979).

Yet there are some whose dependency states, and the facilities which their caring families can offer, are substantially different from the norm. These individuals are those who are able to 'blame' an individual or an event and so claim compensation from the courts.

Early in 1979 a child mentally handicapped by meningitis which his general practitioner failed to diagnose, was awarded £300 000. Yet his needs are no more and no less than those of other equally severely brain damaged children. Under the Vaccine Damage Payments Act 1979 a sum of £10 000 is made available to anyone who has been severely damaged by vaccination against several diseases of which whooping cough is but one. Severe damage is defined as 80% under the scheme for assessing claims for industrial injuries. Receipt of the £10 000 does not prejudice the right of those so damaged to take subsequent court action. Under the Congential Disabilities (Civil Liability) Act 1976 a child born disabled because of the wrongful act of another person can recover damages from that person.

My hope for social welfare improvements in the future lies in hoping that *all* in need will be compensated and provided for, enabling them to live a life without stigma or hardship. The concept of blame which is growing, and with the Acts mentioned above might well accelerate, can only be divisive and hamper the fight for social justice and reduced inequalities that inspired early reformers and brought our present system — with all its faults — into being.

When public expenditure is under attack it is likely both to increase the demands made of the health and welfare services and reduce their capacity to meet these effectively. In the past hostility between the various branches of the caring professions have made the cutting of specific services perhaps easier. It is crucially important that community health staff appreciate the structure and function of the range of provisions affecting their patients, and the implications for their own work of shortage of resources in other related sectors.

REFERENCES

Blaxter M 1976 The meaning of disability. Heinemann Education, London
Central Statistical Office 1979 Social Trends 9 HMSO, London, p 3
DHSS 1969 Report of the committee of inquiry into allegations of ill-treatment of patients and other irregularities at the Ely Hospital Cardiff. Cmnd 3975. HMSO, London
DHSS 1976 Review of the Mental Health Act 1959. HMSO, London (Consultative document)
DHSS 1978 Review of the Mental Health Act 1959. Cmnd 7320. HMSO, London (White Paper)
DHSS 1978 Social Assistance DHSS London
DHSS 1979 Report of the committee of inquiry into Normansfield Hospital. Cmnd 7357. HMSO, London
Field F 1979 The wealth report. Routledge & Kegan Paul, London
Freeman M D A 1979 Violence in the Home Saxon House, Teakfield Ltd Farnborough Hants

Gostin L 1978 The great debate: Mind's comments on the White Paper on the review of the Mental Health Act 1959 Mind, 22 Harley Street, London W1
HMSO 1968 Seebohm Report. Report of the committee on local authority and allied personal social services, Cmnd 3703. HMSO, London
Hunt A 1978 The elderly at home: A study of people aged 65 and over living in the community in England in 1976. HMSO, London
Jones K 1975 The development of institutional care In: Butterworth E, Holman R (eds) Social welfare in modern Britain. Fontana/Collins Glasgow
Jones K 1977 The wrong target in mental health? New Society 39 (3rd March): 438–440
Kempe R S, Kempe C H 1978 Child abuse. Fontana/Open Books, London
McKeown T 1977 The modern rise of population. E Arnold, London
Moroney R M 1976 The family and the state. Longman, London
Opit L J 1977 Domiciliary care for the elderly sick — economy or neglect? British Medical Journal 1 (1st January): 30–33
Parker R 1970 The future of the personal social services. In: Crick B, Robson W A (eds) The future of the social services. Penguin, Harmondsworth
Robson W A 1976 Welfare state and welfare society. Allen & Unwin, London
Sainsbury E 1977 The personal social services. Pitman, London
Seabrook J 1978 What went wrong. Gollanz, London
Titmuss R M 1974 Social policy. Allen & Unwin, London

FURTHER READING

Brearley P, Gibbons J, Topliss E, Miles A, Woods, G. 1978 The social context of health care. Blackwell, Oxford and Martin Robertson, London
Butterworth E, Holman R (eds) Social welfare in modern Britain. Fontana/Collins Glasgow
Holman R 1978 Poverty: explanations of social deprivation. Martin Robertson, London
Parker J 1975 Social policy and citizenship. Macmillan, London
Robson W A 1976 Welfare state and Welfare society. Allen &Unwin, London
Sleeman J F 1973 The welfare state, its aims benefits and costs. Allen & Unwin, London

12

Health and work

Jennifer Barnard

For many men and women work is extremely important. Not only is the income it brings essential to maintain a reasonable standard of living but also it makes them happy: they feel fulfilled and enjoy most aspects of it. Their occupation helps them to achieve a sense of personal identity, status and worth. Such people will often make great sacrifices to get to work despite ill health, transportation difficulties, domestic crisis or personal discomfort. The involuntary cessation of work through injury, illness, pregnancy, dismissal, redundancy or early retirement often comes as a great shock and may be the cause of considerable distress and anxiety.

Since so many men and women spend up to 25% of each week at work, due consideration must be given to those factors at the work place and in the environment which can affect health, behaviour and attitudes. Technology and scientific developments have improved the working and general environment immeasurably during the last century. Some of these developments however have produced their own hazards.

Many health and safety experts, scientists and engineers are now deeply concerned with preventing the occupational injuries and diseases which affect so many people each year causing temporary and permanent incapacity, anxiety, frustration and loss of earnings. Many man hours are lost through sickness and ill-health. By preventing this loss it is possible to raise levels of production, standards of services and to improve the national economy.

In order to understand the working background of her patients and clients the community nurse should be familiar with as many of the work places in her area (and elsewhere) as possible. Without an understanding of the wide variety of jobs, work places and management styles now in existence it is difficult to imagine the nature of many clients' problems.

Some busy employers or managers may need a fairly convincing reason for spending time in showing someone around if there are no advantages to gain for the company or organisation. However, it should be possible to find good reasons for visiting many of the larger work places, especially if a number of potential clients or patients are employed there. The establishment of good relationships with employers, personnel managers and occupational health staff can bring considerable long-term benefits in preventing ill-health and in the provision of health care and advice. In visits to the different kinds of workplace it is important to try to identify why some workers appear happy and fulfilled in dreadful conditions

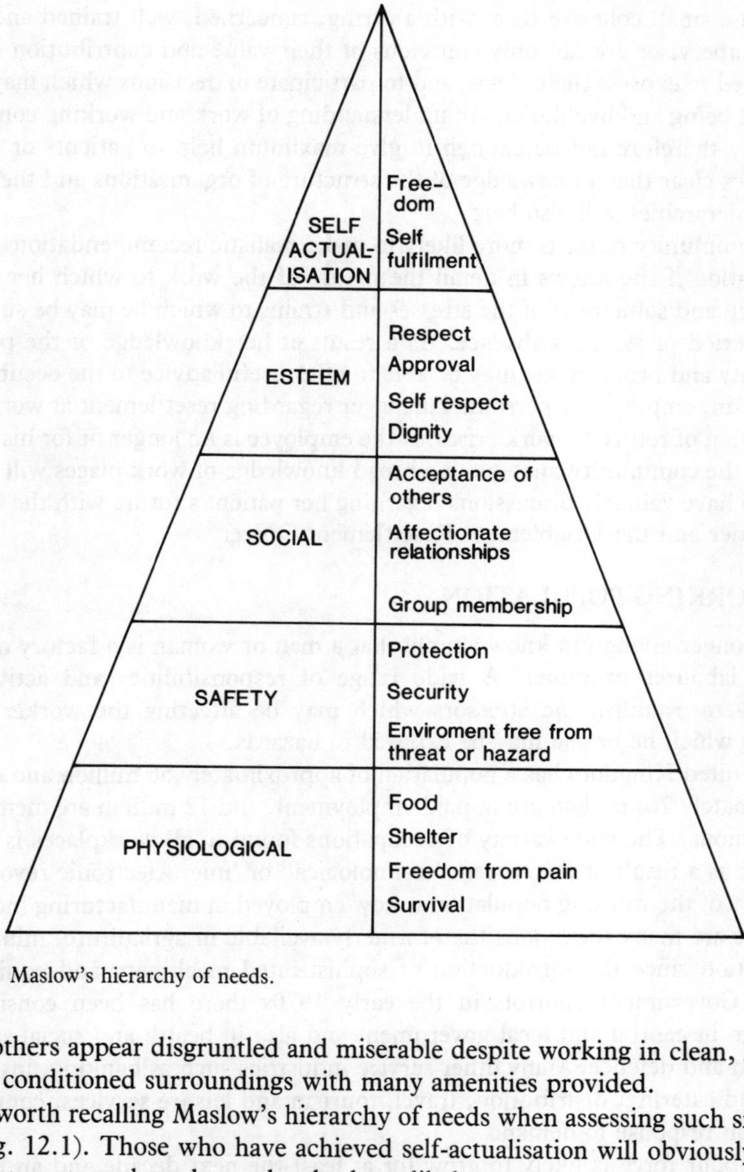

Fig. 12.1 Maslow's hierarchy of needs.

whilst others appear disgruntled and miserable despite working in clean, hygienic and air conditioned surroundings with many amenities provided.

It is worth recalling Maslow's hierarchy of needs when assessing such situations (see Fig. 12.1). Those who have achieved self-actualisation will obviously appear the most contented, and may be the least likely to use any excuse to stay away from work for a day.

Discussions with employed people about their work place and organisation can prove enlightening. A great many people now work in large organisations where decisions regarding individual departments may be taken far from the place of work. For some employed people this can make their contribution seem small and insignificant and their presence or absence at work seem not to be of great importance. Approximately 40% of the working population earn their living in relatively small businesses but the size seems of little significance in such matters. Of greater importance is the size of the working group and the quality of management. Those people in a small cohesive team with a caring, concerned, well trained and experienced supervisor are not only conscious of their value and contribution but are encouraged to express their views, and to participate in decisions which may affect their well being and livelihood. An understanding of work and working conditions alone may therefore not be enough to give maximum help to patients or clients. It becomes clear that a knowledge of the structure of organisations and the nature of their hierarchies will also help.

The community nurse is more likely to make realistic recommendations during rehabilitation if she knows in detail the nature of the work to which her patient will return and something of the stresses and strains to which he may be subjected after a period of sickness absence. As a result of her knowledge of the patient's personality and progress she may be able to offer useful advice to the occupational health team, employer or personnel manager regarding resettlement at work when the question of return to work arises. If the employee is no longer fit for his former job then the community nurse with a broad knowledge of work places will be well placed to have valuable discussions regarding her patient's future with the General Practitioner and the Disablement Resettlement Officer.

THE WORKING POPULATION

It is no longer enough to know simply that a man or woman is a factory or office worker, labourer or miner. A wide range of responsibilities and activities is necessary to establish the stressors which may be affecting the worker or the extent to which he or she may be exposed to hazards.

The United Kingdom has a population of approximately 56 million and of these approximately 26½ million are in paid employment, and 12 million are members of trades unions. The wide variety of occupations found in all workplaces is rapidly changing as a result of the current 'technological' or 'microelectronic revolution'. Only 32% of the working population is now employed in manufacturing industries and there are many fewer jobs than formerly available in agriculture, mining and construction since the introduction of sophisticated machinery and equipment. Despite Government controls in the early 1970s there has been considerable expansion in central and local government and also in health and social services, education and defence. Many other service industries such as banking, insurance, hotels and catering, distribution, travel, tourism and leisure services, continue to develop in response to demand.

The labour force is likely to grow for at least the next decade and an increase of 2 million (or 8%) is anticipated by 1991. The work force will become younger and many more women will be working, albeit part-time. More people are likely to be highly qualified and fewer will have no academic qualifications. By 1991 it is also predicted that between 5% and 6% of the working population will be of New Commonwealth or Pakistani ethnic origin, as compared with just over 3% in 1976. A substantial proportion of these people will have been born in Britain (Dept of Employment 1979).

THE INFLUENCE OF WORK ON HEALTH AND WELL-BEING

It is well recognised that an inappropriate life-style, unsuitable environment, inadequate nutrition, the lack of adequate rest, sleep and exercise, poverty, bad housing and poor personal relationships may all contribute to illness and disease. The influence of factors relating to work and occupation must always be borne in mind too. A recent report (Townsend, 1979) revealed with shocking clarity the unequal conditions in which many blue collar and white collar workers are employed, and the deprivation some employees suffer as a result (see Table 12.1). Through ignorance, carelessness, lack of concern or money, many people are also exposed to a wide variety of occupational hazards which can affect their physical or mental health in the short- or long-term.

Table 12.1 Percentages of men and women experiencing different kinds of deprivation or difficulty at work

	Men (%)	Women (%)
The character of the job		
Working mainly or entirely outdoors (including transport)	31	4
All working time standing or walking about	57	42
At work before 8 a.m. or working at night	36	15
Working 50 or more hours last week	24	4
Security		
Unemployment more than 2 weeks in last 12 months	5	4
Subject to 1 week's notice or less	44	51
Conditions and amenities		
Working conditions very poor or poor	23	15
Welfare or fringe benefits		
No wages or salary during sickness	37	35
Paid holidays of 2 weeks or less	56	61
No meals paid or subsidised by employer	76	69
No entitlement to occupational pension	43	61

Extracted from New Society article P. Townsend 1979

The difficulties, discomfort and physical hardship arising from work problems such as long hours, poor working conditions, and lack of pay during periods off work through illness or injury are unknown to many people. They may find it hard to imagine how it can be to work all day in a hot dusty foundry or deep in a mine kneeling in wet sludge at the coal face with the walk of a mile or more back to the lift shaft before going home. What kind of frustration and fatigue develops in the man who works at a task all day long, exactly as instructed, only to be severely reprimanded at the end of the day for doing it wrong, thus rendering the completed work useless? Can such a person who has been incorrectly instructed and poorly supervised take such criticism on a regular basis without some form of reaction, internalised as stress or externalised as verbal aggression or 'militancy'? How does the asbestos worker stripping lagging cope with his job, if inadequately protected and yet aware of the hazards to his health? How does the trans-continental haulage driver handle his problems — tight time-schedules, foreign languages and street signs, unfamiliar currency, complicated formalities as well as delays at borders and ferries and even picketing at the gates of his destination? The reactions will obviously vary according to the temperament and experience of the worker as well as depending on the state of his health and relationships.

Many of the problems at work arise from the interactions between people at all levels. Frustration, anguish and difficulties occur through misunderstandings, from demands rather than requests, autocracy rather than consultation and faulty communications. Superiors, subordinates and peers may all be affected. Those in the middle often have the most stressful time, suffering pressure from all angles.

The community nurse who finds herself dealing with a patient or client who is obviously having problems arising from work should establish clearly the precise nature of the work by asking a number of searching questions. The questions appearing in Table 12.2 could be introduced into the conversation in a structured manner in order to cover the most important points. If preferred, a written questionnaire along these lines could be devised. The nurse should then ask herself the following questions:

1. Is this person's job likely to be a source (*the* source) of problems now or in the future?

Table 12.2 Questions to ask of patients/clients who work

1a.	What is your job? [Establish category: professional, administrative, skilled (non-manual or manual), partly skilled, manual.]
b.	What precisely do you do in your work?
c.	What are your responsibilities?
d.	How long have you been in this job?
e.	Have you always worked at this level or were you promoted?
f.	What was your previous job? – and before that?
2a.	What hours do you work? (full-time, part-time, shifts, nights, flexitime).
b.	How many days each week?
c.	Do you ever work overtime/or bring work home? If so, how much, how often?
3a.	Where do you work?
b.	How far from home is it?
c.	How do you travel to work?
d.	How many changes do you make (e.g. bicycle, train, bus, etc.)?
e.	How long does the journey take?
4a.	What are the occupational hazards in your work?
b.	Do you work with any known health hazards? (Physical, mechanical, ergonomic chemical, biological, psycho-social)
c.	What substances do you handle?
d.	Is your work physically active?
4e.	Does your job involve lifting and handling items? — or heavy and bulky goods?
f.	Is your work standing, sitting, peripatetic or all three?
g.	Do you work indoors or outdoors?
5a.	Do you occasionally feel stressed at work?
b.	Do you work alone?
c.	If not, how many of you work together?
d.	What is your position in the group?
e.	Do you get on well with most people at work?
f.	Do you have any relationship problems with any particular people?
g.	Are you studying at present?
6	Do you enjoy your work? — if yes — why? if no — why not?

2. Could the job cause (or has it already caused) the present distress/illness/ill-health/injury/disability or handicap?

3. Is the job likely to be aggravating (or to aggravate in the future) an existing medical condition or handicap?

4. Does the illness (physical or mental) or present state of health (or residual disability) affect this person's ability to pursue his occupation effectively? (Include pregnancy).

5. Should he/she be advised to change his/her job or to give up work altogether?

The answers to these questions may not be immediately apparent. On those occasions when it is necessary to make such enquiries the established liaison with employers and occupational health colleagues should prove invaluable. Either a visit to the work place or a discussion with those who know it well may provide the answers.

When the community nurse suspects that the work place is the source of the present health problems and fears that there may be some hazard which may be affecting others, but can gain no information from the employer, then she should contact the area office of the Employment Medical Advisory Service (EMAS) for advice. Since they have access to all work places they should be able to obtain the necessary information.

PREPARATION FOR WORK AND TRAINING

The present information explosion and the phrenetic pursuit of knowledge is not likely to decrease in the next few decades as science and technology continue to make dramatic advances affecting all our lives. New developments in every area of industry, commerce and office life mean that work people have to adapt increasingly to more and more change, to periodic reorganisation, to the redundancy of certain skills, the abolition of many jobs, and the creation and development of new skills and occupations.

The range of occupations now available is constantly extending and changing and many jobs require not only a good basic education but also further education and vocational or special training to develop the necessary skills and knowledge. The proportion of people in unskilled work is now dramatically reduced compared with the first five or six decades of this century. However, some young people on leaving school will continue to go straight into unskilled employment without any preparation or training.

Education and training will soon be necessary for the vast majority of jobs and in the future many people will be required at various stages in their working life and career to retrain for entirely new work or to learn additional skills. Large numbers of working people will undoubtedly take advantage of the Open University, correspondence courses and evening classes to study for further qualifications in their spare time.

The pressure to acquire new knowledge may induce considerable stress both in young people and in the mature student. Many will overstretch themselves as a result of ambition or pressures to succeed from friends, family or employers.

Trainees and students who cannot cope may react by opting out whenever possible or by unusual or aggressive behaviour — 'fighting or fleeing'. Those who have problems or who are frequently 'off sick' may need considerable help and support from college counsellors where these exist, or from tutors, technical training or personnel staff and occupational health doctors and nurses, if available.

During training and retraining those suffering from anxiety and strain will need extra help, guidance and support. Some people may need to be encouraged to lower their sights and to undertake less ambitious programmes or to be chanelled into different work and to develop other latent talents and skills.

REDUNDANCY, UNEMPLOYMENT AND THE SEARCH FOR A JOB

It will soon be unusual for a person to remain in the same job for a working lifetime. The technological revolution, improved education and different expectations have all contributed to job mobility. The search for work and new jobs frequently takes people away from their original home town to other regions where new industries and services may be developing.

People change jobs voluntarily for financial, personal or domestic reasons. They may want different hours, work nearer home, improved wages or salaries, another job because their spouse's work or promotion necessitates a move, or they may just wish a change. Some people seek other work because they can no longer tolerate their working conditions, or because relationships at work have broken down. Those people who leave their jobs before finding another may have considerable difficulty in obtaining suitable alternative employment immediately, unless they possess much sought after skills or are prepared to move to another part of the country.

Unemployment is now a worry for people at all levels and in all sectors of society. The increasing need to improve efficiency and productivity has caused both private and nationalised employers to rationalise their position and to implement redundancy programmes. Whether dismissed or made redundant the man or woman who no longer has a job may suffer considerable distress. Many feel stigmatised and experience a lack of self-confidence, a sense of worthlessness, rejection and hopelessness.

Unemployed people and those threatened with redundancy frequently feel inadequate and develop signs and symptoms of ill-health such as headaches, gastrointestinal disturbances and skin disorders as well as depression. Anorexia or obesity and excessive smoking or drinking may become problems as the unemployed person withdraws into himself and attempts to cope with the social and economic problems he now faces.

The search for a new job may prove long and difficult. Repeated applications for jobs and subsequent disappointment are wholly demoralising. Members of the primary health care team can provide counselling, support and guidance to the whole family when it becomes apparent that unemployment is causing a breakdown in the health of individuals or the family unit. Those community nurses working in regions of high unemployment are particularly likely to encounter problems amongst the unemployed.

Considerable help and advice for all employment problems is obtainable from local Jobcentres or Employment Offices. Jobcentres and private employment agencies offer a service both to employers and to those seeking employment by bringing vacancies and suitable applicants together. The Government's Job Search Service run by the Manpower Services Commission will also assist unemployed people in finding work beyond daily travelling distance of home. Under the Employment Transfer Scheme it is possible to obtain grants and allowances for transfers to take up such work for a period of up to two years. The staff in local Jobcentres are also able to provide details of other forms of assistance including training at a Skillcentre or elsewhere through the Training Opportunities Scheme (TOPS).

Many people who have been unemployed for long periods have great difficulty in facing up to the physical and mental adjustment of returning to work again, particularly if their absence was due to a debilitating or handicaping illness or injury. Courses are provided at Employment Rehabilitation Centres to help such people with an assessment of the type of work to which they are suited to regain their self confidence and to become familiar again with the daily routine of work. Vocational guidance is given and if necessary appropriate training can be arranged in industry, at a technical or commercial college or at a Skillcentre. Certain voluntary organisations provide special rehabilitation for specific categories of people such as the blind, mentally disabled and young spastics.

Particular difficulty in obtaining employment is often experienced by physically or mentally handicapped people, despite the fact that research has shown that employed disabled people frequently are more conscientious and attend more regularly than their able-bodied colleagues. Both the Disablement and Blind Persons Resettlement Officers (DROs and BPROs) are available through local Jobcentres to give assistance. They will provide advice and guidance on financial assistance, rehabilitation, training and suitable employment. For some handicapped people it may be appropriate to recommend application for employment in sheltered workshops run by the local authority, a voluntary organisation or in a Remploy factory. Remploy Ltd. is a company operating as a commercial concern under the direction of the Department of Employment and employs approximately 8000 disabled people in 90 factories throughout Britain.

HOME WORK

Many people's work is in their home, unpaid, as housewives and mothers. They may also be caring for dependent relatives and friends or paid as industrial outworkers or homeworkers. Some manufacturers find it economic to distribute to people in their homes small parts assembly work or machining tasks for the clothing industry. Large numbers of women and some disabled and retired people undertake such work regularly. The dearth of nursery schools, creches at work places and day care facilities for the handicapped and elderly prevent many people who would otherwise like to go out to work from leaving their homes. Social and cultural pressures to remain at home cause certain women including members of the Asian and Cypriot communities, in particular, to undertake such work. Unfortunately many home workers run the risk of serious exploitation. Extremely poor pay, production pressures and health hazards associated with assembly and other work all need close observation to ensure that these men and women do not suffer from such problems. In 1980 the Health and Safety Commission published proposals for new regulations to replace legislation dealing with the registration of homeworkers. It is intended to safeguard homeworkers from potential risks to their health and safety arising from the processes used.

Where work is undertaken at home involving the use of glues, solvents and paints, particular attention needs to be paid to instructions and warnings on containers and to the ventilation of the workroom as well as to the effects on other members of the household including children. Symptoms of ill-health amongst otherwise healthy homeworkers and those who are 'do-it-yourself' enthusiasts or keenly active in making items for a hobby should always cause suspicion to be cast on the activity. The health visitor or district nurse when visiting such homes should always issue warnings regarding the hazards to health and safety when using unfamiliar materials, liquids and solids including pesticides. The workroom, garden shed or garage frequently contains particularly hazardous items. In the event of a crisis or symptom arising from an unknown agent advice should be obtained from the general practitioner, the Employment Medical Advisory Service, the nearest poisons centre or an experienced occupational physician or occupational health nurse who may help to identify the cause, and recommend appropriate action.

HOURS

Many people work permanent or regular overtime. These employees and those who take second jobs are likely to be subject to extreme fatigue as well as to problems in their family or domestic circumstances as a result of being out of the home so much. Health problems may develop in the course of time, arising from prolonged physical activity and inadequate sleep and rest. Complaints of digestive troubles arising from stress and rushed or missed meals, insomnia, and palpitations, may arise initially and lead on to hypertension, angina and chronic anxiety states. Pressures from the spouse or family to increase the household's income may prevent certain individuals from heeding nature's warnings and taking action to reduce the pressure. Others may have become so accustomed to working long and hard that they cannot imagine how they will occupy themselves if they return home after only eight hours work and insist that they must continue. Those on regular overtime may hesitate to discuss their problems with their employer and to mention the possibility of reducing the hours worked for fear of losing their job, since others may be more prepared to undertake the extra work.

Increasingly people are going to have to learn how to make good use of their leisure time, for there are now many pressures to reduce the working week, to abolish overtime and to encourage early retirement. In this way it is hoped to help create more jobs for the unemployed and for school leavers. The community nurse has a role both in schools, with the workers and parents of tomorrow, and with the families of today, to teach people how to make sensible use of their time and retirement years.

Many people who undertake office work have the opportunity to work flexible hours or 'flexitime' enabling them to avoid the worst of 'rush hour' travel if they wish to, or to fit in with home and other commitments. Providing they attend for the obligatory core period during the day and complete their work in the number of hours required of them, their employer allows them to come and go as they please.

With the continuing introduction of automation to the work place involving highly expensive equipment and machinery, employers frequently maximise their use by ensuring their continuous activity. Hence shift work and night work are introduced and are often frequently necessary in industry and also in other undertakings where a continuous process or a 24 hour service is provided. Many variations exist including rotating and split shifts. Approximately 20% of male manual workers and 10% of female manual workers are employed on shift systems while only 4% to 5% of non-manual men and 7% to 8% of non-manual women work on shifts. 'Twilight' or early evening shifts are popular with many married women enabling them to get out of the house for a break and to earn some money of their own, whilst their husband or other members of the family cares for children or dependent relatives. Many women undertaking full- and part-time work develop a wide variety of health problems since they are effectively carrying out two jobs and may have little respite from work all day long and seldom have sufficient rest or relaxation.

Night workers and those on rotating shifts which include periodic night work may remain in such a routine for years. Those who cannot tolerate the changes in life style which shift work or night work necessitate or who have difficulty in physically adapting, soon leave and return to 'normal hours'. Certainly working such hours can create havoc with social and family life and may create great difficulties with interpersonal relationships where these may already be strained.

The community nurse who identifies those who are having family problems or who are suffering ill-health possibly as a result of excessive hours or unsuitable shifts should, where possible, advise the individual affected of the future implications for his or her health and should suggest that consideration should be given to reduced or altered hours or even a change of job. Where the employer has an occupational health service the community nurse or general practitioner may wish to discuss the problems of the employee, with his consent, in order to establish the best course of action.

JOB SATISFACTION AND COMMUNICATIONS

A day at work is likely to be a source of stimulus and enjoyment for many people but for others it can be the casue of frustration, anger and annoyance. There are many reasons why people work and considerable research has been undertaken this century on work motivation. Contrary to popular opinion, financial reward is not necessarrily the principal reason why a person enters employment, starts up his own business, decides to become an author or to seek promotion. Companionship and job satisfaction for many people are more relevant factors.

Companionship at work is extremely important for many people and the relationships established with colleagues at all levels contribute a great deal towards their attitude to life at the end of the day. Unfortunately, although many people work in groups on production and assembly lines, in a maintenance team, or in an office department, noise, work pressures and other factors may prevent the type of communications which the prospective employee had in mind.

Communications have never been so sophisticated or important as now, but the human element inevitably causes failures. When communication fails and misunderstanding arises great harm may occur to the individual's mental health. Anxiety may develop and if not resolved can lead to insomnia, strain, a lack of concentration, accidents, mistakes and reprimands, further perpetuating the cycle.

Many people work alone as self employed people or in lonely or isolated jobs. Certain personalities can cope with spending long hours without the companionship of others, especially if working at home and during their leisure they have a full and socially active life. However the tedium of certain jobs such as security staff or guards on long distance freight trains may prove too much, causing them to leave to seek a job with more activity and human contact. Those such as coastguards and process operators monitoring dials whose work gives them regular radio or telephone communication with others, as well as considerable responsibility, may claim to achieve considerable job satisfaction. The community nurse may occasionally be in a position to advise employees when seeking new work, particularly those who have suffered from mental ill-health such as depression and other psychiatric states. These people should be discouraged from working in lonely and isolated jobs with the reminder that their condition will not be helped by being alone for long periods.

Job satisfaction is a vital factor in any person's employment. Owing to the increasing tendency, in the interests of speed and efficiency, to break jobs down into their component parts, leaving operatives and others to undertake the same task repeatedly, any sense of reward and pleasure has disappeared from the work place for large numbers of people. However, increasing automation, the use of robots and the introduction of computers and microprocessors is taking the tedium out of some work. Some of the boring jobs have been abolished altogether and in other areas new employment opportunities are being created which are more interesting and challenging. Considerable concern has been registered on this subject by occupational psychologists and others and job enrichment programmes have been consciously developed in certain companies. Recent evidence suggests that most jobs can be made more satisfying without losing efficiency. This means completely redesigning jobs and is time consuming, expensive and a difficult task. However in some companies serious efforts have been made to overcome the problems. Volvo, the Swedish car and truck firm, Volkswagen and the Philips organisation have all become particularly well known for their job enrichment programmes. These have included a return to unit production by groups of workers and participation in decision making by the workers themselves, based on the belief that the humanisation of work and efficiency can be compatible. Many of those companies who have achieved such changes have been able to show a reduction in labour turnover and absenteeism, better industrial relations, easier recruitment, greater flexibility and an improved quality in the product or service.

THE FUTURE

The search for new products and services and the creation of personal and national wealth means that scientists and others will continue their explorations for new techniques, developments and processes. Employers will continue to strive for success, greater financial returns and profitability. Meanwhile the introduction of new technology will inevitably cause the fear of redundancy for many people as has happened, for example, in the newspaper industry. As jobs change so it seems inevitable that social mobility will increase. Roots will not be set down deep and individuals may need a great deal of help, support and guidance, as they cope with new surroundings, new people and situations.

The increase in leisure means that the leisure industries will themselves expand dramatically and people will have to learn how to make good use of their free time and how to communicate effectively with each other. They can no longer consider spending all their free time in front of the television if they are to remain healthy and capable of work. Voluntary work in the social services sector and other areas will inevitably increase. Judicious guidance of the right personalities into such work could prove a valuable community service. The community nurse's knowledge of those people requiring particular help and assistance will be of value in encouraging those who would not otherwise entertain the idea of voluntary work to contribute some of their skills and talents to helping others.

The explosive growth in the number of workers whose sole activity is to handle paper-based information is likely to continue. At the beginning of this century about 10% of the working population was employed in handling information, now it is 50%. As the data processing industry develops further this will inevitably increase for we are now in an era in which the electronic transmission of documents is becoming commonplace and will ensure improvements in the quality of information exchanged.

It is difficult to ascertain whether the large numbers of jobs which will be created as a result of new technology will outnumber the many jobs which will be lost in more traditional occupations. Electronic systems will definitely change the patterns of employment, and much manual work and uninteresting clerical work will be taken over by machines and microprocessors.

Since communications will become ever more important, a reasonable standard of literacy will become essential for most work people. At present amongst an Asian population in Britain of 340 000, some 200 000 have only the most elementary working knowledge of English. Attendance at general education and literacy classes is necessary for all those who have problems with the language or who have failed to benefit from the education system.

Few people now or in the future, except craftsmen, will be able to take pride in a product made entirely themselves. Therefore the sense of purpose which may have been lost in making things may be regained as people find the true purpose to life in serving others either in the service sector or during their own leisure hours.

Within the next 30 years it is likely that 90% of people in employment will be working in the service sector and only 10% in materials production. Our view of occupations and their hazards will have to change. During this period increasing knowledge, discoveries and new technology should ensure that hazardous processes are carefully contained with minimal risk to workers. Many people will be faced with a constant hazard to their mental health and the need for change and adaptation. The speed with which changes are now taking place in many work places involving the introduction of new machinery, microcomputers, visual display units, word processors, automatic typewriters and millions of microprocessors all of which are gradually taking over the work of human beings, is terrifying to many people and is hardly likely to slacken. However, the rate of change is made tolerable for some people by the gradual effect of the media on their attitudes to the inevitability of change.

By 1985 the standard working week is likely to be reduced to 38 hours and there will probably be restrictions on overtime. By 1990 it may be down to 35 hours and by the years 1995 to 2000 to 21 or 20 hours only. By this time the 3 and 2 day week and the 5 day weekend may be commonplace. Robots will have taken over much of the drudgery in jobs which now require skilled workers to carry them out.

Job opportunities will be created in other areas as many trades and skilled occupations disappear, unneeded. Education and the transmission of information will become more important than ever before. Devices for storing and retrieving information will be everywhere, in the home, in our pockets and on our desk tops. We shall become increasingly dependent upon computer technology.

But as work decreases and more leisure is created and jobs change, go out of existence and are recreated, how will people cope? The health workers of the 1980s will have to concentrate far more on the mental health problems of their patients and clients than hitherto. Medical technology will develop apace but will the intangible factors which could relieve the mentally sick, the frustrated, unhappy frightened and depressed worker of their problems, be improved at the same rate?

CONCLUSION

Many men and women may work for as much as 40 to 50 years of their lives. Depending upon the nature of the work, its hours and its hazards as well as the attitude of the worker, it may exact a considerable toll on his health and his family. During periods of sickness, unemployment or retraining, people will worry not only about the present, but about future prospects, possible limitations and their potential loss of earning power. Such worry and strain may affect recovery rates and mental health and will have repercussions for the entire family unit. The community nurse can often help a husband or wife to understand why it is that his or her spouse is suffering or reacting the way he is, why he is so tired and has little inclination for conversation or family activities.

Without an idea of how each person requiring help spends his or her week it is very difficult to identify those factors which may be preventing the maintenance of health or return to normality.

A knowledge of the implications of the various types of work and the changes and developments within work places as well as the many sources of help and information now available is also necessary in order to give appropriate advice and guidance during sickness, rehabilitation and pregnancy and to direct patients and clients to the appropriate agencies for further help. Health workers may find that many employers, employees and self employed people may initially present their work problems in the form of deviations from normal health. Their signs and symptoms may signify stresses which are becoming intolerable.

The community nurse can help people physically to get better by giving appropriate advice. She can also help them mentally and emotionally to come to terms with their problems and circumstances by giving them an opportunity to talk through their problems in confidence and to make relevant enquiries or referrals.

The community nurse has potential contact with people at all stages in their lives. Young people, the physically and mentally handicapped and mothers returning to work after bringing up their family all require particular assistance. Those facing redundancy or retirement and the unemployed need special understanding, guidance and support. Liaison with employers, and occupational health staff, in particular with occupational health nurses, will obviously enhance the value of advice given to working people and will avoid misunderstandings and conflicting recommendations.

Work in the future will be very different for many people. However, it will continue to affect the physical and mental health of work people in all types of occupation. We must learn to understand the problems of those whose occupation lacks the variety and numerous changes between tasks which exist in our own work. Our job is to help improve the health of those placed in our care, to prevent ill health and to encourage positive attitudes to work and living. We must ensure that work proves a favourable influence upon the working population enhancing the quality of their own and their families' lives. Our observations, knowledge and actions can also ensure that complications and handicapping conditions are minimised and that the length of people's lives is not shortened as a result of the many potential influences and health hazards at work which can affect their physical, mental, emotional and spiritual health.

REFERENCES

Bassett P 1979 Labour and the microchip. Office Equipment VI. Financial Times Oct 23rd

Bosworth D L Dawkins P J 1978 Proposed changes in the extent and nature of shift working. Some important policy issues. Personnel Review 7(4) Autumn 1978: 32–35

Department of Employment 1979 Employment Gazette. Changing composition of the labour force 1976–1991. June 87(6): 546–551

Department of Employment 1979 Employment Gazette October 87(10). (Figures obtained and calculated from Employment Statistics)

Maslow A H 1968 Toward a psychology of being. Van Nostrand Reinhold, New York

Townsend P 1979 Inequality at the workplace: How whitecollar always wins. New Society 18th October: 120–123

FURTHER READING

Argyle M 1974 The social psychology of work. Pelican, London

Brown J A C 1954 The social psychology of work. Pelican, London

Buchholz Rogine A 1978 The work ethic reconsidered. Industrial and Labour Relations Review 31(4): 450–459

Department of Employment 1973 On the quality of working life. Manpower Papers No 7. HMSO, London

Scott D 1970 The psychology of work. Duckworth, London

Davis E, Taylor J C (eds) 1979 Design of jobs. In: Herzberg F One more time: How do you motivate employees? Goodyear, London, ch 10

Dean A 1979 A survey of the current employment situation. Management Decision March 17th 1979

Equal Opportunities Commission 1979 Report and Recommendations: Health & Safety Legislation: Should we distinguish between men and women? Equal Opportunities Commission, London
Goldring M 1979 Into the electronic eighties. *The Listener* May 24th 699–701
Goldthorpe J H, Lockwood D, Bechhofer F, Platt J 1968 The affluent worker: Industrial attitudes and behaviour. Cambridge University Press, Cambridge
Hall E M 1979 Rudiments of care 3. Helping the patient with work or productive occupation. Nursing Times June 21st
Harrington J M 1978 Shift work and health A critical review of the literature. HMSO, London
Jahoda M 1979 The psychological meanings of unemployment. New Society Sept. 6th: 492–495
Maddock I 1978 The future of work. Beyond the Protestant ethic. New Scientist Nov 23rd: 592–595
Social Trends 1979 Mass unemployment into the eighties. New Society Feb. 18th: 252
Toffler A 1970 Future shock. Pan Books, London
Toffler A 1980 The third wave. William Collins, London
Turner P 1979 Easiest to exploit. Morning Star January 31st
Walker J 1978 The human aspects of shiftwork. Institute of Personnel Management, London
Warr P B (ed) Psychology at work. In: Blackler F, Williams R People's motives at work.
Wigham E 1976 Protecting the army of home workers from exploitation. The Times May 4th
Wilson N A B 1973 On the quality of working life. A report prepared for the Department of Employment. Manpower papers No. 7. HMSO, London

13

The politics and economics of health care

Jane Salvage

Tower Hamlets is a borough and health district in the East End of London. Many of its residents are among the most deprived in the United Kingdom: the number of registered unemployed approaches 20% of the working population in some areas, at least 700 families were homeless in 1979, and the number of children in care and households with more than one person per room was over twice the London average. Many homes still lack hot water and inside lavatories.

The low social and economic status of Tower Hamlets residents is reflected in their morbidity and mortality rates, which are higher than the national average in every respect. The crude death rate in 1976 was 23% above the national norm; there is an increasing proportion of elderly people and an above average number of disabled people. These facts are carefully set out in the Tower Hamlets Health District Plan, which lays down a strategy for the development of health and some social services. Yet a comparison of the extent and nature of the services provided with those in a more prosperous district would not reveal striking differences.

With a large number of people in need of support services and home visits rather than long-term inpatient care, it is perhaps surprising to find that 'whereas the acute services in the district are allocated a substantially greater proportion of the budget than occurs nationally (nearly 74% compared with 56% in 1976), community services receive roughly one half of the national figure (4.6% compared with 9.1%) (Yudkin, 1978). The reasons are partly historical, including the large number of acute hospitals set up by charitable bodies to serve the poor at a time when the population was at least three times as large, and the presence of a major teaching hospital. As a result there is extensive provision of acute services, rudimentary primary care and little provision for those people needing long-term institutional care or supporting services. The teaching hospital, taking a large share of the annual revenue and capital expenditure, sprawls amid appalling social conditions to which patients are discharged to 'convalesce'. Conventional health education is entirely unable to tackle the prevention of ill-health in the district, with its tiny budget and inadequate conceptual tools.

Tower Hamlets is not typical of all health districts but its patterns of ill-health reflect those of society at large; increased life expectancy, through better standards of living and the ability to keep alive those who would once have died, is creating demands for health services which do not necessarily cure but provide care and support.

This prompts two questions. If the community's health depends largely on factors such as housing, nutrition and safe working practices, how appropriate is the curative emphasis of modern health care — and the training of those who deliver it? And if this awareness of the changing patterns of ill-health is as widespread as it appears, why is the shift of resources from cure to care not taking place more quickly?

The tension between chronic health needs and acute medical care is clearly displayed in Tower Hamlets and may help us to discern similar patterns elsewhere. Understanding the dynamics of that tension, and the reason why there is so little effort to seek out and prevent the chief causes of ill-health, forms the foundation of that rather airy concept, 'the politics and economics of health care'.

THE SHIFT OF RESOURCES

Successive governments in recent years have declared their intention of shifting resources from the acute sector of the National Health Service to the Cinderella services, a policy reiterated in the document *Care in Action* (1981). 'The main emphasis of our priorities continues to be along the lines on which our predecessors were working, and includes giving a high priority both to the prevention of ill health and to the so-called Cinderella services for people who are mentally ill and handicapped, and those who are elderly,' Social Services Secretary Patrick Jenkin wrote to the chairmen and members of district health authorities.

There has been much discontent with the slow rate of these proposed changes, and some scepticism about their ability to cope with demographic trends such as the growing number of frail elderly people. 'Many of the areas to which the DHSS professes to be giving priority are not to receive any increase in their percentage share of the total budget,' wrote the Radical Statistics Health Group in 1976. 'Some of the proposed 'growth areas' for expenditure will have such a slow growth rate that the targets set by the DHSS will take many years to achieve, even if the population remains static.'

Matters have been complicated since 1976 by a deepening economic recession and the election of a government committed to reducing public spending. Strict cash limits mean that any large shift of resources will rob Peter to pay Paul — a move which the acute services will fight tooth and nail. Meanwhile acute medicine and surgery continue to enjoy the lion's share: the inequitable nature of resource allocation is most vividly shown in a comparison of inpatient costs per day at different types of hospital (Table 13.1).

Policy documents, then, may try to influence decision making but they are little more than window dressing. What are the forces which actually determine policy? N.H.S. staff on the whole know and care little about the mechanism of decision making, and in one sense their scepticism is based on a realistic awareness that the real decisions are made somewhere else. This is not to say there is no point in trying to influence bodies like health authorities and community health councils, which have nominal powers, and it is not to deny that democratic advances have been made. But fundamental change is unlikely to occur unless we come to grips with deeper forces.

Table 13.1 Cost per in-patient week of different services in different types of hospital, as percentage of cost in acute non-teaching hospitals.

Type of service	Long stay	Chronic	Mental illness	Mental handicap
Medical	27	13	26	13
Nursing	65	66	45	40
Domestic	58	60	27	27
Catering	55	48	45	43
Cleaning	68	55	35	32
Total net costs	44	39	32	30

Source: DHSS 1974 Hospital Costing Returns. HMSO, London

The economic system

The most obvious and at the same time most hidden influence on health care, because it is so pervasive as to seem natural, is the economic system of the Western world, capitalism. The priority of this system, despite the modifications of a mixed economy and the undoubted improvements in living standards it has made possible, is to make profit for those who control it. This is most clearly shown in a recession, when many of those who have sweated for capitalism find themselves redundant, sick or old — and lacking the economic support the system is prepared to give in wealthier times.

Health care is often assumed to be separate from politics, as though we can extract money from the system for our own particular concerns without considering or being affected by the reasons why it is given. But I make no apology for my crude description: health care is not a right but a luxury in the eyes of capitalism. Even when the nation is prosperous there are many people whose needs are barely met, or are met in a way which should shame a supposedly civilised country — because the elderly or the handicapped have no economic power and few strong allies.

Capitalism also affects health care in more specific ways, through the intervention of profit-making companies. The use of increasingly complex technology, for example, is encouraged by supply companies, as the use of a pill for every ill is encouraged by pharmaceutical companies; the market is booming and they are only too willing to find new products and techniques, often justified by 'medical science' in the shape of a doctor on the payroll. These commercial groups would have little to gain, and perhaps much to lose in a shift of resources from the acute sector.

The reduction of health care to a commodity to be bought and sold has the effect of distorting people's expectations, whether they are delivering it or receiving it. Seduced by the prospect of miraculous high-technology cures, patients abdicate their own responsibility for their health, as though their bodies were machines to be serviced — and they fail to identify the social causes of their health problems when the remedy seems to be available on an individual level. As Doyal (1979) puts it, 'the defining of health and illness in a functional way is an important example of how a capitalist value system defines people primarily as producers — as forces of production . . . The medical model limits people's own expectations of what it is to be healthy and is thus significant in keeping sickness (and also the demand for medical care) under control.'

Private medicine

The supremacy of curative medicine is reinforced by the expansion of private medicine, another increasingly important element in the politics and economics of health care. Its emphasis on the easily curable and therefore profitable acute illnesses of the body is reflected in the sophisticated advertising for private health insurance, which reinforces the public's image of health care as acute medical treatment.

The advances made by the N.H.S in planning a comprehensive range of health services within a defined geographical area, and in trying to distribute resources more fairly, are threatened by the largely uncoordinated growth of private services. This could cause many problems. Should representatives of private firms participate in N.H.S management teams? And if private facilities were planned as part of a full range of services, what would happen if they had to close for any reason? The intervention of market forces in health care needs careful consideration.

It is argued that the private sector will 'save' public spending on acute services, releasing funds for the deprived areas, but there are few signs of this happening, particularly under a government which wants to reduce public spending. Moreover, many of its critics point out that it *relies* on public spending, indeed could not exist without it: 'At present the N.H.S has a lot of resources which the private sector badly needs. The private sector lacks technical and nursing skills,' Bosanquet said in 1979 — skills which public money pays to develop but whose fruits are then lost to the public in general.

The medical establishment

Doctors often complain that their decision making powers in planning matters have been usurped by administrators, but they are still the most potent interest group in modern health care. Much of their status derives from the profession's success in securing a monopoly of authority in 'medical matters' — matters which almost always, in fact, need to be defined more broadly. The position of the medical profession was convincingly analysed in the 1980 Reith Lectures by Ian Kennedy: 'If we are to take back power to control our lives, we can and must examine (doctors') judgments and evaluations,' he concluded. 'We must become the masters of medicine, not its servants.'

Not all doctors have the same influence, however. The hierarchy of prestige within the N.H.S reflects the hierarchy within medicine, with teaching hospital specialities at the top and geriatrics and mental handicap at the bottom. The system encourages doctors to practise acute, curative medicine, a tendency instilled during the long training when medical students concentrate almost exclusively on the disease model. The almost sacerdotal authority they enjoy depends heavily on their curative function, and the temptation to play God is one few have the ability or desire to resist: its consequences have been provocatively discussed by Illich (1977).

The 'clinical freedom' which doctors claim so vigorously is a manifestation of their freedom to make independent decisions, and it causes particular problems in the planning of community services, where it is linked to the general practitioner's role as an independent contractor. The G.P.'s financial and decision-making independence is merged in an ethical construct which becomes a justification for maintaining his separation from other practitioners. Until this is demystified and family practitioner services are planned alongside other community services, the primary health care team will be little more than a myth and community care will lack integration and coordination.

Sexual divisions and 'medical need'

The sexual division of labour in our society is exemplified in the work of nurses and doctors and their relative influence in decision making. Nursing is still widely thought of as 'women's work', a caring rather than skilled job which can be performed by women almost instinctively; whereas medicine claims the hard edge of masculine objectivity. The doctor is the man of science who can judge his patients' best interests without becoming 'too' involved. Inside the professions it may be felt that the division is becoming blurred, but it is still potent.

The feminine/caring and masculine/curing division plays an important role in the planning process, especially on bodies like health authorities which have a number of lay people as members. 'Logic' is often equated with 'medical need' in discussions preceding priority decisions; medical and administrative staff become allies in their ability to make 'tough' decisions, with their apparently hardnosed objectivity taking precedence over the feminine, feeling aspects of health care. Very often, of course, this objectivity is simply a way of expressing particular interests in disinterested terms; but it has succeeded in discrediting other forms of expression.

Of course attempts must be made to evaluate decisions in an objective way. But caution is needed in dealing with those who claim objectivity as their justification, who appear to cut a swathe through the emotionalism which is always supposed to engulf those who fight passionately for less powerful interests.

I have tried to outlined some of the reasons for the overemphasis on acute services in modern health care. Let us now look at the causes of ill-health, and the reasons why they receive little attention.

RADICAL PREVENTION

The prevention of ill-health is not generally seen as a major part of the N.H.S's function; it is usually consigned to the fringe area of health education. Yet doctors are regarded as authorities on prevention, and writing self-help manuals on avoiding heart attacks and hypertension is a popular medical sideline: the experts on sickness are also regarded as experts on health. Consideration of the causes of ill-health nevertheless has little influence on health care policy, a deficiency which needs correction.

Every disease process is subject to individual variation, and 'personality' may always have an indefinable effect on prognosis. Broad patterns of susceptibility to ill-health and ability to overcome sickness can, however, be discerned, and it is increasingly obvious that these patterns lie outside the domain of medicine. The decline in tuberculosis and diphtheria, for example, may owe more to improved living standards than to medical intervention. The enormous improvement in the population's health in the last 50 years is largely due to better housing, safer and shorter working hours, better nutrition and so on. As Doyal (1979) states 'this is not to suggest that the physical and chemical laws governing disease mechanisms can simply be abandoned, but rather that they must be seen to operate within a social and economic context which is constantly changing.'

That changing context is evident in the new patterns of disease in Western societies, where the latest epidemic killers are cancer, heart disease, accidents and mental illness. Medicine is as much at a loss in coping with them as it was in dealing with epidemic infectious disease in any large scale way.

Some causes of ill health are clearly visible when morbidity and mortality rates are classified not only according to the part of the body concerned, as in 'heart disease', but according to the social/economic/occupational class of the sufferers. Not only in Tower Hamlets but everywhere else, the rates are worse for those in the poorer classes: the statistics in the Black Report (*Inequalities in Health*, 1980) dispel the myth of equality of opportunity in Britain today. 'Mortality tends to rise inversely with falling occupational rank or status, for both sexes and at all ages. At birth and in the first month of life twice as many babies of unskilled manual parents as of professional parents die, and in the next 11 months of life 4 times as many girls and 5 times as many boys, respectively, die.'

Providing more special care baby units is one answer — but would not make a significant difference to those statistics. The only way to eradicate those appalling inequalities is surely to attack them at root, that is in the mode of organisation of our society. Health care in that sense is a highly political issue.

If the N.H.S does have only a marginal effect on the nation's health, there might be a case for reducing it to a much smaller, mainly curative national sickness service. Other agencies could then undertake the increasingly important caring and support functions, perhaps through extended social services. This would remove them — and, particularly, those people training to work in them — from the distorting and enveloping influence of the acute sector. Nurse training, for instance, might develop along the lines suggested in the Jay Report (1979), if indeed there would be any place for nursing as we know it.

Certainly prevention is an 'in' word and epidemiology is an 'in' subject, but the general approach to prevention is still individualistic. We know that cancer is not an act of God, but is highly likely to be caused by external triggers such as smoking or exposure to certain substances. Yet the individual smoker is condemned far more vigorously than the refusal of many employers to introduce absolutely safe working conditions. It is easier to characterise smokers' inability to stop as irresponsibility, lack of willpower, failure to deal with stress or whatever, than to adopt a more political approach. But it should be apparent that the victim-blaming of conventional health education does not work very well. Hospital nurses know more about the effects of smoking than most people, and nurse patients dying from it, but half of them smoke.

Adopting a 'life-style' approach takes us further in understanding the causes of ill health, but even this can be condemnatory rather than analytical. Obesity, coronary heart disease and bowel cancer are often cited, but our overindulgent Western habits cannot be changed just by exerting the will and eating unsaturated fats. Our politics of health and health care must be developed on a far more questioning and complex level if the fight against ill health is to be anything other than token.

This battle cannot be fought by health workers alone. I have hardly touched on the involvement of lay people but this is not a reflection of their lack of importance. The public's desire for information and participation is voiced increasingly often. Partly it is a challenge to professions which guard their knowledge as a weapon of superiority rather than sharing it freely and enabling clients to make their own decisions. It is also evident in a more general desire to participate in decisions about priorities and resources, a desire which must be taken into account in providing health services which meet people's needs in a manner acceptable to them.

The nurse's role

It may be argued that the nurse's role is to care for those who are already ill, rather than to worry about the politics of ill health. There are, however, several reasons why nurses should be actively involved in prevention.

The first is their own claim to be health educators, an explicit part of the health visitor's function. Those working in curative fields can also communicate with their patients on health matters in an intimate and responsive atmosphere; and people who are sick or disabled may be more receptive to ideas about ill health than the healthy, for whom the notion of sickness is usually academic.

Nurses must transform the lipservice they pay to their educative role into informed pressure. They have a duty to share their knowledge with their patients but they also have a responsibility to society to use their influence and understanding, which they have often been reluctant to do. They must refuse to allow important decisions about health care to be made by a powerful minority, or to be based on inappropriate criteria. Who better to speak for the users of the service, especially if they cannot speak for themselves, than nurses?

Identifying and preventing the causes of ill health may in any case be a more effective use of resources than fighting an often losing battle against disease when the problem may already be past remedy, or require expensive, labour intensive treatment and care — although it is impossible to make accurate cost comparison. More importantly: nurses choose to help relieve suffering. How much better to forestall it, to try to eradicate the causes of so much misery. It sounds simple, and on humanitarian grounds the choice before us *is* simple, even if acting on that choice is fraught with difficulty.

Finally, understanding the causes of ill health should be an absolute prerequisite to determining the nature of health services. Health care cannot be separated from general social policy, as the solutions to many health problems are outside the scope of health care policy alone. The first requirement is simply to put health and health care on the political agenda — to accelerate the current recognition that the N.H.S., for all its advantages, has not solved the problem of ill health, and to find the reasons why. The task is one all health workers should be engaged in, and if that means stepping outside the boundaries of what is generally held to be their proper concern, it is a step they must be prepared to take.

REFERENCES

Bosanquet N 1979 Health for sale? Socialist Medical Association, London

City and East London Area Health Authority (Teaching) 1977 Tower Hamlets Health District Plan, 1978–9, London

City and East London Area Health Authority (Teaching) 1979 Tower Hamlets Health District Plan. 1980–3, London.

Committee of Enquiry into Mental Handicap Nursing and Care (Jay committee) 1979 Report. HMSO, London

Department of Health and Social Security 1981 Care in action. HMSO, London

Department of Health and Social Security 1980 Inequalities in Health. DHSS, London

Doyal L with Pennell I 1979 The political economy of health. Pluto, London

Illich I 1977 Limits to medicine. Penguin, Harmondsworth

Kennedy I 1980 The Reith Lectures: Unmasking medicine. The Listener November 6, 13, 20, 27, December 4, 11

Radical Statistics Health Group 1976 Whose priorities? Radical Statistics Pamplet 1, London

Yudkin J S 1978 Changing patterns of resource allocation in a London teaching district. British Medical Journal 2: 1212–1215

FURTHER READING

Chronic and Critical 1980 A discussion document commissioned by community health councils in London. South Camden CHC, London

Doyal L with Pennell I 1979 The political economy of health. Pluto, London

Ehrenreich B, English D 1976 Witches midwives and nurses. Writers and Readers Publishing Coperative, London

Politics of Health Group 1979, 1981, Food and Profit; Cuts and the NHS; Going Private, POHG, London

Radical Statistics Health Group 1980 The unofficial guide to official health statistics. Radical Statistics, London

Widgery D 1979 Health in danger, Macmillan, London

SECTION THREE

Clients

This section of the book is concerned with people and their problems. There is a developmental strand from birth to old age and the section ends with a consideration of certain issues within the context of family life and a final chapter on the family role in care. Many of the issues debated by Chris Sage in her chapter on home or hospital confinements are probably equally relevant to health care throughout life. There are psychological as well as economic reasons why we should be encouraging patients to be cared for at home where this is possible. Resources, both cash and personnel, are becoming more limited and it is likely that an increasing proportion of total health care will, in the future, be delivered by community nurses working in collaboration with other professionals. New approaches to health care must be explored, with the emphasis on the individual supported by his or her family. We must develop a family-centred approach, taking into account the needs of all members of the family and the interaction between them.

Today when we speak of a family, we are generally referring to the nuclear family, a married couple and their children. However, with the merging of different cultures and the development of a variety of styles of communal living, the reality is more complex than this and encompasses other small social groups who live together with a high degree of intimacy and who are not necessarily even blood relations. More numerous than this are one-parent families and single women with dependants. This latter group are much neglected and their problems are outlined by Sheila Quinn.

The change from hospital to community care also necessitates a change in the nurse's approach. We are catering for an increasingly sophisticated public with infinite demands who regard health care as a right. On a home visit it is the patient and not the nurse who has territorial rights. The didactic approach is, therefore, no longer acceptable. Nurses must become more knowledgeable, not only in their own area of expertise, but in cultural concepts and interpersonal skills. This will help them to communicate better, for example, with parents who have just experienced the sudden death of their baby, with an individual who has become an alcoholic because the stresses of life have become intolerable, or with a 95-year-old who is living on childhood memories of the 19th century.

These and other examples of the health and social problems which are experienced by individuals and their families are presented. However, as this is a book of readings and not a textbook, the section does not claim to be comprehensive.

Contributions have been selected as representative of particular areas of importance. The essays are descriptive but present current debate where this is relevant.

In the words of Leo Tolstoy from *Anna Karenina* (1877): 'All happy families resemble one another, but each unhappy family is unhappy in its own way'. If the community nurse can learn to understand the individual and his or her family and so attempt to alleviate unhappiness in some measure, her work will not have been in vain.

14

Birth: Debatable issues

Christine Sage

The aim of this chapter is to try to look objectively at the various arguments for and against a) home confinement versus hospital confinement; b) natural childbirth versus induction and active management.

HOME CONFINEMENT

The number of babies born at home has been declining since the late 1960s. This has been due to a variety of factors, but not least due to the acceptance of The Report of the Standing Maternity & Midwifery Advisory Committee (DHSS, 1970) which recommended the provision for 100% hospital confinement, hospital being regarded as the safest place in which to have a baby. Since then many people have questioned the reasoning of Peel and his colleagues, not least the members of the pressure groups which have formed to resist the move towards 100% hospital confinement. These include the Association for Improvement in Maternity Services (AIMS), the Society to Support Home Confinement, the International Childbirth Association, and Sheila Kitzinger and the National Childbirth Trust.

Advantages of home confinement

According to the advocates of home confinement, the advantages are as follows:

(a) The mother is attended by a team known to her
(b) The mother remains in familiar surroundings
(c) The mother receives the continuous support of family and friends
(d) There is total involvement of the family
(e) Obstetric interference is limited
(f) There is greater professional satisfaction.

The mother is attended by a team known to her

How important is this factor? Does it have any relevance to the outcome of labour? The answer to both is probably yes. Obviously, it is a very attractive idea to know the people who will attend you during one of the most important days in your life, but does it stop there? A mother who relates well with her midwife will build up trust in her. The midwife who really knows her client will respond quickly to non-verbal communication. This could be vital to the early detection of abnormalities. Many mothers seem to know intuitively when there is something wrong. The midwife will know when to listen and when to take action. Communications between adults are seldom straightforward and time is needed with each individual so that total understanding of the language he or she uses can begin. This may be a partial explanation of the fact that even skilled consultants cannot divide their patients into high and low risk groups successfully, as shown by the research of Cox (1976). In this small piece of research, patients delivered in the West Middlesex Hospital and its catchment area, were divided into two groups, 61 in the high risk group and 91 in the low risk group. The number of birth and neonatal problems which actually arose were almost equal in the two groups. A consultant who only sees a patient once or twice during pregnancy will not be able to pick up the finer and perhaps more important aspects of the conversation with his patient, hearing only the answers given, which may be what the patient thinks the doctor wishes to hear rather than the full facts.

The domiciliary team also has an opportunity to know the other members of the family and the type of support they may give or additional stress they may cause. This enables the team to assess the patient's needs and plan accordingly. If the hospital team know the facts, then they too can make plans, but often the mothers do not want to bother the nurse in case they are busy.

The mother remains in familiar surroundings

The main advantage of remaining in familiar surroundings is that it reduces the stress caused by fear. Stress has many unwanted side-effects, including rise in blood pressure and increased intolerance of pain, both of which are important factors in obstetrics. The amount of pain relief required by mothers in their own homes is significantly less than that required by their counterparts in hospital (Cartwright, 1979; Kitzinger, 1979).

The mother receives the continuous support of family and friends

This is probably as much of an advantage for the family and friends as for the mother herself. There is no doubt that a mother who has a baby at home needs a strong support team surrounding her. Such an event may help to unite the extended family. However, if not wisely handled, family rows can arise between the mother's mother and her mother-in-law.

There is total involvement of the family

Probably all professionals would agree that this is important. A lot has been written about bonding and the need for infant/mother contact but not much has been written on the father's role. It is known that some fathers, as well as siblings, can suffer jealousy at the arrival of a new baby. If the total family are included in the preparation, the birth, and the early post-natal care of mother and baby, this jealousy can at least be reduced if not eradicated. The father can be a great asset at delivery but there are still some hospitals which exclude him from this important occasion. Why should the father not be present at delivery even if it is a Caesarean section carried out under epidural anaesthesia?

Obstetric interference is limited

This is mainly because of lack of equipment and facilities in the home. Whether the lack of interference is an advantage or not is another question and discussed later in the chapter.

There is greater professional satisfaction

Some may question the right to seek professional satisfaction as one is trained to give a service. However, a worker who derives satisfaction from the job will give more to it. Most professionals would agree that there is a greater sense of satisfaction derived from being able to follow a client's course through from beginning to end, whatever the type of work. In the hospital this is impossible and may be the reason why more professionals are prepared to walk out on a job when duty is over rather than see it through to its conclusion as used to be the case.

The advantages of home confinement can perhaps be summarised by quoting some satisfied clients:

> The midwife was with me from eight in the morning until midnight (the baby was born at ten at night) never did she try to hurry things or force me to accept drugs or gas and air, which I wanted to try and do without. The atmosphere was calm but exciting all the time. She must have been very tired but she didn't rush at all.
>
> It was such a family affair. The children had got to know the midwife well during the pregnancy. They were able to come and see the baby just after she was born and thoroughly enjoyed themselves helping the midwife to bath and dress their new baby sister.

Disadvantages of home confinement

(a) lack of facilities in an emergency
(b) the increasingly few appropriately experienced midwives
(c) the cost to the family.

Lack of facilities in an emergency

The problem lies in that no-one is able to guarantee that labour will be normal or that the baby will be fit and healthy. A good practitioner will observe early deviations from normal and act accordingly but post-partum haemorrhage and neonatal asphyxia remain, to a large extent, unpredictable. This is a risk that the family will have to accept if they wish for a home confinement. The practitioner(s) in attendance at the birth are trained to deal with such emergencies but they will lack equipment and so the client may need to be transferred to a specialised unit. This may result in delay which could prove fatal. However, Barron Thomas & Philips (1977) in their research carried out in Newcastle-upon-Tyne and Tew (1977) in a national survey, showed that stillbirth rates among patients delivered in hospital are higher than those delivered at home. The differentials are remarkably uniform when high-risk and low-risk groups are compared. Barron and his colleagues concluded that the trend towards increasing hospital confinement is possibly dangerous and wasteful.

The risks cannot however be ignored and careful selection is essential if perinatal and maternal mortality figures in the community are to remain at an acceptable level.

During the period 1970–1972, 254 521 women delivered at home, of this number 44 women died. Of these 26 were true deaths and 18 were associated deaths, which represents a maternality mortality of 0.17 per thousand maternities. However 12 (27.27%) were the direct result of poor selection. Three women who died were expecting their fifth or subsequent child and nine women were over thirty-five years of age (DHSS, 1975).

An ante-natal prediction score has been outlined by the authors of the British Births 1970 Survey, which serves as a useful guide to selecting clients suitable for home confinement (Butler, 1969).

The increasingly few appropriately experienced midwives

With the increase in hospital confinements community midwives find themselves carrying out fewer and fewer deliveries each year. In some areas a midwife may have only one home confinement a year. This naturally results in the midwife losing confidence. This problem may be partly overcome if there is a general practitioner unit at which the midwife may practise. The safety of home confinement is very dependent on the experience and confidence of the practitioner.

The cost to the family

The additional cost that has to be borne by the family can be quite considerable. In the home they have to cope with the inevitable mess created at delivery. However careful the family and the midwife may be, mattresses can be soiled and wall-paper and ceilings marked!

A mother is given a long list of things to provide for the midwife; most are common household items like a nailbrush, but many families will buy new items for the occasion.

For the mother in hospital food and care are given free for eight days. In the home the family have to pay for her food and care. The husband may need to take time off work or pay for a home help if there is no suitable relative to take control. However, if a family wishes for a home confinement, they rarely count the expense involved.

The advantages of hospital confinement

(a) It is cheaper for the family
(b) It is safer for mother and baby.

Cheaper for the family

This is a natural corollary if the previous paragraph regarding the cost of home confinement is accepted. However, account must be taken of the cost to the family of travelling to the hospital for visiting time.

The emotional cost can be considerable in units where the family are made to feel that they have only been allowed into the inner sanctum as a special privilege, they must not touch anything, let alone the baby.

> The babies were kept in the nursery except for thirty minutes at each feed. There were constant injunctions 'not to touch that baby', 'put it down' and so on. Consequently I left hospital with a strange baby. It certainly left me feeling totally inadequate as a mother, and really unused to physical contact with my baby.

An extreme example as far as mother and child go, but a common state for relatives of the child.

The last thing that any responsible consultant would wish to do would be to lay his patients and their offsprings open to severe infections. Should such a situation arise whereby an infection such as gastroenteritis swept through the nurseries there would soon be a hue and cry for a public enquiry. However, what evidence have we that this would be the outcome of relatives handling their new member of the family. Could it not be tried in a small way, carefully monitoring the outcome?

Safer for mother and baby

There is little doubt that the safest place, physically, for the mother to have her baby is in a fully equipped consultant obstetric unit which has a well-equipped special care baby unit attached to it. The unit should contain the latest technological aids to assist diagnosis and be able to offer a wide number of treatments. For mothers at risk, either medically or obstetrically, this will help to ensure a safe delivery and a healthy mother and baby.

Can the government afford to provide this type of service for every mother? Is it really necessary or should we reserve such specialist services for those mothers in high risk groups?

It has already been acknowledged that it is difficult to isolate the high risk group, possibly because the categories are drawn so broadly.

The disadvantages of hospital confinement have been covered by the discussion on home confinement, but a summary of a study by O'Brien (1978) may highlight some factors. In this study women who had been delivered in 24 different health districts reported on their experiences of delivery in hospital as compared to home. The following facts are included in the findings:

1. Labour lasted a considerably shorter time at home
2. Fewer women were left alone at home
3. Fewer women had episiotomies at home
4. Husbands played a more important role at home
5. 76% of husbands were present at the birth at home while only 30% were present at the hospital delivery
6. 57% of mothers at home were able to hold their babies for as long as they wanted compared with only 29% in hospital.

This spells out very clearly the need to improve the qualitative aspects of delivery in hospital.

NATURAL CHILDBIRTH

Pregnancy and birth, for the majority of women, is not a sickness but a natural process. Protagonists of natural childbirth would like women to learn about their bodies and to understand the various sensations felt as their body changes during the menstrual circle and subsequently in pregnancy. The mother and father attend classes where they are taught the techniques for coping with contractions, backache, cramp, leg trembling and overbreathing. They are both taught the breathing patterns so that the husband can encourage his wife in labour, using the words which will be familiar to her. This enables them to work together towards relaxation which may help to shorten labour and ensure an adequate oxygen supply to the mother and baby. All this is achieved without the use of drugs which themselves could have an adverse effect on mother and baby. The very act of working together in love may arouse sexual feelings. Such arousal causes the production by the body of oxytocin, which enhances labour.

The freedom that natural childbirth gives the mother means that she is able to walk around while in labour. Research has shown that ambulation during labour results in less uncomfortable contractions, a shorter labour, significantly fewer fetal heart abnormalities, with improved apgar scores at one and five minutes (Flynn, Kelly, Hollins, Lynch 1976 & Mendez-Baker 1973).

Natural childbirth can easily incorporate Leboyer's technique of delivery. Theories on the effect of trauma of birth have been developed by many psychologists including Jung (1961) and Laing (1967). These psychologists have set out their theories of how and why birth affects us so deeply and sets up patterns of behaviour for our entire lives. In therapy this knowledge is used to enable people to relive their birth experiences in order to change the negative imprint which may be adversely affecting their lives.

To Leboyer the newborn infant is technically hypersensitive through the skin, eyes and ears, and so needs gentle handling in an atmosphere of calm silence and shielded lights. The first sensations experienced by the child should be joy and relief at this new found freedom and space, along with the security felt as the child is placed next to the mother's bare, warm flesh, hearing again the rhythmic thump of her heart beat.

For the Leboyer method to really work, the mother needs to be actively participating in a calm, relaxed way, which would not be possible if she was half unconscious from drugs.

The advantages of natural childbirth not already spelt out include the deep feeling of satisfaction felt by the mother, the close involvement of the father, the elimination of the risk to mother and infant from the use of drugs, and the less traumatic delivery for the infant.

However there are disadvantages to natural childbirth of both an obstetric and a psychological nature. If the mother who has received this training finds that she cannot cope when it comes to the actual birth, she can feel devastated, a total failure. Such situations need careful and sensitive handling. Problems can also be encountered should obstetric intervention be necessary for the health of the mother or child.

Induction and active management of labour

In recent years obstetric practice has become increasingly interventionist as the figures in Table 14.1 show.

There are possibly three reasons for the increase in active management of labour. Work carried out by Tipton & Lewis (1975) led them to believe that induction reduced perinatal mortality, led to shorter labours and healthier babies. Baird (1960) claimed that investigations suggested that there was much to be said for induction of labour to avoid the risk of placental insufficiency which increases with prolonged labour. Such observations encouraged other obstetricians to embark on a programme of induction.

Table 14.1 Numbers of obstetric operations per 1000 deliveries in N.H.S.

	1968	1969	1970	1971	1972	1973
Forceps	82.8	85.4	86.2	85.3	92	102.3
Episiotomy	223.9	232.8	242.8	261.7	335.4	369.8
Ceasarean section % of all births in England and Wales	4.0	4.4	4.3	4.6	4.9	
Active management of labour	15%					41%

The second factor may be that by inducing the patient, the doctor feels that he has closer control over the situation. It can also give him a feeling of employing scientific methods.

The third factor, which led to a public controversy in late 1974, was that of social convenience to achieve daylight delivery: 'Technology is now being used in some hospitals to induce births routinely, not primarily for the baby's safety or the safety of the mother, but in order to create a production line system where, women have their babies by clockwork during daylight hours' (Gillie & Gillie, 1974).

The incidence of induction remained fairly low until 1964 because of the fear of failure. Turnbull & Anderson (1968) published a series of papers describing a more effective means of induction. From then on the percentage of inductions has steadily increased.

Advantages of induction and active management of labour

There is no doubt that induction of labour reduces perinatal mortality in certain groups of women, including primaparae over thirty-five years of age in whom pregnancy has continued for forty-two weeks or more, rhesus isoimmunisation, diabetes mellitus, essential hypertension, renal disease and intra-uterine growth retardation.

Prolonged dysfunctional labour which may lead to maternal and fetal distress can also be successfully treated by the active management of labour. Few obstetricians would hesitate to induce labour where the mothers life was at risk if pregnancy was allowed to continue, for example in eclampsia.

In active management of labour, labour is accelerated by the use of drugs which improve the efficiency of the uterine action. This enables obstetricians to be sure that the baby will be born within twelve hours, even if it is the mother's first child. Such techniques, provided that they have been carried out by a fully prepared team in a well equipped unit, have made a valuable contribution to reducing the incidence of prolonged labour with its attendant hazards of maternal distress and fetal asphyxia.

Some mothers have a strong desire to arrange the day of the child's birth. This may be for an acceptable reason such as the wish for her husband to be present, or it may be associated with superstition. For these women the idea of a planned delivery, be it for social convenience, is very attractive.

Disadvantages of induction and active management of labour

The disadvantages of induction of labour are mainly those of the hazards that such interference may cause. These include prematurity, fetal distress, a higher Caesarean section rate, uterine rupture and neonatal jaundice.

Many women are unsure of dates, which makes the reliability of assessing fetal maturity by dates hazardous and can lead to women of 42 weeks gestation by dates delivering a premature infant with the attendant problems. Therefore, ideally, before induction is carried out the women should be sent for ultrasonography and perhaps, in addition, the lecithin/sphingomyelin ratio in the amniotic fluid should be assessed, both of which will help to ascertain the maturity of the fetus.

Very few reliable, controlled experiments have been carried out to assess the true impact of induction and accelerated labour on the fetus. From a knowledge of the physiology of labour it would appear logical to assume that the fetus is deprived of oxygen, as the length and strength of a contraction is in direct relationship to the reduction of blood flow. Accelerated labour has been described by some as short and fierce but, as already stated, research is required to substantiate such a hypothesis.

Maternal problems are most likely to arise when induction has been carried out on patients with an unripe cervix.

A higher incidence of neonatal jaundice has been reported by some as a result of induction using oxytocinon (Ghosh & Hudson, 1972; Davies, 1973). However, whether such jaundice has any lasting effects on the infant has not yet been established.

When labour is being accelerated, the mother is confined to bed as she is most likely to be attached to an intravenous infusion. This of itself is not a pleasant experience but the main problem is the increased pain felt by non-ambulant patients. The advantages of ambulation during labour have already been briefly mentioned. Mendez-Baver (1973) compared the supine with the standing position in labour and not only found better uterine action while standing, but also found that the patient experienced less pain with the contractions and was more comfortable in this position.

Assessment of pain is of necessity very subjective. Of the mothers interviewed by Cartwright (1979) 44% said that the pain they experienced following induction of labour was worse than for a previous spontaneous delivery. Many practitioners would agree that mothers in whom labour is induced require more drugs. In some maternity units epidural anaesthesia is offered routinely to mothers who are to be induced. The increased use of drugs and regional anaesthesia bring with them their own inherent problems.

Some mothers in whom labour is induced feel that they are no more than part of the machinery to which they are attached, that the whole process of modern obstetrics is inhuman. It is this factor that has led to the increase in the demand for home confinement. In the research carried out by Chalmers et al (1976) on obstetric practice and the outcome of pregnancy in Cardiff residents from 1965 to 1973, the following comment is contained in the summary:

> Hospital delivery became almost universal, monitoring the fetus during pregnancy was introduced, and induction and acceleration of labour became commonplace. These developments were not associated with any striking change in either the death rate, or the timing, or the cause of perinatal death.

All professionals should make a very real effort to treat their clients or patients as human beings. This means taking each person, as they present themselves to us for consultation, as an individual, taking into account their total circumstances, feelings, beliefs and desires. On the basis of this assessment, it is then possible to discuss with them the pros and cons of the various actions that could be taken, allowing them to decide which course to take and then supporting them in their decision, whether or not we think it to be a wise one.

REFERENCES

Awais G M, Lebherz T B 1970 Ruptured uterus. A complication of oxytocin induction and high pariety. Obstetrics and Gynaecology 36: 465–472
Baird D 1960 The evolution of modern obstetrics. Lancet 2: 557–564, 609–614
Barron S L, Thompson A M, Philips P R 1977 Home and hospital confinement in Newcastle upon Tyne 1960–1969. British Journal of Obstetrics and Gynaecology 84: 401–411
Beazley J M, Alberman B 1975 Neonatal hyperbilirubinaemia following the use of oxytocin in labour. British Journal of Obstetrics and Gynaecology 82: 265–271
Brook D 1976 Naturebirth. Penguin, Harmondsworth
Butler S 1969 Perinatal problems. Livingstone, Edinburgh
Cartwright A 1976 The dignity of labour. A study of child bearing and induction. Tavistock, London
Cartwright A 1979 The dignity of labour: A study of child-bearing and induction. Tavistock, London
Chalmers I, Zlosnik J E, Johns D A, Campbell H 1976 Obstetric practice and outcome of pregnancy in Cardiff residents 1965–1973. British Medical Journal 1: 735–738
Chard T, Richards M 1977 Benefits and hazards of the new obstetrics. Spastics International Medical Publications
Cox C A, Fox F S, Zinkin P M, Matthews A E B 1976 Critical appraisal of domiciliary obstetric and neonatal practice. British Medical Journal 1: 84–86
Davies D P, Gomersall R, Robertson R, Gray O P, Turnbull A C 1973 Neonatal jaundice and maternal oxytocin infusion. British Medical Journal 3: 476–477
Department of Health and Social Security 1970 Report of the Standing Maternity & Midwifery Advisory Committee (Peel Report). HMSO, London
Department of Health and Social Security 1975 Report on Confidential Enquiries into Maternal Deaths in England & Wales 1970–1972. HMSO, London
Ghosh A, Hudson F B 1972 Oxytocic agents and neonatal hyperbilirubinaemia. Lancet 2: 823
Gillie L, Gillie O 1974 The childbirth revolution. And the vital first hours. The Sunday Times, 13th and 20th October
Jung C 1961 Freud & psychoanalysis vol 4. Routledge & Kegan Paul, London
Kitzinger S, Davies J A 1978 The place of birth. Oxford University Press, Oxford
Kitzinger S 1979 Birth at home. Oxford University Press, Oxford
Laing R D 1967 The politics of experience. Penguin, Harmondsworth
Leboyer F 1977 Birth without violence. Fontana, London
Lloyd G 1977 The case against home confinement. Update 574–577
O'Brien M 1978 Home and hospital: A comparison of the experiences of mothers having home and hospital confinement. Journal of the Royal College of General Practitioners 28: 460–466
Roberts G, Weaver A 1974 Labour and neonatal jaundice. Lancet 1: 935
Tew M 1979 Home versus hospital confinement: the statistics. Update 1317–1322
Tipton R H, Lewis B V 1975 Induction of labour and perinatal mortality. British Medical Journal 1: 391
Turnbull A C, Anderson A B M 1968 Induction of labour, part III, results with amniotomy and oxytocin titration. Journal of Obstetrics and Gynaecology of the British Commonwealth 75: 2–41
White T G E 1977 The case for home confinement. Update 571–572
Zander L 1976 Home versus hospital delivery. The Journal of Maternal and Child Health 14–20

15

Sudden unexplained infant death

Deborah Holroyd

Sudden unexplained infant deaths are the single largest cause of death in the under two-year-old age group. One in 500 infants die as a result, 3000 per annum (Camps, 1970). In terms of loss of life years it is more serious than carcinoma of the lung. From reading these figures, the size of the problem is obvious.

WHAT IS KNOWN ABOUT SUDDEN INFANT DEATH SYNDROME TO DATE?

First, a clarification of what is meant by the term 'sudden unexplained death in infancy' or 'cot death' is needed. Beckwith (1969) has used the definition: 'The sudden death of any infant or young child which is unexpected by history and in which a thorough post-mortem fails to demonstrate a cause of death'. This definition has been queried for several reasons. First, it does not specify an age limit although this is generally accepted to be from about the age of two weeks to two years. The reference to 'unexpected by history' is dubious in the light of recent knowledge. We know from research that many of these children did suffer from symptoms, but that the symptoms were not recognised or acted upon. However, if we think of sudden infant deaths as deaths occurring between the ages of two weeks and two years, suddenly and unexpectedly, either at home or hospital, with no apparent pre morbid symptoms, this definition will be adequate for our present purposes.

Children have always died in this manner. However, before specific study of this syndrome began, it was really not separated from other causes of death. Large, poorly spaced families were the norm and high perinatal and infant mortality rates were expected. The deaths were accepted as 'God's will' or 'nature's way'. However in 1890, Templeman, noted this group of babies who were one day apparently well and the next found dead. He sought an explanation for this and formulated the theory that suffocation was to blame. The less sophiscated post mortem techniques then available indicated asphyxia as the cause of death and this supported his theory (Canadian Foundation for the Study of Infant Deaths, 1974).

Another theory appeared in 1941 when a pathologist stated 'dried milk kills babies' (Canadian Foundation for the Study of Infant Deaths, 1974). This statement received much publicity and the Department of Health investigated the claim. His theory was that the milk produced a 'carburretor effect on the larynx' which effectively drowned the baby. This theory was disposed of by Dr Barnett of Cambridge University who believed milk could be associated with the deaths but not in the manner claimed. He pointed out that in many anoxic deaths, the stomach contents are regurgitated and hence the mere presence of milk in the air passages at post-mortem is of little significance (Canadian Foundation for the Study of Infant Deaths, 1974).

In 1951, a memorandum was submitted to the Ministry of Health by Professor Sir Samuel Bedson, Professor of Bacteriology, London and Professor Francis Camps, Home Office Pathologist. Several questions regarding sudden infant deaths were posed.

In 1952, a committee of investigation was set up by the Ministry of Health under the Chairmanship of Professor A. C. Barber. As a result, much study was undertaken into this problem and many theories were suggested. By 1965, the committee reported no firm conclusions but a tendency toward respiratory infection was found.

In 1970, a seminar was arranged by Professor Camps and others of the 1952 committee. At this seminar many theories were discarded, such as paraffin heaters, lack of ventilation, pet viruses, disease spread by birds and vermin, innoculation, vaccination and such theories associated with a history of eczema or family history of allergy which were considered valueless after the studies done in London and Cambridge. The methods used in the study performed were outlined. The study was undertaken in two main areas; Cambridge, and one-third of London. All children dying unexpectedly were considered and a post-mortem was performed on each child to elicit cause of death. The study indicated that a significant proportion of the infants had suffered from symptoms of respiratory illness prior to death. The incidence of death was found to be greater during the winter months and this confirmed the findings of the Cleveland survey which indicated a peak between November and April. In some years the pattern is much flatter than others. Most of the deaths were discovered between first thing in the morning and a little later in the morning which is in agreement with a later study undertaken in Newcastle during the period 1974–76 which put the most common time between 6 a.m. and 12 midday. The study indicated a sharp peak at the age of three months with the numbers tailing off at two years. This finding also is supported by the Newcastle study which indicated a peak between two and four months.

There was nothing new to the post-mortem findings Camps reported, all that was found was a picture of general asphyxia. This, however, conflicts with the findings of Emery's study in Sheffield (Emery, 1977). However, Bodian and Heslop did suggest at the time that if the specimen of lung is 'fixed' intact before section an explosive desquamation of the bronchial epithelium could be demonstrated. The study indicated that boys were more susceptible than girls. It also emphasised the sociological background of infants who died in this way. Most cases were found amongst social classes IV and V, among families generally suffering from overcrowding and illegitimacy. It was found that 56% of the babies who died and 70% of the babies in the control group had been breast-fed. The last feed before death was found to be a breast feed in only 5% of the cases as opposed to 4% of the babies in the control group. As a result of these findings, the seminar group decided to advocate breast feeding for at least the first two weeks of life.

Professor Coombs formulated the theory that deaths could be due to anaphylactic shock caused by an antibody to cow's milk (Emery & Carpenter, 1974). He said that if infants develop antibodies to milk protein they become allergic to it, in other words they have an altered reactivity to milk which they did not have before developing these antibodies. This may cause a hypersensitive reaction which could be fatal. An infant who has just had a cow's milk feed is winded and put to sleep. While he is asleep, some milk may be regurgitated and this could be aspirated into the lungs. This milk has a high antigen potential and sets up an antigen-antibody response with the milk antibodies which results in an anaphylactic reaction. The experiments to prove it have, however, only been carried out on lightly anaesthetised guinea-pigs.

The fact remains that some infants who died in this way are totally breast-fed. However, research has shown that there are other good reasons for breast feeding. Gunther (1975) has pointed out that colostrum contains immunoglobulins, lysosym, lactoferrin and interferon, all of which constitute a vital part of the infant's immune responses. Emery's Sheffield study (1977) confirms that breast-fed babies are less susceptible to cot deaths than bottle-fed babies for this and other reasons.

Gunther also points out that babies are less susceptible if the mother's blood is Blood Group A. If the mother's blood is Group O or B, the anti A antibody may be reaching and impairing the lymphoid tissue of the fetus (if his blood is A Group), thus impairing the late immune response.

Gunther also supports Emery's view that drugs used in pregnancy, particularly antibiotics, may interfere with the immune response and she notes in particular the drugs given for urinary tract infections which are common in pregnancy (Emery, 1974). In support of her theory of immune responses she states that premature babies are likely candidates for sudden infant death as they are known to have low amounts of positively acquired antibodies and immaturity of immunologically competent tissue. She also thinks that younger mothers are more likely to have babies who die, especially if they have several children in quick succession and this is coupled with poverty and over burdening. This is likely to result in dietary insufficiency, especially protein and folates.

The combined evidence shows that sudden unexplained deaths in infancy could be due to anaphylactic shock and that the antigen may be produced as a result of an infecting agent such as blood.

A study undertaken in Sheffield during the period 1963–72 (Smith, 1974), found that of 302 mothers using powdered milk, 87% were making up the feeds at too high a concentration. These feeds were sampled when mothers came to the clinic; they were not told in advance of the study. These mothers were found to be giving sodium to their infants at up to three times the acceptable level: 23% of the infants had blood urea 10 mmol/L over the normal. The urea levels of the breast-fed babies were found to be much lower. Despite repeated instruction by midwives and health visitors, the mothers were still giving feeds which were too concentrated. This is disturbing as in a study of 40 infants suffering sudden infant deaths, over half had severe hypernatraemeic uraemia at post-mortem. It should be noted, however, that all proprietary baby milks are now modified to reduce the sodium content.

The main conclusion of the 1980 seminar was the fact that post mortem revealed little, but three possible causes were suggested:

(a) Infection
(b) Anaphylactic reaction
(c) Suffocation was thought unlikely, but a rare possibility

This seminar also resulted in the establishment of the Foundation for the Study of Infant Deaths.

The next theory to be investigated was the 'carry cot theory'. The theory was that the carbon dioxide breathed out became trapped in the carry cot (due to the high sides) and eventually the baby suffocated due to lack of oxygen. This was, however, disproved when workers at the London Hospital showed that when carbon dioxide is expired at body temperature, it does not sink but rises.

Breathing patterns in the two weeks to two year age group were investigated. It was found that it was normal and characteristic for infants to be apnoeic for up to 15–20 seconds at a time. In other experiments related to breathing, it was shown that the breathing patterns of lambs who had been given cow's milk were different during the period after a feed from those of lambs who had been fed sheep's milk. The same reaction can be demonstrated in babies and it is due to the activity of certain tiny receptors situated around the epiglottis (Camps, 1970).

Studies in Newcastle showed that over a two year period, one in every three cot death babies was found to have a viral infection of the lungs, the most common causative organism being respiratory syncytial virus (Camps, 1970).

Cross (Camps, 1970) suggested that because babies are characteristically 'nose breathers', if a nasal infection occurs, the response is physiologically different from an adult. Babies are not good at breathing through their mouths. If this difficulty is coupled with a cool environment (i.e. during the winter months) the oxygen requirement is increased and in a cool environment hyperventilatory response to hypoxia is not maintained. With increased metabolic demand and diminished ventilation, lethal asphyxia may well occur without crying (Symposium, 1974). This view is disputed by Gunther (1975) who points out that sudden infant death occurs in hot countries just as often as in cooler lands.

Another theory put forward at about this time was suggested by Porter (1970). He suggested that the syndrome was a result of an inborn error of metabolism present in a heterozygous form, possibly an amino acid metabolism disorder which could result in hyper amino-acidaemia due to the extra protein in cow's milk. This is also coupled with the deamination of amino-acids which occurs as a result of immaturity of the liver. If the mother introduces cereals or other milk thickeners with the aim of increasing the interval between feeds, hypo-insulinaemia is likely to occur. She is most likely to do this at night. If this child has, in addition, a slight upper respiratory tract infection, he is less likely to be hungry so will, therefore, go longer without a feed. Hypo-glycaemia will result and this, coupled with the fact that the infant will not be able to move his head, will produce at post mortem a picture of death by asphyxia.

As a result of the setting up of the Foundation for the Study of Infant Deaths in 1970, a study financed by the Foundation and organised by the London Borough of Camden was undertaken in North London (Camps, 1970). The aim was to interview all parents whose babies had died suddenly and unexpectedly between the ages of two weeks and two years. The study commenced in February, 1972 and was completed in February 1974, covering only one complete calender year — 1973. Post-mortems were also carried out on the babies involved. The interviews were carried out by a medical officer and a health visitor using a structured interview schedule. Two interviews were made, the first to ask key questions and the second to fill in any necessary data missed in the initial interview. The results identified the following factors:

(a) Low socio-economic group
(b) Low birthweight
(c) Death occurring most commonly at night during sleep
(d) Greater incidence during winter months
(e) Below average standard of mothering
(f) Illness symptoms prior to death

The first four findings reinforced what was already known. However, the last two factors did seem to throw new light on the situation as they could be shown to be preventable by good post-natal support.

Concurrently with the interview investigation, Professor Cameron had been undertaking the post-mortem examinations. His findings were that out of the group of 62 children only five showed no signs of obvious physical disease.

At about the same time two further studies were undertaken in Sheffield and Newcastle (Watson, 1975).

THE NEWCASTLE STUDY

This study was undertaken between 1974 and 1976. All the early childhood deaths occurring within a total population of 297 000 were investigated. During the study period of 27 months, there were 70 deaths of children aged one week to five years: 36 children died at home, 27 suddenly and unexpectedly. Detailed post-mortem examinations were carried out on these children and in half of the cases of sudden and unexpected death, a disease process which was clearly or probably related to the death was demonstrated. The remaining children exhibited no recognised disease process. It should, however, be noted that some viruses kill so rapidly that no extensive histological changes take place.

The events preceding the sudden infant death and the child's environment were investigated by interviews with parents. Symptoms of serious illness occurring within 24-hours of death were identified in 9 out of 29 children. However, in the majority, symptoms were absent or negligible and rather similar to the control group. A very different result emerged from the Northern London Study (Watson, 1975). Most children with major symptoms had been seen by a doctor within a few days prior to death. The two most striking findings were that 16 out of the 29 sudden infant deaths occurred at a weekend or bank holiday and that 45% occurred in three adjacent city wards which contain only 13% of the under-five study population. These three wards constitute a very socially deprived area. Sudden infant death was also found to be more common among families where the mother was aged 21 or under.

THE SHEFFIELD STUDY

At about the same time, a study was taking place in Sheffield led by Professor Emery (Emery & Carpenter, 1977). This study was slightly different from all the previous studies in that it tried to assess the groups considered most at risk of sudden infant death and to prevent it occurring. In order to do this a group of 100 children whose deaths had been described as 'cot deaths' were selected and as much information as possible was gathered to try to gain a picture of their background. The mother's obstetric history, labour, age, the child's sex and blood group, were all explored. As a control to each case, the next child born in the hospital was compared. In all, about 200 pieces of information were collected about each child. When this data was analysed, 19 factors were identified as being statistically different between the two groups of children. These factors were rated and assigned a score. The aim of this procedure was to define a group of babies in whom the likelihood of death was such that it justified close supervision.
The most important factors were the following:

Maternal age (under 21)
Birth order (large family)
O, B, AB } Blood group
Absence of intention to breast feed
Prolonged second stage of labour
Urinary tract infection in pregnancy (treated)
Polyhydrammios
Prematurity (below 2500 kg and/or below 37/40 weeks gestation).

When these factors were scored, the results identified a high risk group comprising 15% of the population which was expected to include 60% of the sudden infant deaths and to have a relative risk 8.6 times the rest of the population.

The scores of all babies born in a defined area were evaluated within 24 hours of birth. Scores greater than 85 were called Group A. Scores less than 85 were called Group B. Half of Group A were selected at random and similarly half of Group B. Those selected were then examined at 48 hours and five weeks old. They were visited ten times by specially trained health visitors during the first twenty weeks of life. By 1973, 6003 births had been screened (19 less than had been registered in the area).

In 1977 figures were published which suggested that increased surveillance of high risk groups could reduce infant mortality and particularly sudden infant deaths. The results showed that the unexpected death rate in the high risk control group was six times greater than the low risk group. Mortality of infants from one week to one year in age from 1908–1942 in Sheffield was 8.2 per 1000 live births (England and Wales 7.6 per 1000). During the study period, the rate dropped to 5.2 per 1000 live births (England and Wales 7.4 per 1000). Calculations imply that had the surveillance and advice been extended to all the high risk group this mortality rate could drop to 4.8 per 1000 live births.

At this point let us review the evidence and consider whether we are any nearer to a solution. Emery (1978) has suggested five factors which are currently under discussion as possible causes of sudden infant death.

(a) Children suffering from some type of sub-clinical abnormality, either arising *in utero* or in the perinatal period. Often these children are premature or light for dates.

(b) An abnormality in the maturation of the child's physiological reflexes, particularly related to inhalation avoidance and sleep patterns.

(c) An abnormal reaction to infection, either anaphylactic or by the induction of a particular reflex such as the diving reflex inhibiting breathing.

(d) Some deficiency in the mother/child mutual stimulation which is essential for healthy growth of the child.

(e) Parents' knowledge of disease in children. Their standards of health, the threshold of illness which makes them call for help, and use of the health services.

We now have a picture of not just a single cause as was earlier thought but of a multitude of possible causes and of a number of factors which, when they occur togehter, suggest a high risk group. The factors are low social status, poor housing, poverty, multi-parity, young mothers, poor mothering, small babies who are bottle fed and prone to infections.

THE EFFECT OF SUDDEN UNEXPECTED DEATH IN INFANCY ON THE FAMILY

'I don't think the horror of turning my baby over and realising he was dead will ever leave me': a sentiment often expressed by mothers and fathers suffering a sudden infant death (Limerick, 1978). The loss of a baby so young seems so unfair and cruel. The endless question 'why us?' seems unanswerable. The suddenness of the loss coupled with the fact that the infant was apparently well prior to death make the tragedy all the more unbearable. Death from a long illness, accident or old age seems more acceptable. The death of an apparently healthy infant inevitably leaves the family numbed by shock, but guilt and bewilderment are more severe and prolonged where the death was so unexpected and not even understood. 'If only I hadn't left him' or 'I wish I hadn't gone out' make the parents feel doubly guilty, especially if the death occurred whilst the infant was with the baby sitter or neighbour. Consider also the effect on the neighbour.

Cot deaths tend to be rather shrouded with suspicion especially when the neighbours see the policeman go into the home, a statutory duty when any death occurs in suspicious or unexplained circumstances. Talk of battering or neglect creeps in and parents may feel cut off and shunned.

Other family members, grandparents, brothers and uncles, may not really understand. They may offer sympathetic advice. 'At least it was only a baby'. This sentiment, whilst meant kindly, implies that the infant by virtue of the fact that it is young, is possibly not such an integral part of the family as an older child. Siblings may feel frightened, particularly very young children who may feel that they too may disappear. Siblings will also grieve although they may show this in a different way from an adult. They may exhibit behavioural problems and symptoms of insecurity. Occasionally they feel the need to compensate for the lost child and may be confused by the parents unstable emotional state. Such a death may have either a positive or a negative affect on the marriage. Some parents grow closer together, however, feelings of blame and guilt may be a threat to harmony and divorce and separation does sometimes occur as a result (Limerick, 1977). The fact that most cot deaths occur at home means that the parents are generally alone to cope with this tragedy.

WHAT HAPPENS AFTER A SUDDEN INFANT DEATH

When a sudden infant death occurs, the family unit is threatened. The mother has probably still not fully recovered from pregnancy, childbirth and the traumatic weeks of early motherhood. The father has had his hopes destroyed, his child is dead. The siblings are alone, numbed and frightened. It is in this state that the family is subjected to the full brunt of police enquiries, the coroner's court, post mortems and investigations.

Emery (1972) has summarised the sequence of events* after the death as follows:

1. The baby is found dead.
2. The baby is either rushed to hospital or the general practitioner is called and then death is confirmed.
3. The parents are told that the doctor cannot give a cause of death and the case will have to be referred to a coroner.
4. The police officer visits. An inspection of the cot and the surroundings is made. A police report is made.
5. The infant is transferred to the mortuary for post-mortem.
6. The parents attend the police station and make a statement.
7. Delay of two to three days.
8. After the post-mortem, an inquest is held.
9. Immediately prior to the inquest, the parents have to identify the body.
10. Inquest. Parents have to attend to confirm their previous statement and listen to evidence of identification. They hear the pathologist's report and the coroner's verdict.
11. Usually a Disposal Certificate is given. A Death Certificate may be obtained from the registrar of births and deaths if needed.

This sequence of events itself creates considerable trauma on top of the existing shock.

It is vital that the police visit should be made by a woman police officer in plain clothes. At this initial visit, she could also take the statement. She should make all her information immediately available to the pathologist to help his work.

If possible, the inquest should be informal and this is now sometimes done. The press should, however, be allowed reporting rights so that any blame can be dispelled from the parents and the community can read this in the press. The parents need to be told and helped to understand the reasons why there has to be an inquest and why the coroner has to be involved before they have to face what will, inevitable, be an ordeal. The leaflet 'Information to Parents Whose Child Has Died Suddenly and Unexpectedly in Infancy', which is available from the Foundation for the Study of Infant Deaths, is useful for this purpose. This explains the coroner's role. The identification procedure is extremely unpleasant for the parents.

It is important that, at the inquest, the cause of death should be made clear to

---

* Applies to England and Wales only

the parents to allay any feelings of guilt. Emery maintains that, in most cases, a cause can be found at post-mortem if the examination is undertaken by a skilled paediatric pathologist. However, he concludes that a very small group of babies do not appear to exhibit any cause at post-mortem. For these babies, the phrase 'Sudden Infant Death Syndrome' should not be on a Death Certificate as the cause of death, as this tells the parents nothing.

SUPPORT FACILITIES AFTER THE SUDDEN INFANT DEATH

At this vulnerable time, a family is in great need of support from professionals as well as friends.

For a good percentage of parents, the first line of action is to go to the hospital. Here they should be told promptly but kindly of the death. If only one parent is present, then the other should be contacted immediately. It should be possible for the parents to see the infant and, if they want, to hold him. The doctor should make himself available to answer the inevitable questions. The hospital doctor should inform the health visitor and the general practitioner as soon as possible to arrange for continued support. Many general practitioners will not have come across a sudden infant death before and will probably be as baffled and distressed as the parents.

Because of the baby's age, the health visitor is likely to have been involved quite closely with this family before the death, possibly more so than the general practitioner. As a result of her established relationship with them, she may be able to help by just listening to the parents. As a professional who was involved with the baby, she may have developed quite a close relationship with the mother. She may have known the mother before the baby was born and may be involved with siblings, who may also be glad of a familiar face. The health visitor has a unique role to play in re-establishing the mother's confidence in herself and, indeed, the whole family's confidence. At such a time, the mother will feel a sense of failure in motherhood.

It is important that the health visitor has a knowledge of the phenomenon of sudden infant death and she should also know something of the psychological impact of bereavement. Many parents are frightened by the intensity of their reaction and need considerable reassurance. The period of intense grief may last for several months and the acute phase is prone to recur annually on anniversaries of the death and birthdays. The family will need support throughout this time. Grief is never cured by drugs. The pressure placed on the general practitioner to prescribe anti-depressants is often great. A sedative to aid sleep temporarily is often helpful, but the long-term use of anti-depressants is not to be recommended. On a practical level, advice about suppression of lactation is often needed. It is a very distressing experience to the mother to continue to produce food for a dead baby. Disturbances in the siblings may need practical advice which the health visitor can also give.

The Foundation for The Study of Infant Deaths provides an excellent support system for parents and will put them in touch with other parents who have experienced a similar situation. It provides invaluable advice and newsletters on the subject and can, in conjunction with the health visitor and general practitioner, provide the vital support to the parents. It can ensure that the parents know that they are not alone in this problem.

It would help both the primary health care team and the parents, if the parents could be referred to a paediatrician who would be able to give genetic counselling and professional support. A paediatrician is in a strong position to explain the cause of death.

I would suggest that if the health visitor, the general practitioner and the paediatrician all work together, preferably in conjunction with support from the Foundation for The Study of Infant Deaths, the family who has suffered a sudden infant death could be helped considerably. To do this, communications need to be improved, especially between hospital and community, and there needs to be a greater awareness of the facilities which exist to help the family. The Church should be called in where appropriate, involving ministers with families to whom this sort of help is useful.

The most important need is to listen and to reassure the parents that they are not failures and that they need not bear this tragedy alone.

THE FUTURE — WHAT IS TO BE DONE?

Although considerable research has been undertaken into a syndrome which is the commonest cause of death among children under two years and may contribute to the fact that Britain has the worst infant mortality rate in Western Europe, we still do not know enough. Studies seem to show an association between sudden infant death and legitimacy, size of family, maternal age, type of housing, quality of motherhood and social class. These associations suggest a great variety of possible contributory factors. The realisations are difficult to interpret, for example, low social class is very highly correlated with poor housing.

In Britain in the 1980s, the practice of bottle feeding babies is more prevalent among mothers of low social class. This is a reversal of the pattern of 30 years ago when the move towards bottle feeding was led by middle class mothers. The decision to bottle feed has been implicated as a possible causative factor in sudden infant death and this suggestion is substantiated by the research in Sheffield (Emery & Carpenter, 1977) and by the work of Gunther (1975). However, some of the babies who die suddenly and unexpectedly and with no apparent cause are breast-fed.

Another factor which has been tentatively suggested is a defect in the process of bonding and mothering. One would think this factor unlikely to occur in a breast-fed baby where bonds of physical closeness and eye contact have maximum chance for expression and establishing a bond early.

Prematurity is also cited as a possible cause. It is suggested that the premature baby is less able to support itself in the extra-uterine environment and is more likely to succumb to infection, and also that a bond is more difficult to form between mother and baby if the baby has been in an incubator or hospital for a prolonged period.

Bowlby (1976) placed great emphasis on early bonding for the development of a good relationship between mother and baby, but is this bond so important that if it is not established then death can result? One would expect poor bonding to produce poor mothering and this is also a factor which has been suggested as a possible cause. This particular factor is most certainly not confined to social classes IV and V, although its manifestation in higher social classes is perhaps more subtle.

Factors such as polyhydramnios in pregnancy and a prolonged second stage of labour were cited by Emery (Emery & Carpenter, 1977). Polyhydramnios may indeed be an indication of a congenital deformity such as neural tube defects and other disorders. However, most infants who die, have no such abnormality. A prolonged second stage of labour may produce cerebal trauma in the baby and excessive moulding to the fetal skull. Most of the babies who exhibit signs of cerebal irritation are 'cot nursed' (i.e. handled as little as possible) for 24 hours and apparently recover. Both these factors may be a clue.

I am suggesting that, in spite of the variety of factors which have been considered, we still do not know why sudden infant deaths happen. Patricia McWeeney (1977), in writing about the Sheffield Study, differentiates certain areas where she sees 'successful' parents differing from 'unsuccessful' parents (successful in this context means those who have not experienced sudden infant death). First, the 'unsuccessful' parents' perception of disease was altered. They may have observed symptoms but not recognised them as needing treatment. The 'successful' parents noted these symptoms and recognised them as needing attention.

The health visitor can help by teaching parents to recognise dangerous or potentially dangerous signs. Symptoms such as croupy coughing, difficult breathing, prolonged crying and drowsiness and more urgent symptoms such as convulsions, excessive feed refusal, quietness, vomiting and diarrhoea, discharging ears, floppiness and excessive mucous secretion from the mouth, should all be reported and medical help should be sought.

Secondly, 'unsuccessful' parents were found to be far less efficient at using resources if they were worried. They did not seem to summon help from their general practitioner or hospital. Moreover, it was noticed that once they did call in help, if the treatment was unsuccessful, they would not recall the doctor but would resign themselves to waiting for the condition to clear up spontaneously. The health visitor may be the family's only link with the health service on a regular basis. The impression of accessibility which she gives may colour the family's way of approaching the other resources. If their relationship with her is good, then the family may be more able to approach other professionals in a crisis.

The Foundation for the Study of Infant Deaths has produced a leaflet on what signs and symptims parents should worry about with an infant. This leaflet, coupled with health visiting support, could help.

McWeeney (1977) also suggests that failure to diagnose correctly accounted for a considerable proportion of the deaths. This appears to confirm the suggestion that we really do not know enough, or is the problem that we are simply not aware enough?

Until we do know the cause, the health visitor must use existing theories and advise accordingly. Practical advice such as:

1. The advocation of breast feeding.
2. Instruction on correct bottle feeding practices.
3. Discouragement of the use of pillows for babies.
4. Encouragement of the use of a well-fitting mattress for baby.

5. Advice on sleeping positions and the dangers of the baby sleeping on his back.
6. Advice regarding warmth and not to let the baby sleep in a draught.
7. The use of adequate and safe clothing and blankets.
8. Advice on the mother's rights regarding child benefits and family income supplements, free milk and vitamins if the family is below the poverty line.
9. Help for families to use the services offered.
10. Assurance that the parents understand the advice given.

For the future, it is clear that there is a lot to be done. There is a real need to channel government resources into research into this field which hitherto has been largely sponsored by the Foundation for the Study of Infant Deaths. Money is needed to make available more manpower to allow the intensive visiting needed in the first vital months of life to high risk groups. Only with a joint concerted effort of research, improved communications and a spirit of caring can we hope to solve the problem which causes heartbreak to 3000 parents every years.

REFERENCES

Camps F E 1970 Sudden unexpected deaths in infancy. Report on the proceedings of the Sir Samuel Bedson Symposium. April

Canadian Foundation for the Study of Infant Deaths 1974 Proceedings of the Francis Camps International Symposium on Sudden & Unexpected Deaths in Infancy. Canadian Foundation for the Study of Infant Deaths

Dounham M A P S 1978 Support for a family bereaved by cot death. British Medical Journal June 10

Emery J L 1972 Welfare of families of children found unexpectedly dead. British Medical Journal March

Emery J L 1978 Cot deaths handling the family. Johnston's Baby Newsline Number 10

Emery J L, Carpenter R G 1974 Identification and follow up of infants at risk of sudden death in infancy. Nature August 250: 729

Emery J L, Carpenter R G 1977 Final results of infants at risk of sudden deaths. Nature August 25

Gunther M 1975 The neonates immunity gap, breast feeding and cot deaths. Lancet February 22 1977

Limerick S 1977 Cot deaths, bereaved parents need for support. Midwives Chronicle and Nursing Notes October

McWeeney P 1977 The use of child care facilities related to sudden infant deaths. The Institution of Health Education Journal Number 15

Newcastle Survey on deaths in Childhood 1974/1976 with Special Reference to sudden unexpected deaths 1977 Archives of Disease in Childhood p 828-n835

Smith B A M 1974 Feeding over strength cow's milk to babies. British Medical Journal December 28 p 741–742

Watson E 1975 An analysis of the findings of the inner North London sudden death in infancy project. Public Health. May vol 89

FURTHER READING

Bowlby 1976 Child care and the growth of love.

Chambers 1973 Sudden infant deaths. Health Visitor. October vol 46

Foundation for the Study of Infant Deaths Newsletters Numbers 12 13 and 14

Lancet 1975 Cot deaths. November p 1024

Limerick Lady 1976 Support and counselling needs of families following cot death. Proceedings of the Royal Society of Medicine Vol 69 No 11 November

16

Childhood accidents

Jean Gaffin and Hugh Jackson

INTRODUCTION

Over the past few decades there has been a gradual change in the causes of death in childhood and accidents to children are now the largest single cause of death. Table 16.1 shows childhood deaths from accidents and violence in the years 1968–74 and includes accidents in the home, on the road and elsewhere.

Table 16.1 Childhood deaths from accidents and violence 1968–74 in England and Wales

Diagnosis	Age in years Under 1 year	1–4	5–9	10–14	Total aged 1–14 years	Total aged under 15 years
Accidents and violence (E800–999)	3206	4371	3712	2796	10 877	14 083
All causes	91 568	16 071	9611	7519	33 201	124 769
Accidents and violence as a percentage of all causes	3.5	27.2	38.6	37.2	32.8	11.3

Source: Population Trends No 12 Summer 1978
OPCS (Reproduced with the permission of Her Majesty's Stationery Office)

Figure 16.1 clearly shows the age related nature of accidents, and the way in which boys predominate in both age groups and in relation to all types of fatal accident.

Accidents are not only the major single cause of death of children after the first year, they cause one in five admissions to hospital and result in the attendance of one in six of all urban children at the Accident and Emergency Department of their local hospital. Figure 16.2 shows the hospital discharges of children treated for the effects of accidents and violence, 1968–78. The figures were derived from the Hospital Inpatient Enquiry, based on a 10% sample of the forms completed for every patient discharged from or dying in an N.H.S. hospital in England and Wales.

However, national data on non-fatal childhood accidents are woefully deficient, although the Home Accident Surveillance System run by the Consumer Safety Unit of the Department of Trade collects information about certain types of home accidents from 20 different hospital Accident and Emergency Departments, and

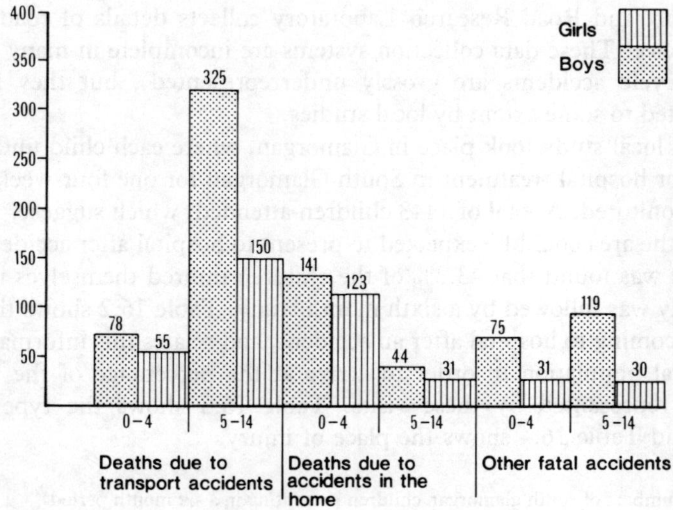

Fig. 16.1 Child deaths related to place of accident, age and sex. Source: 1978 Mortality Statistics Accidents and Violence Series DH4 HMSO (OPCS)

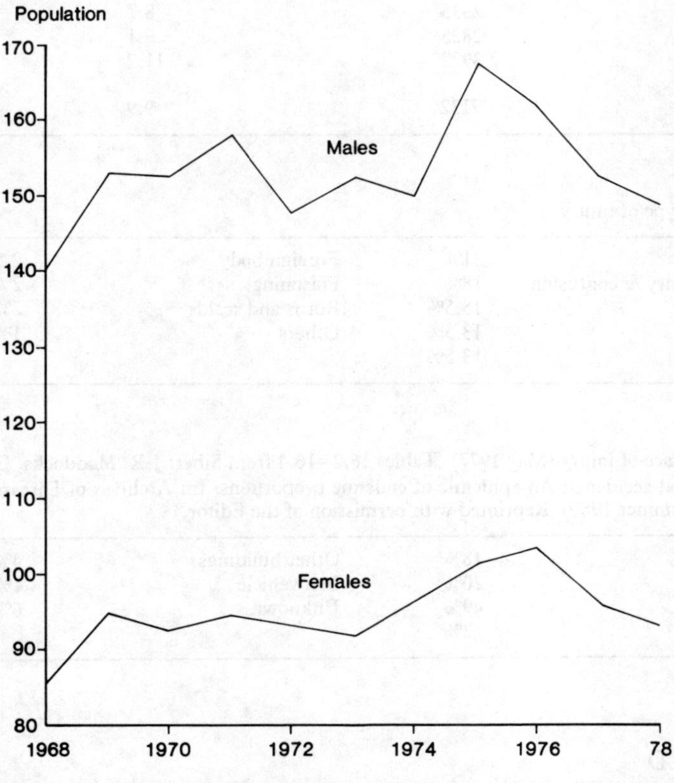

Fig. 16.2 Discharges from and deaths in hospital due to fractures, dislocations and sprains and other injuries and reactions, children aged 1–14 years, 1968–78, England and Wales, rates per 10 000 population. (From Hospital Inpatient Enquiry. Reproduced by permission of Her Majesty's Stationery Office).

the Transport and Road Research Laboratory collects details of road accidents from the police. These data collection systems are incomplete in many areas, (for example bicycle accidents are grossly underrepresented), but they have been complemented to some extent by local studies.

One such local study took place in Glamorgan, where each child under 16 who presented for hospital treatment in South Glamorgan for one four-week period in 1976 was monitored. A total of 1443 children attended, which suggests 17% of the children in the area could be expected to present to hospital after accidental injury in a year. It was found that 43.3% of the children injured themselves in falls.

This study was followed by a sixth month study. Table 16.2 shows the number of children coming to hospital after an accident, and relates this information to the relevant total population in order to arrive at the percentage of the total child population represented by these visits. Table 16.3 shows the type of injury involved, and Table 16.4 shows the place of injury.

Table 16.2 Numbers of south glamorgan children presenting in a six month period

Age group	Numbers presenting in 6 month period May–October 1977	% of child population presenting in a 6 month period
0– 4 years	2335	8.7
5– 9 years	2825	9.1
9–14 years	3972	11.7
Total 0–14 years	9132	9.9

Table 16.3 Type of injury

Lacerations	31%	Foreign body	2.5%
Superficial injury & contusion	18%	Poisoning	2%
Head injury	15.5%	Burns and scalds	2%
Sprains	13.5%	Others	1%
Fractures	13.5%		

Table 16.4 Place of injury (May 1977) (Tables 16.2–16.4 from Sibert J R, Maddocks, G B, Brown B M Childhood accidents: An epidemic of endemic proportions. In: Archives of Diseases in Childhood (Summer 1980). Reprinted with permission of the Editor.)

At school	18%	Other buildings	4%
At home	20%	In a vehicle	1%
Out of doors	49%	Unknown	6%
Sports areas	2%		

THE CHILD

An obvious factor relating to the child is the effect of sex upon accidents. Boys begin to have more accidents than girls by the age of 8 or 9 months, and this preponderance of boys continues throughout childhood. Figure 16.3 illustrates this

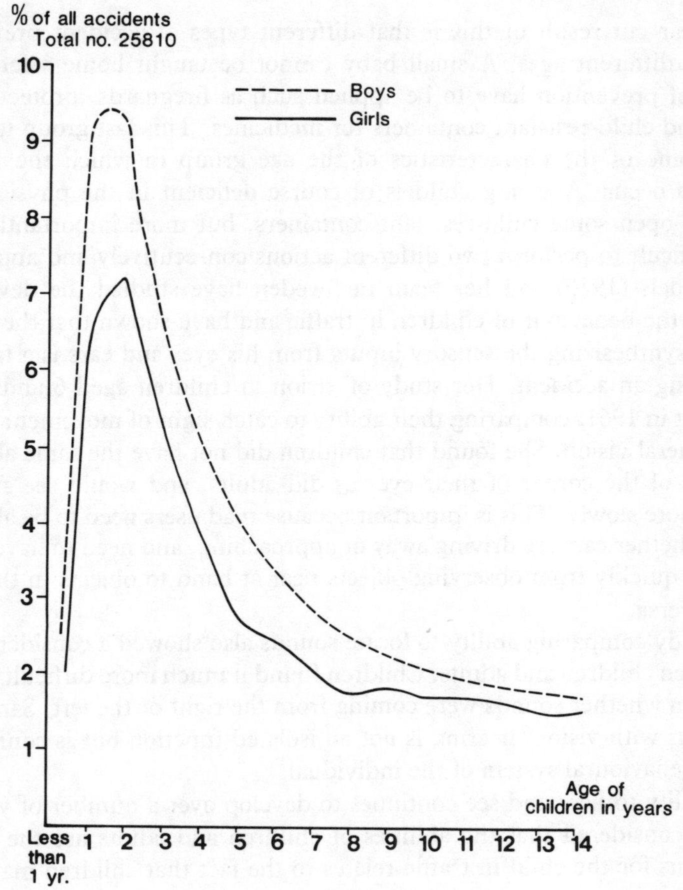

Fig. 16.3 Home accidents to children by age and sex (Based on data published in the Home Accident Surveillance System: Analysis of Domestic Accidents to Children. Consumer Safety Unit; Department of Trade. London 1979)

difference in relation to home accidents. Interestingly, it is not only in the number of accidents that boys exceed girls, but in their severity as well: for example, the ratio of boys to girls admitted to hospital with head injuries is about 2 : 1, but this rises to 5 : 1 when only serious head injuries are considered. It is, of course, usually said that boys are more adventurous than girls, but analyses of risk-taking behaviour are not easy to carry out, although one such study is referred to later.

Childhood is that period of life characterised by growth and development, and the question of child development is one of the most important factors in accidents. Children have different accidents at different ages. A young toddler of 2 or 3 explores his environment and has generally minor accidents in and about the home where he spends most of his time. A young school child of 5 or 6 has more serious accidents caused by his immaturity, impulsivenes and lack of appreciation of danger, such as 'dashing-out accidents' in traffic. A young adolescent of 12 or 13 has adventure accidents. He needs to test himself almost to the limits of his skill and endurance, and, therefore, has accidents such as falls while climbing.

One clear cut result of this is that different types of accident prevention are needed at different ages. A small baby cannot be taught home safety. Physical methods of prevention have to be applied such as fireguards, protection around cookers and child-resistant containers for medicines. This last group takes advantage of some of the characteristics of the age group in which the majority of poisonings occur. A young child is of course deficient in the physical strength needed to open some child-resistant containers, but more importantly, children find it difficult to perform two different actions consecutively and appropriately.

Dr Sandels (1975) and her team in Sweden have studied the developmental aspects of the behaviour of children in traffic and have shown that the child's difficulty in synthesizing the sensory inputs from his eyes and ears is a factor in the child having an accident. Her study of vision in children aged 6 and adults was carried out in 1961, comparing their ability to catch sight of movement at the side, i.e. peripheral vision. She found that children did not have the same ability to see traffic out of the corner of their eyes as did adults, and would see approaching vehicles more slowly. This is important because road users need to be able to grasp quickly whether cars are driving away or approaching, and need to have the ability to change quickly from observing objects near at hand to objects in the distance, and vice versa.

The study comparing ability to locate sounds also showed a considerable difference betwen children and adults. Children found it much more difficult than adults to ascertain whether sounds were coming from the right or the left. Sandels points out that, as with vision, hearing is not an isolated function but is connected with the total behavioural system of the individual.

The ability to hear and see continues to develop over a number of years before it can be considered that the abilities of children and adults are the same. The implications for the child in traffic relates to the fact that children may appear to look about them quite correctly and watch out for traffic situations but in fact are looking at entirely different objects, and in the same way, may appear to be listening to relevant traffic sound but in fact are not doing so.

Sandels has also shown that children's understanding of road signs and of traffic nomenclature is deficient. Some children interpret the pedestrian crossing sign as meaning 'only adults may cross here' or 'people must walk down the middle of the road so as to be safe', and the school crossing sign as meaning 'children must run across the road quickly so as to avoid being knocked down by cars'. Even phrases such as 'to cross the road' or 'one-way street' are not clearly understood by quite a high proportion of 8–10-year-old children.

A very good example of research into children's behaviour in traffic is that done by Professor Howarth (1974) of Nottingham. He studied the behaviour of boys and girls of different ages in traffic, and showed that boys' increased liability to accidents was not merely because they spent more time playing in the street, but because they had twice as high a rate of injury per road crossing as girls at the age of 5. However, by the age of 9 or 10 both sexes had an equal risk when crossing roads. This approach teaches us a great deal about what we do *not* know as well as what we *do* know. It shows us a group of children, namely boys of 5, to whom we must pay particular attention in our traffic education, but it also shows that we have got to analyse their behaviour and perceptual ability in greater detail in order to understand why they have this high risk of accidents when crossing roads compared to girls. Accident prevention in this age group clearly involves teaching children in a positive sense and accident prevention, part of health education as a whole, should be part of their education for life.

Perhaps we need to remember that educating children is but one part of the problem. As Howarth & Repetto-Wright (1978) remind us:

> We have recently been made aware of the danger of rearing children in impoverished environments. High rise flats and concrete jungles are now believed to be unsatisfactory places in which to bring up children because they do not provide places for play or for constructive pursuits. But even in modern housing developments intolerably dangerous roads are still the most attractive, and in some cases, the only places for children to play. The motor vehicle is not only killing our children, it is also having a major effect on the quality of their lives. Should the motorists not recognize this responsibility also?

Education of the adolescent is paradoxically more difficult in some ways than that of the younger school child. He resents adults trying to teach him how to behave and his need for risk and adventure is part of his breaking away from the family which comes with increasing independence. So far as accidents are concerned he has got to learn by his own mistakes to some extent. An adult whom he trusts, who may be in his own family but who is often somebody outside the family such as a scout or youth leader or a teacher, may be able to persuade him about the wisdom of using proper equipment in his adventure sports, sailing, climbing, canoeing and so on, but by and large safety comes from self discipline rather than imposed discipline at this age.

An interesting facet of the human aspect of accidents is that of the child's personality and his intelligence. Much work has been done on the question of accident proneness. Is there a group of children who have more accidents than one would have expected by chance and, if so, what are the characteristics of this group?

In order to compare such children with children who do not have more than their share of accidents, it is necessary to have a large enough group of children who are a fully representative cross-section of the population and who are kept under observation long enough to find out how many children have how many accidents and at what ages. The thousand family survey group in Newcastle upon Tyne, were a group of this size, which included all the children born in the city in a period of two months in 1947 who were followed from birth to school-leaving age. As part of the survey they all had intelligence tests and a personality inventory done, partly by a psychologist and partly by the teachers. A correlation of intelligence with the accidents experienced by these children during their school years shows that there was very little effect so far as small numbers of accidents were concerned. However, when children having larger numbers of accidents are considered, there is a statistically significant difference with an excess of accident repeaters among the less intelligent children. When children who had large numbers of accidents were compared with those who did not, it was found that the children involved in accidents were below average in concentration, reliability, initiative, neathandness and ability in craft-work whereas those who avoided accidents, on the whole, tended to be above average in these characteristics.

The material on accidents in childhood collected in the National Child Development Study (1958 Cohort) has not been fully analysed. Preliminary analysis of the 1970 cohort, under the supervision of Professor Neville Butler of the Department of Child Health, Bristol University, points to the age of the mother at the time of the child's birth as being relevant to childhood accidents.

One final point about the child himself is his need for play. This must be provided for, and we must learn to expect children to behave unpredictably in play. Playgrounds must be designed and play equipment installed in such a way as to minimise reasonably the child's risk of an accident without dampening down entirely the risk he takes and the fun he gets from his play activities. Nevertheless, bizarre accidents will occur and some accidents will occur in the natural environment as well as the man-made one.

THE PARENTS

Probably the most important single factor in the human environment which bears directly upon a child's accident is the question of his parents' competence and skill in child rearing. There is, of course, no direct relationship between parental competence and social background. Some well-to-do parents may be bad parents from the point of view of the child. The vast majority of poorer parents are excellent. Nevertheless, overall socially deprived and under privileged children are more likely to have accidents. This relationship in the United Kingdom between social class and death rates has been clearly demonstrated by Adelstein (1976). As Table 16.2 shows, the death rates rise steadily in pre-school, school and adolescent children as socio-economic status falls.

Table 16.5 Number of deaths and rates per 100 000 per year from accidents, poisonings and violence (ECD E800–E999) 1959–1963 England and Wales. (From Adelstein & White (1976) Reproduced with the permission of Her Majesty's Stationery Office)

Age		Social class I	II	III	IV	V
1–4	Numbers	60	231	1169	598	443
	Rates	9.50	12.77	16.87	24.00	44.86
5–9	Numbers	40	227	1002	480	323
	Rates	6.28	9.37	12.68	16.10	28.90
10–14	Numbers	43	231	858	405	208
	Rates	7.36	8.09	9.70	11.23	15.50

There are two particular ways in which parents are liable to fail their children in a way which will lead to an accident. First, parents often underestimate their young child's abilities or fail to understand their behaviour at certain stages of their development, e.g. a young child reaching out at a cup of coffee and getting scalded, or a child's ability to climb to reach some medicines kept in a cupboard, or to fall out of a window as a consequence. Second, parents unfortunately fail to use safety devices which are already installed, or are easily obtainable, such as window catches or guards in front of electric fires.

These failures also relate to aspects of the physical environment which are not pursued further here, but it is right to mention one more aspect of the family background which has been shown to be associated with an increased liability to accidents, namely the emotional situation within the family at the time. Many studies, such as the well known paper of Backett & Johnston (1959) have shown that accidents are more liable to happen when the mother is under stress because of some family or personal crisis. Backett & Johnston's study was of children involved in road accidents, but the clinical impression that family stress is a factor in other types of accident has been amply confirmed by many studies in America (Sobel 1971), as well as by Sibert (1975) in respect of poisoning in childhood in the U.K.

Equally relevant is the work of Brown & Davidson (1978). They showed that the accident risk to the children of a random sample of 458 women living in Inner London was associated with both a working class status and the presence of psychiatric disturbance, usually depression, in the mother. The presence of the psychiatric disorder greatly increases the likelihood of accidents to children. They found that it was only during a period of psychiatric disturbance in the mother that children had an accident rate above normal. The accident rate before onset or after recovery was similar to that in families of women with no psychiatric illness. They estimated the accident rate in any one year, per 100 children, to be 20.7 in the week when mother was disturbed, 4.8 in the weeks before onset or after recovery, and 5.4 in women with no psychiatric disturbance.

SOCIETY AS A WHOLE

We live in an adult world, designed by adults, for adults.

There is no doubt that the environmental aspects of accidents are of great importance, and the Swedish State Commission for Investigation of Childhood Accidents (1979) goes so far as to say that the main cause of such accidents is the physical environment, which has been constructed mainly by adults. The needs of children have had far too little consideration in the shaping of the physical environment.

Society as a whole is responsible for designing the environment in which our children are brought up. The safety of the major environment of city, town or village, of the local environment of the home, and of the products brought into the home are to a large extent the responsibility of individuals other than the family such as town planners, architects, builders and designers. National governments and local authorities have an important responsibility here too, particularly by setting and implementing safety standards.

Besides designing the environment, society has a second responsibility. This is in the education of its members in matters relating to accident prevention. At the present moment a great deal of effort goes into the training of children in road safety, whether as pedestrians or cyclists, but adult members of society also need to be educated in the use of safety measures and, particularly, in the needs of young children and in the way they are likely to behave. The health visitor has a particularly important role here, as does the family doctor, the community midwife, district nurse and other health care staff.

Sandels (1975) has said that, in the end, accidents to children in traffic are always an adult responsibility. This is true in the main for all accidents to children wherever they occur.

REFERENCES

Adelstein A M, White G C 1976 Causes of children's death analysed by social class. In: Child health a collection of studies. OPCS Studies on Medical and Population Subjects No 31. HMSO, London

Backett E M, Johnston A M 1959 Social patterns of road accidents to children. British Medical Journal 1: 409–413

Brown G W, Davidson S 1978 Social class, psychiatric disorder of mother, and accidents to children. Lancet 1 (8060): 378–381

Howarth C I, Routledge D A, Repetto-Wright R 1974 An analysis of road accidents involving child pedestrians. Ergonomics 17 (3): 319

Howarth C I, Repetto-Wright R 1978 The measurement of risk and the attribution of responsibility for child pedestrian accidents. Safety Education, Autumn Issue (144) 10–12

Office of Health Economics (September 1981) Accidents in childhood. OHE briefing, no. 17.

Sandels S 1975 Children in traffic. Elek Books, London

Sibert J 1975 Stress in families of children who have ingested poisons. British Medical Journal 2: 87–89

Sobel R 1971 Psychiatric implications of child poisoning. Paediatric Clinics of North America 17: 653–6

Spence J et al 1974 A thousand families in Newcastle upon Tyne. Oxford University Press, London

Swedish Government 1979 A Report of the State Commission for Investigation of Childhood Accidents. Swedish Government

FURTHER READING

Burman S, Genn H (eds) 1977 Accidents in the home. Croom Helm, London

Jackson R D (ed) 1977 Children, the environment and accidents. Pitman Medical Tunbridge, Kent

Nelson A (ed) 1972 Medical aspects of home hazards. The Medical Commission on Accident Prevention, 50 Old Brompton Road, London SW7

The Facts about Accidents 1976 Royal Society for the Prevention of Accidents. Birmingham

Safety Education Published each term by Royal Society for the Prevention of Accidents, Birmingham

17

The healthy school child

Patricia Slack

School days should be happy. They should be full of vigour and joy, a time of discovery and rapid learning the start of a life of success and fulfilment. For many children they are a time of misery and unhappiness. Their inadequacies are reinforced as they fail to learn. They withdraw or they are bored and find other outlets start truanting and perhaps even get into trouble with the police.

Children fail to learn for various reasons. It is the teacher's task to see that her teaching is at the right intellectual level and related to the children's previous experiences. However, her efforts are useless if a child cannot hear or see properly. Equally a child who is in pain or not feeling well, unhappy or afraid, will be less likly to learn. The school health service exists to find and treat such problems and to explain the effects to parents and teachers.

HISTORY

The school health service first appeared along with other major public health services at the turn of the century. Doctors were employed in schools to find physical disease and handicap and to ensure that children were fit to benefit from their education. As families could not afford treatment, a free school health service was developed. Nurses were particularly involved in the treatment of children and this was probably the service's most successful period. When hospital and family doctor care became free to everyone in 1948, they gradually took over all the treatment. Health screening was left to the school doctors but as it was not attractive to the medical profession it was seen as low priority and status.

From 1945 school nursing was supposed to be the job of health visitors but they too regarded it as secondary. Most of their school work was delegated to SRNs or SENs who, until latterly, had no training in school work. During this time malnutrition and physical disease in school children have given way to the far more difficult psychological and social illnesses. School doctors and nurses have not adapted to this and seldom provide the most helpful service to the children.

HEALTH PROBLEMS

Our knowledge of health problems in primary schools has increased over time. Sensory defects of vision and hearing are the most common complaints. Indeed, it is estimated that 7% of new entrants have a vision defect. 6% of boys are likely to be colour blind and 12% of eleven year olds with normal vision show a defect at 16 years (Peckham, 1979). Five per cent of primary school children are also likely to have a hearing loss (Rutter et al, 1970), though this may be temporary following respiratory illness, otitis media or glue ear. To ensure early discovery, vision should be reviewed yearly and hearing twice in the primary school.

Primary children also suffer respiratory complaints and their side-effects, bed-wetting, infectious diseases, skin complaints and poor sleep. A survey of the 9–12 years age group (Rutter et al, 1970) suggested the following breakdown of difficulties:

Intellectually retarded	2.6%
Educationally backward	7.9%
Psychiatric disorder	6.8%
Physical	2.7%

Very little work has been done on adolescents. A study of 16-year-olds (Fogelman, 1976) suggests that headaches, menstrual pains, acne, asthma and wheezy ronchitis are common complaints. One per cent of 16-year-olds are still bed-wetting and the accident rate is very high, particularly among boys.

Adolescence is often a time of stress as children become adults. Coping with sexuality and an adult identity can be difficult and confusing, especially as this occurs at the same times as there is pressure to pass examinations and decide on a future career. Such anxiety on top of unresolved childhood problems, which have been ignored or mishandled, can lead to truancy, drug-taking, early pregnancy, petty theft, violence and abusive language. These are all typical expressions of unsolved childhood problems. Schools cope with this in a variety of ways.

All schools have some sort of pastoral care system and some have full or part-time counsellors. Sometimes a full-time school nurse is employed and expected to include counselling in her work. Until recently this was not considered part of the school nurse's responsibility and consequently head teachers financed this out of their own budget. As there was and is no appropriate training, it is left to the nurse's own discretion as to how she carries out this task.

ACCIDENTS AND FIRST-AID

These are technically the responsibility of the head teacher and school first-aider. The responsibilities of the school health service have always been unclear and occupational health in the school health service needs to be defined. Record keeping is poor. No attempt is made to analyse the aetiology of school accidents or first-aid demands and to link this to an individual child or to the school environment. It is unlikely that any head teacher has ever involved the school health team in planning the length of lessons, the timetable or alterations in the buildings.

HANDICAPPING CONDITIONS

Physical or mental handicap may be discovered during school life but severe handicap should be diagnosed either at birth or during the pre-school surveillance. The

Warnock Committee suggested that 1 in 5 children have a handicap sufficiently severe to interfere with their learning and each child needs education tailored to the handicap. Assessment for this should be shared between parents, doctors, teachers, social workers and educational psychologists. They then decide where and how the child can be educated depending on the degree of handicap and the facilities available. Where possible the child attends ordinary school and he may have the support of a peripatetic special teacher, a resource room or a special class or unit. He may attend a special school either full-or part-time or he may live in a residential special school. The doctor and nurse must see that both parents and teachers know how the handicapped child is to be treated. They also need to know the side-effects of any treatment and what the child can be expected to manage.

EDUCATING FOR HEALTH

Plenty of time and effort is devoted by discovering illness or handicap but teaching children how to be healthier has not had the same attention. The old Chinese proverb 'give a man a fish and you feed him for a day. Teach a man to fish and you feed him for a life-time' can surely be applied to health.

Although good health is essential to the quality and happiness of life it is not a compulsory school subject. Whether it is taught depends on the whims of the head teacher and a health visitor, school nurse or teacher may undertake it. Too often there is no rationale behind the choice of teacher, topic or the length of time allocated. However the Schools Council has produced excellent teaching materials which are being used in schools and gradually teachers are taking more interest.

Similar progress has not happened in the school medical room. The doctors' and nurses' health checks are seldom used as a time for teaching. Children have their eyes and ears tested without knowing why and they are not taught to do this themselves. But why not? This is a first step in taking responsibility for their own health.

In the U.S.A there are exciting developments in teaching children to be 'active health consumers'. They learn to weigh and measure themselves and to judge their progress on the results. They learn to complete their own health history — they even keep a copy of it. Compiling a health history includes discussing the self-medication they use at home and through this they are learning to make choices about drugs as well as something of the kind of useful discussion they can have with their doctor.

American school nurse practitioners have introduced these programmes in Colorado, New York, North Dakota and Utah. They are funded by the Robert Wood Johnson Foundation and are being evaluated by the University of California Los Angeles. These innovations are worth considering and some British school nurses have visited these programmes since they were first reported (Slack, 1980)

THE CHILDREN'S VIEW

The children's view on school health shows that innovation and change in approach is overdue. A survey of fifth and sixth form attitudes found that they had some knowledge of curative medicine and visited their family doctor but the concept of prevention meant little or nothing to them. Most participants did not know a doctor with whom they felt they could discuss their problems. Nurses were more approachable and met some of their needs but were seen as mainly concerned with headlice and asprins (Court, 1976).

Another study (Whitmore unpublished) which questioned parents and teachers found that parents had few expectations of the service. Head teachers found it helpful but class teachers had great difficulty in extracting information relevant to their classwork. In an age when project work is prolific in school it seems a pity that the children do not investigate their school health service. Their involvement could help to give a more relevant service as well as being a useful learning exercise.

RECENT CHANGES

During the last decade a number of event have taken place which seem bound to culminate in an altered and improved service. Firstly a study of the service in the 1960s (Rutter et al, 1970) suggested that doctors could use their time most usefully with children who have complex health problems. As a result routine medical examinations at 5, 7, 11 and school leaving age were abandoned in favour of an extensive medical examination on children at five years. These are followed by selective medicals on children with problems and a school leaving interview at about 13 years. School nurses have the task of identifying problems in all normal children over the age of six years.

Another important influence for change came with the National Health Service reorganisation in 1974. A senior doctor and nurse known as the Area Specialist and the Area Nurse (child health) were appointed in each Area Health Authority to be responsible for school and child health services and answerable to the education authority. This was the first time that a very senior doctor had primary responsibility for schools. It was also the first time that senior nurses attended education authority meetings on behalf of their own profession. These appointments had a considerable effect on improving the service. 1974 was also the first time that school health was represented in the children's division of the Departmet of Health and Social Security. It was the first time that school nursing had a voice at government level.

Our national approach to child health was changing and in 1973 a Government Committee chaired by Professor Court was set up to consider the future of the child health services. The Court Report (C, 1976) was the most comprehensive review of child health in this century and viewed the 'connection between health and education as one of the most important aspects of paediatrics'. Their recommendations on school health constituted a national guideline to the service, and their definition of educational medicine outlined the service very clearly:

> Educational medicine is the study and practice of child health and paediatrics in relation to the processes of learning. It requires an understanding of child development, the educational environment, the child's response to schooling, the disorders which interefere with the child's capacity to learn, and the special needs of the handicapped. Its practitioners need to work co-operatively with the teachers, psychologists and others who may be involved with the child and to understand the influences of family and social environment.

It was proposed that prevention and treatment be combined and that, as group practice attachment seemed the most desirable pattern of primary care, it should

Fig. 17.1 School Health Service Structure

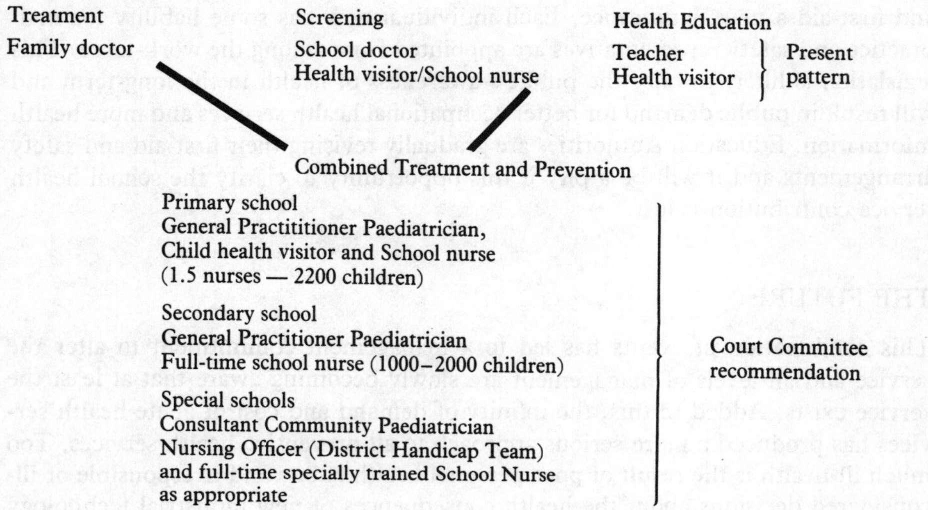

include school health. This would be the responsibility of one doctor in the practice who should be specially trained in child health, and known as a General Practitioner Paediatrician. The attached health visitor, whom they felt should be solely concerned with children 0–16 years (Child Health Visitor) would have overall responsibility and be assisted in schools by a school nurse. This nurse would have a statutory training and certificate in educational nursing (see Fig. 17.1). All of this, other than the principle of training for school nurses, was rejected. Nevertheless, there are examples of this method of working and many believe that it will be adopted eventually.

What has been accepted and has grown is the recommendation to set up District Handicap Teams to be responsible for the assessment and care of handicapped children. The nuclear team consists of a senior Community Paediatrician (Consultant status), Nursing Officer, Social Worker, Principal Psychologist, and Teacher, with other specialists as required, depending on the handicap. It was envisaged that the Community Paediatrician and the Nursing Officer for the team would act as school doctor and Health Visitor for some special schools.

There are also exciting developments among school nurses. Those without a Health Visitor Certificate have long been a neglected group. Working alone and often isolated from each other, their task is a difficult and lonely one. First and middle nursing management has been generally poor and there are many nursing officers who do not know the schools for which they employ staff. They have done little to provide suitable induction courses or introduce the staff properly into the schools. School nurses initially dissatisfied with salaries and working conditions have started to meet together in groups and held their first national conference in 1979. There is enthusiasm and impetus which may be the beginning of a new era in school nursing and a new look for school health. This coincides with a fall in the recruitment of doctors to the service because of uncertainty following the Court Committee proposals. On balance this may mean that school health becomes a predominantly nursing responsibility.

Finally, the Health and Safety at Work Act 1974 gave responsibility for safety and first-aid a new significance. Each individual now has some liability for malpractice and safety representatives are appointed from among the work-force. This legislation is likely to raise the public's awareness of health in the long-term and will result in public demand for better occupational health services and more health information. Education Authorities are gradually revising their first-aid and safety arrangements and it will be a pity if this opportunity to clarify the school health service contribution is lost.

THE FUTURE

This combination of events has led to a management commitment to alter the service and all levels of management are slowly becoming aware that at least the service exists. Added to this, the infinity of demand and cost of acute health services has produced a more serious approach to all preventive health services. Too much ill-health is the result of poor personal health habits and irresponsible or ill-considered decisions about the health consequences of new industrial technology and changes in the environment. As we cannot afford the treatment costs of chronic illness and preventable handicaps we must look for new approaches. School has a considerable influence on the thinking of the future generations and is the most likely place to try to prevent the repetition of poor practice from one generation to the next. Perhaps it is a fitting conclusion for those who may dismiss this importance,to make a final quote from Court 1976:

> The greatest single need in medicine in the next 25 years is to give prevention the degree of scientific and educational attention that has been given in the last 25 years to treatment.

REFERENCES

Court Report 1976 Fit for the future. Report of the Committee on Child Health Services. HMSO, London

Fogelman K ed 1976 Britain's sixteen-year-olds. National Children's Bureau, London

Peckham et al 1979 Vision screening of adolescents and their use of glasses. British Medical Journal 1: 1111–1113

Rutter M, Tizard J, Whitmore K 1970 Education, health and behaviour. Longman, London

Slack P (1980) School Nursing in the USA (series of five articles) Nursing Times V 76 (9): 365–366, 420–421, 468–469, 521–522, 557–558

Warnock 1978 Report of the Committee of Enquiry into The Education of Handicapped Children and Young People. HMSO, London

FURTHER READING

DES 1977 Health education in schools. HMSO, London

Fitzherbert K 1977 Child care services and the teacher. Maurice Temple Smith, London

Illingworth R S 1974 The child at school. Blackwell Scientific, Oxford

Slack P A 1978 School nursing. Balliere Tindall, London

Varma V B 1973 Stresses in children. ULP, London

18

Becoming adult — health problems and implications

Alexander D. G Gunn

In physiological terms, and still today in primitive social communities, the passage from childhood to adult is relatively simple and takes place over a short period of time. In the young female it is marked by the development of the breasts, the change in fat distribution and skeletal growth that produces the widened hips, the expected adult female contours of the body and the onset of menstruation. In a well-nourished community these changes occur on average between the ages of 11 and 13. In the male an increase in height, shoulder girth and generalised musculature development is accompanied by a deepening of the voice tone, a length increase in the penis and the production — though unrecognised at the time — of active spermatazoa in the seminal fluid, and these changes typically occur between the ages of 10 and 14. In the male in all societies the duration of the change, which is medically termed puberty, takes longer than in the female. In addition to these physical changes, brought about by the release of growth hormone from the pituitary gland and influenced by the hypothalamus, there are considerable psychological and social adjustments for the individual.

In an undeveloped agricultural society the period of adjustment is shorter, often marked by certain cultural 'rites de passage' that recognise the change and create a new status of adulthood for the individual. In contemporary developed society the physiological changes are relatively unmarked by society which has created new criteria for adulthood associated with the requirements of education, learning to drive, earning a living independently of the parents, and the legal right to marry, reproduce and own a home. These requirements are entirely artificial in terms of the human's anatomical and physiological development but they are reflected in the use of the term 'adolescence' to describe this period of life. Not surprisingly, therefore, since it is a cultural phenomenon and not a biological one, adolescence is a time when many social problems emerge both for the individual and society.

It is convenient to regard 'becoming an adult' as lasting from the age of 15 to 25. At the earlier age, for most, the changes of puberty are under way, complete or well advanced, and at the later age educational training is completed, marriage and parenthood commenced and the last bone in the body to ossify — the clavicle — has done so, completing the growth cycle of the human skeleton.

Contemporary western society often sees its young people as being uncooperative, angry, surly, unkempt, rejecting the standards of the older generation, disregarding the morality of their seniors, and causing invariably 'problems'. Talk of the 'generation gap' is engendered by the apparent inability of the young to conform to any behaviour patterns other than ones they invent for themselves — and 'peer group influence' is the hallmark of changes that occur. Commercially this is the time of life in which the individual has the maximum amount of disposable income — for expenditure on leisure, clothes, alcohol and social activities — since the home and essentials of life are most commonly provided by the older generation. Constant visible indulgence in such apparent non-essentials acts as a further irritant to the parents, who are themselves at this time economically most deprived, and so envy and resentment form part of the changing relationship between parent and former child.

Medically, however, where in former years the problems of tuberculosis, contagious disease and sepsis would have occupied the majority of the written texts about this age group, today the common concerns are glandular fever, acne, sports injury, contraception and acute depressive illness. The 'captain of the army of death' is no longer the tubercle, but the motor-cycle. In terms of infective illness most of the life-threatening diseases have been virtually eradicated by improvements in public health, food provision and immunisation. Poliomyelitis, for example, has not broken out in epidemic proportions in the United Kingdom since 1957. Awareness of the need for constant reinforcement of 'herd immunity' is, however, lacking and social failure to take up, or worse to reject, opportunity for vaccination against tuberculosis, polio, rubella — and perhaps in the near future gonorrhoea — requires considerable effort in terms of health education. If the community's protection rate ever fell below 60%, then epidemics would recur.

Health education has not so far succeeded in its attempts to reduce the unwanted pregnancy rate in this age group. Despite free access to medical advice and the free prescription of effective contraception (U.K.) there is still an annually increasing incidence of unmarried pregnancy (currently, 1979, 11% of all children born) and abortion (currently 120 000 per year). There has been described a five year 'gap' between the first experience of sexual intercourse and a regular commitment to the use of contraception (Schofield, 1973) and the occurrence of sexual activity is taking place earlier. One in every hundred terminations performed by one of the largest Pregnancy Advisory Agencies in the United Kingdom in 1979 was carried out on girls below the age of 16. The commitment to contraception is thus being delayed and is brought about by knowledge of a contemporary who has become pregnant, by peer group influence, or by the development of an apparently stable relationship that involves regular sexual activity. Large differences exist between ethnic groups in the age at which sexual experience begins. Caribbean and African origin groups find that their teenagers not only mature physically earlier than the Caucasian but also become involved in sexual activity earlier, whilst Asian and Oriental ethnic groups, perhaps because of the characteristic family patterns, are not exposed to the opportunity until a later age. Nevertheless, by the age of 17 to 18 few of today's adolescents are sexually inexperienced.

No doubt as a consequence of this pattern of sexual behaviour, the incidence of venereal disease, and notably gonorrhoea, is rising. With a quarter of a million new cases a year occurring in the under-25-year-old age group in the United Kingdom, and in the United States where sexually transmitted diseases now form one of the highest causes of consultation in the college health services, there is no room for any complacency. Some European countries (notably West Germany, Sweden and Holland) have found that the free availability of the condom — in all colours thus recognising that sex is a 'fun thing' for youth — has been the most effective public health measure that has had any impact on these statistics and those of unwanted pregnancy. The development of a vaccine against gonorrhoea offers the prospect of a major reduction in one sexually transmitted disease — but the problems of non-specific urethritis, trichomonas, monilia and herpes remain.

The older generation's morality that was based on the imposition of chastity — because of the fear of pregnancy — was outdated by the development of the oral contraceptive and access to termination. Behavioural change is rarely effected by information alone, but only by motivation. It has to be accepted that the motivation of the developing adult for sexual activity, personal and mutual exploration of gender identity and the formation of physical as well as emotional relationships with a member of the opposite sex, is high. Preventive medicine has inadequately recognised the need for research in this area of adolescent sexuality, and most of the published material has been derived from sociologists whose work, as yet, has failed to change established medical practice. Only in the development of voluntary organisations, such as the youth Advisory Clinics, Counselling Services and, to some extent, the work of the Family Planning Association, has there been any marked change in the care available to this age group in the last decade.

Sexual identity is sought by the growing adult as a natural development of personality, and homosexuality is an expression of the same search. For some this is the conclusion of their personal satisfaction, for most it is a natural stage in their progress, and the liberation of attitudes towards homosexuality is the most welcome of recent changes in society's attitudes to sexual behaviour. Nevertheless, illogical barriers exist, some created by statute, that still place restrictions on non-procreative relationships, and these, as well as the constantly changing pattern of an adolescent's personality development, prove a source of neurosis, depressive reaction and unhappiness.

Some subscribe to the view that outdoor physical activity — in the form of sport — leads to health of mind and body, as well as perhaps providing an outlet for aggression, competitiveness and self-glorification. As currently some 7% of all cases seen by the casualty, or accident and emergency departments of all general hospitals in this country originate from so-called sporting activity, this view might well be re-evaluated. For example, the highest cause (apart from road traffic accidents) of cervical spine dislocation and subsequent paraplegia in this age group is the playing of rugby football and other sports. Amendment of the rules by the Rugby League will go some way to reducing this toll but the concept of sport for all, without physical training for all, has inherent dangers.

It is not the regular athlete, committed sports player or club member who heads the list of injured, it is the untrained casual player. The same is true for mountaineering, caving, sailing, swimming, power-boat racing, skiing and hang-gliding. Physical fitness in terms of physical education for the proper use and protection of the human body is distinctly lacking in the provision of this country's formal educational structure. The virtual dissolution of the school medical services may bear some responsibility for this, but this country's provision of gymnasia, swimming pools, athletic tracks and training facilities is now the worst in Europe. When over 500 young adults and children drown every year in the United Kingdom because they cannot swim there is room for serious concern. If the same number died from T.B. every year it would give cause for justifiable national outrage — yet such deaths are largely preventable. Contemporary medicine and care have to move from their disease-orientated background to recognise that modern problems are not always associated with therapeutics derived from pharmacy. The single most important contribution that could be made to the health of the nation, at least in respect of this age group, would be the eradication of the motor-cycle, since in 1979 it led to over 50 000 severe injuries and over 1700 deaths.

In general, however, the greatest concern is expressed over less significant issues. For example, major concern has been repetitively, and ineffectively, expressed over this age group's use of 'drugs'. Cannabis has excited more comment from those who have had no experience of its use whatsoever than masturbation did in Victorian times — and the same dread prospects of indulgence have been described. Hallucinogens (LSD) are no longer a contemporary fashion, access to amphetamines as stimulants is now virtually denied by legislation and restriction on manufacture, whilst heroin, cocaine and morphine derivative usage, although subject to the vagaries of illegal importation, remains a 'problem' for some 2000 or so adolescent individuals a year (of the 12 000 000 at risk). 'Glue sniffing', or inhalant abuse, is an increasingly serious problem. All of these indulgences share one characteristic, apart from being physically harmful — they are social or group activities. Abusers and addicts belong to peer groups whose need for expression is not met in any other way. It is not a 'drug problem' but a personal problem of the individuals who find either solace, adventure, rebellion, escape or relief. If there were less concentration on the pharmacology and more on the characteristics of the individuals who become involved, the prospect of prevention of that which becomes dangerous would be greatly enhanced. Cure for the addicted individual is despairingly almost impossible — the identification of the prone might be a much more effective tool in dealing with the problem.

The young adult's dose of alcohol, as the most widely available, advertised, cheap and encouraged drug of contemporary society, should excite much more concern. Some young adults have been spending more than 40% of their disposable income on alcohol (Gunn, 1977). More young adults were convicted of drunkenness in this country in 1979 than at any time since records have been kept by the Home Office (nearly 120 000 cases in one year). One in eight young men are regularly drinking alcohol in sufficient quantities to harm their present health and to damage their livers in the future if the habit is maintained (Office of Censuses 1980). One in every four young male drivers (and one in thirteen young women) drink more than the legal limit of alcohol, regularly, before driving home. The law is ignored, yet the danger is widely advertised. Again, the example of behaviour being little influenced by the availability of information is presented. Alcohol has been, throughout mankind's history of evolution, the most widely used of all social drugs. Drunkenness, ill-health and crime following its use have caused legislation that has ranged from the ridiculous (Prohibition Act, U.S.A., 1932) to the barbaric (eg. Islamic Law in Saudi Arabia 1980), with varying degrees of constant ineffectiveness. Alcohol supports the State through taxation revenue and, used in moderation, it is safe, pleasant, relaxing and often beneficial in certain of its effects.

The problem, therefore, is not the drug, but its use, and until society defines how it should be used in the interests of greater safety and the preservation of health, the contemporary pattern of misuse will grow. The hard-drinking adolescent of today is the cirrhotic patient of tomorrow if current social trends are not abated.

The same grounds for concern exist with regard to the current pattern of adolescent disturbance expressed through the consumption of tranquillisers, antidepressants and hypnotics. Drug prescriptions for the young adult are annually increasing throughout Western Europe and North America as neurosis, anxiety, conflict, depression, despair and misery — albeit the characteristics of variation in the normally labile emotions of the adolescent — are presented to the medical profession by ever more and more individuals. It may be as a consequence of the pressures of society, fewer outlets for emotional expression, the adult body ruled by the socially immature mind, contemporary prolongation of the artificial state of adolescence — the causes are probably legion, but the effect is disastrous. At least one in every ten young adults shows some sign of psychological distress, and one in a hundred comes under the care of a psychiatrist (Gunn, 1976). Fortunately, only one in a thousand is psychotically ill, regardless of socio-economic background, educational achievement or ethnic origin. It is the large number of unhappy, malajusted, insecure, immature and behaviourally disordered young adults who need help with the difficulties and recurrent crises of growing up that reflects society's inadequacies in providing properly for this age group. In the U.K. deliberate overdosage is now the single most frequent cause for admission to a hospital in the 15–25-year-old age group. Fortunately the death rate is low, but as an index of personal despair it is a major epidemic that shows no sign of abatement. Voluntary organisations have created counselling services — the Samaritans now get one-third of all of their telephone calls from this age group —, hospitals arrange psychiatric referral before discharge, self-help organisations have sprung up to 'befriend' the sufferer, and researchers blame unemployment, sex, parents, doctors and 'cultural isolation' singly or together. There is little evidence for consolation apart from the fact that on average an adolescent makes three times more 'gestures', 'cries for help' or 'hysterical attention-seeking devices' than any other age group and only succeeds — if that is the term to use — in genuinely harming himself permanently, or dying, at a rate that is one-tenth of any older age group. If the cultural context meant that they made the 'gesture' with firearms, as they do in Scandinavia, then the death rate would be twenty times higher. Is this preventable? Not entirely, since there will always be individuals who cannot cope with the normal and inevitable stress of growing up. The great majority, however, should be enabled to cope without the dramatic and personally degrading effect of publicly exhibiting their despair. Peer groups are usually supportive, but sometimes rejective. Parents are sympathetic, but sometimes demanding. Personal relationships are satisfying, but sometimes disruptive. Health professionals are often understanding, but sometimes disapproving — and life is full of variations in response to the individual.

That, however, is what becoming an adult entails, responding constantly to variations in experience. Adolescence is the testing time for the foundations laid in childhood as the personality inherited is shaped and equipped to grow. It is a time of life in which there have always been, and always will be, some casualties. The role of those charged with health care is to mitigate the penalties, reduce the casualties and advise from experience those who will be the adults of the future.

REFERENCES

Gunn A D G 1970 The privileged adolescent. Medical & Technical Publishing, Lancaster

Gunn A D G Brown C B 1977 Alcohol consumption in a student community. Practitioner 219: 238–242

Office of Population Censuses and Surveys (1980) Report on the Drinking of Alcohol. HMSO, London

Schofield M 1973 The sexual behaviour of young adults. Allen Lane, London

FURTHER READING

Alcohol and alcoholism 1979 Report by Royal College of Psychiatrists. Tavistock Publications, London

Emotional problems of childhood and adolescence 1973 Collected articles, British Medical Journal, B.M.A. Publications, London

Gunn A D G 1970 The privileged adolescent. Medical & Technical Publishing, Lancaster

Haslam M T 1975 Psychiatric illness in adolescence. Butterworth, London

Schofield M 1973 The sexual behaviour of young adults. Allen Lane, London

19

The health of the worker

Jennifer Barnard

The risks inherent in each job and work place vary according to the nature of activities undertaken, the attitudes and knowledge of management and workers and their compliance with health and safety guidance, codes of practice and legislation. The risks to each individual will also depend upon the individual's state of health and well-being and suitability for the job he or she is required to do.

Preventive action to ensure that exposure to hazards is abolished or reduced to a minimum must now be seen as a priority. It is essential not only to minimise the effects of occupational hazards upon individuals whose quality of life may be severely affected, but also to help cut the consequential costs to society as a whole. Such costs include lost productivity and reduced services, as well as the expenditure of a great deal of taxpayers' money on the provision of services for accidents and emergencies, hospital treatment, after care and rehabilitation, as well as social and welfare services, social security, sick pay and insurance schemes.

LEGISLATION AND WORK

A great deal of legislation has been passed in Britain this century to reduce the toll of human suffering and to make working life safer, healthier and more tolerable for able-bodied and disabled people of all ages and to protect their rights as citizens, workers and members of trades unions (see Table 19.1).

The most important statute ever passed to safeguard the health and well-being of all people at work in Britain is the Health and Safety at Work Act 1974 (HASAWA) which became effective in 1975. It supercedes all previous health, safety and welfare legislation in its scope and protects all people at work except domestic servants in the home.

Particular attention has been paid over the years in the various Factories Acts to the protection of women and young people at work. A report published by the Equal Opportunities Commission (1979) the Working Party reviewed the legislation to see what should be done to eliminate, where appropriate, different treatment of men and women. The Commission recommended that legislation on night work, shiftwork and maximum numbers of hours where men and women are treated differently should be repealed, and that provisions should be made instead in relation to job security and accommodating the temporary needs of parents. They also recommend that legislation specifically favouring women should be repealed or amended to afford equal treatment to men and women, and that guid-

Table 19.1 Important legislation related to work and health

1920	Employment of Women, Young Persons & Children Act
1933	Children and and Young Persons Act
1938	The Young Persons (Employment) Act
1944 & 1958	Disabled Persons (Employment) Acts
1944	Education Act
1954	Mines & Quarries Act
1954	Baking Industry (Home & Work) Act
1956	Agriculture (Safety, Health & Welfare Provisions) Act
1957	Occupiers Liability Act
1957	Nurses Act
1960	Professions Supplementary to Medicine Act
1961	Factories Act
1962	Education Act
1963	Offices Shops and Railway Premises Act
1964	Industrial Training Act
1965	Redundancy Payments Act
1969	Employers (Compulsory Insurance) Act
1969	Employers (Defective Equipment) Act
1969	Children and Young Persons Act
1970	Nurses Act
1970	Chronically Sick and Disabled Persons Act
1970	Equal Pay Act
1971	Industrial Relations Act
1971	Mines Management Act
1972	Contracts of Employment Act
1972	Redundancy Payments Act
1973	Employment of Children Act
1973	Education (Work Experience) Act
1974	Health and Safety at Work Act
1974	Trade Union and Labour Relations Act
1974	Rehabilitation of Offenders Act
1974–1976	Trades Union and Labour Relation Acts
1975	Social Security Act
1975	Finance Act
1975	Sex Discrimination Act
1975	Limitation Act
1975	Employment Protection Act
1976	Congenital Disabilities (Civil Liability) Act
1976	Race Relations Act
1976	Fair Employment (NI) Act
1976	Fatal Accidents Act
1977	National Health Service Act
1977	Unfair Contract Terms Act
1977	Safety Representatives and Safety Committees Regulations
1978	Employment Protection (Consolidation) Act
1979	Nurses Midwives and Health Visitors Act

ance on manual lifting and handling should be produced, instead of legislation specifying separate maximum weights for men and women.

Young people under 18 and over the minimum school leaving age (between 15.8 and 16.3 years) are protected by the Factories Act 1961 and the Employment of Women, Young Persons and Childrens Act 1970. Where legislation provided different provisions for male and female young people it is now recommended that they be treated equally. Children and young people who are still at school are protected by the Children and Young Persons Act 1933 (Fife & Machin, 1976) which states that no child may be employed:

1. so long as he is under the age of 13 years
2. before the close of school hours on any day on which he is required to attend school
3. before 7 a.m. or after 7 p.m. on any day
4. for more than two hours on any day in which he is required to attend school
5. to lift, carry or move anything so heavy as to be likely to cause injury to him.

Each local authority is entitled to make its own byelaws with respect to the employment of children and young people under the age of 18 years.

Working people of all ages are protected by the Health and Safety at Work Act of 1974. Under this Act the Health and Safety Commission and Health and Safety Executive were established in 1975. The Health and Safety Commission (HSC) comprises between six and nine members appointed by the Secretary of State for Employment, representing employees, employers, local authorities, professional bodies and others. The Health and Safety Executive (HSE) consists of three people appointed by the Commission, the director of which is approved by the Secretary of State (Fig 19.1). The Secretary of State has powers to make health and safety regulations and to repeal or modify any of the existing legislation. The Commission's powers include the direction of investigation and inquiries and the approval of Codes of Practice. The Executive controls the activities of its professional inspectors, doctors, scientists, administrative, executive and other staff who carry out the functions laid upon them by the Health and Safety at Work Act.

The Act lays a duty upon employers, employees and the self employed to accept responsibility for the health, safety and welfare of themselves and others. It also requires all undertakings employing five or more people to have a written policy for health and safety and that this policy and the arrangements made for carrying it out should be brought to the notice of all employees.

The employers' responsibilities under the Act include providing and maintaining:

1. a safe and healthy work place and working environment
2. plant and systems of work that are safe and without risks to health
3. safe means of entering and leaving any place of work
4. adequate facilities and arrangements for the welfare of people at work
5. arrangements to ensure safety and the absence of risks to health in connection with the use, handling, storage and transport of articles and substances
6. information, instruction, training and supervision to ensure safety and health at work.

Since 1975 when the Health and Safety at Work Act was implemented, the Health and Safety Executive and local authorities have been responsible for enforcing statutory requirements on safety and health. Appointed health and safety inspectors visit work places and can seize, render harmless or destroy any substance or article which they consider to be a cause of imminent danger or personal injury to work people and others. They also have the authority to issue Prohibition Notices, to prohibit the carrying on of an activity giving rise to risk, or Improve-

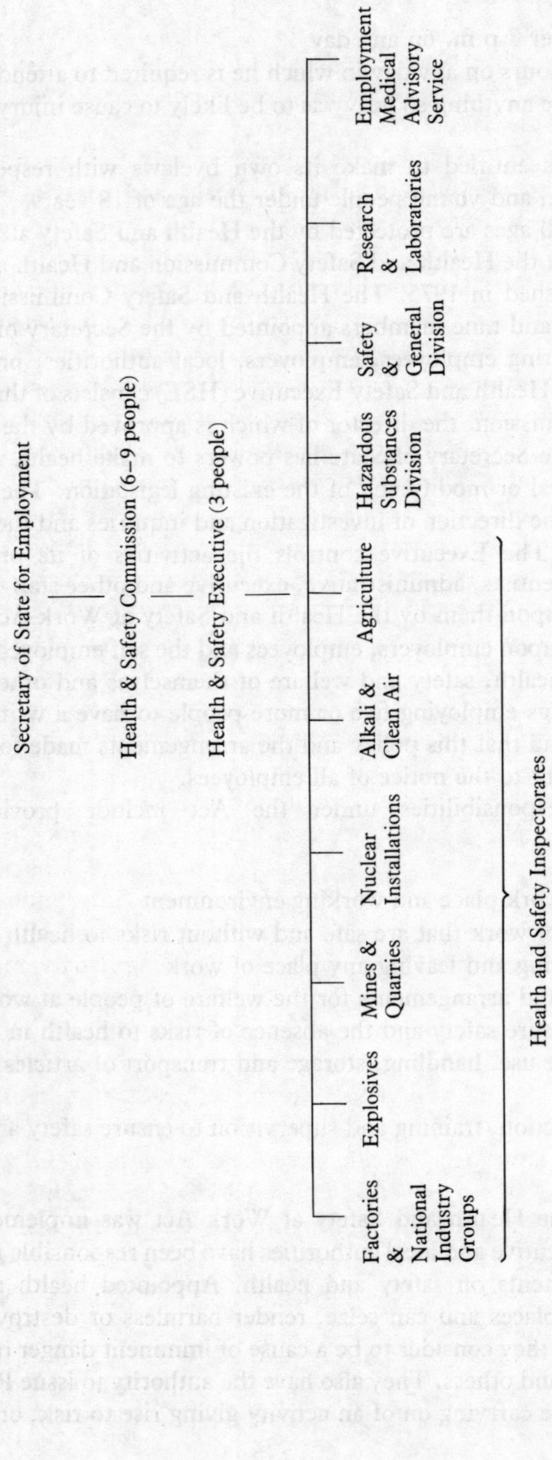

Fig. 19.1 The British Government Health and Safety structure.

ment Notices, requiring remedial action to comply with legislation. Employers are at liberty to appeal to an Industrial Tribunal against such Notices. Contravention of legal requirements may lead to summary prosecution in the Magistrates Court in England and Wales or the Sheriff Court in Scotland or on indictment in the Crown Court in England and Wales or the Sheriff Court in Scotland. Penalties include a fine or imprisonment for up to two years for certain offences.

Safety representatives have now been appointed in many work places by recognized trades unions. Employers are required to consult them whenever they are promoting and developing measures to ensure the health and safety of employees. They are also required to establish safety committees within three months if requested to do so by at least two safety representatives.

The Employment Medical Advisory Service (EMAS) which was established in 1973 is now part of the Health and Safety Executive. EMAS provides an advisory service to employees, employers, trades unions, physicians, nurses and others. Its staff comprises scientists, statisticians, occupational physicians, known as Employment Medical Advisers, and occupational nurses known as Employment Nursing Advisers, and others, all of whom are concerned with the occupational health of people at work (i.e. the safeguarding and improvement of the health of employed people and those in training for employment). Advice can be obtained from staff in its regional and area offices on any subject relating to work and health and frequently the medical and nursing advisers are called upon by health and safety inspectors, employers, employees and others to visit work places, undertake surveys, identify the source or cause of ill-health, to give advice and to recommend appropriate action.

THE EMPLOYER AND THE WORK PLACE

The unconcerned employer who neither complies with legislation nor gives appropriate attention to the people he employs exposes himself to many problems. These may include disgruntled or uncooperative employees, accidents, illness, frequent sickness absence and a high turnover of staff. He may also suffer industrial relations problems and occasional stoppages. Such problems may cause him to receive visits from his insurers, health and safety inspectors, union officials, members of the advisory, conciliation and arbitration service and others and may even result in litigation. Recommendations for remedial action may prove costly in terms of time, effort and lost production. In extreme cases prosecution may arise affecting the reputation of the company or organisation and its product or service causing subsequent recruitment difficulties.

The employer must now make every effort to eliminate from the work place those materials and substances, known to be serious hazards to health and safety. He must seek advice from engineers, research and development staff and from other experts if necessary to discover ways and means of carrying out manufacturing and other processes using less harmful materials, substances and techniques.

As a result of health and safety legislation and the introduction of safety representatives and safety committees into the work place in 1978 there is an increasing awareness of the need to establish safe practices and working procedures and 'permit to work' systems as well as an environment free from hazard. Training and instruction in various aspects of health and safety are obviously essential if people are to work effectively and to understand the reason behind the development of such codes of practice and specific procedures. They must be encouraged to change their attitudes towards risk taking and to become more responsible towards other people, within and outside their work place. The employer cannot confine his energies to his product or service alone, he must now carefully consider his employees. He must look at the effect their work may have upon them and assess the costs and benefits of making improvements. However, when it comes to allocating resources the employer may be faced with the need to choose between improving production or service levels and creating a healthier and safer work place. The competing claims of health and safety legislation, the demands of employee representatives, and shareholders' directions to increase production may cause considerable conflict. Improvements may thus be delayed for long periods unless employee representatives apply pressure, or health and safety inspectors draw upon their statutory powers to issue an Improvement Notice or a Prohibition Order to rectify standards of health, safety and welfare provision which are below minimum legal requirements.

THE NEW EMPLOYEE

The average worker seeking a new job generally hopes for an interesting occupation in a safe and healthy environment. He relies on the employer to provide information about it and from this information makes his decision to accept or reject the post if offered it. Unfortunately a few are prepared to take any job and to accept 'danger' money for extremely hazardous occupations.

Most employers ask at least a few basic questions about health, but not all ensure that where there are or have been health problems an appropriate assessment of the state of health is undertaken by a suitably qualified person, such as an occupational physician or occupational health nurse. Helping to fit people appropriately to occupations, and to make recommendations regarding the adaptation of work to their capabilities, limitations and needs are all part of the proper activities of occupational health personnel.

Those companies and organisations who have a well established occupational health service generally ensure that each new employee completes a comprehensive health questionnaire before commencing work. Some then have a health interview and assessment conducted by the occupational nurse. Many firms employ only a part-time doctor and in these cases new employees may be seen by him. Where a trained occupational nurse is employed she is likely to refer only those cases about whom she is doubtful to the company physician in order to finalise the decision regarding suitability for a specific job.

Before starting work the new employee should be given three types of information relating to his health and safety. He should know in some detail about the hazards he may encounter. He should be told about those health and safety measures which have been adopted for his protection and of procedures which he must adopt. He should also be told about action which is being taken to control or deal with hazards which are relatively new or inadequately contained. Without such information he cannot be expected to act responsibly as an employee or colleague.

THE DISABLED EMPLOYEE

Unfortunately there are a number of people who, as a result of congenital abnormality, birth injury, or subsequent illness or injury, may have a handicapping condition or some residual disability. Employers often find it difficult to acknowledge or accept that disabled people can prove excellent, conscientious and loyal employees. Obviously their choice of work may be limited by the lack of suitable facilities such as ramps, handrails, lifts and internal transport if there are long distances to walk or many stairs to climb. However, some employers are willing to make adaptions and to improve access to toilets, canteens and administrative offices. In many cases it is the ignorance and prejudices of the employer and his managers which cause discrimination against the disabled, although they will often accept back a former reliable employee who has become disabled, whilst not having the confidence to take on someone they do not know.

ACCIDENTS AND INJURIES

Accidents and dangerous occurrences at work are unplanned and unforeseen events which may be caused by many factors and are the result of unsafe acts, unsafe conditions or unsafe people. Unfortunately they continue to result in many serious and incapacitating injuries, disablement and a substantial number of deaths each year.

In 1978 amongst those people covered by existing health and safety legislation, 750 people died as a result of accidents at work and there were over 340 000 reported accidents (Financial Times, 1980). Obviously minor accidents are not reported officially, and statistics were based on those which were sufficiently severe to cause the absence of 3 days or more from work. Employers are now required to report major injuries and fatalities to the Health and Safety Executive, in order that investigations can be instituted where necessary and steps taken to prevent further incidents. The notification of Accidents and Dangerous Occurrences Act (1980) also requires employers to notify dangerous occurrences which include acute poisoning and gassing incidents.

Accidents caused by unsafe acts may be the result of human error, faulty judgement, inexperience and lack of training. Unfortunately recent trends towards piece work and bonuses with the emphasis on speed and high productivity may mean that certain safety rules are overlooked. Guards and safety devices may be removed or tampered with, defective tools and equipment may be used to save delays in finding a replacement or waiting for repairs. Personal protective devices such as goggles, gloves, visors, aprons, and safety boots or shoes may be cast aside in favour of comfort or speed. Essential routines for certain work may be abandoned, or unfamiliar work carried out without authorisation, just 'to be helpful'. The energy and enthusiasm of youth is often relieved in monotonous conditions by practical jokes and horseplay. Unfortunately such activities may result in serious accidents and injury.

The employee who is preoccupied with domestic worries, the nervous trainee terrified of making a mistake, and the man or woman who is feeling strong emotional feelings of anger or fear may be particularly vulnerable. Employees who are generally unwell, in pain, discomfort or running a fever will be unlikely to concentrate totally on their work. Employees who have been prescribed certain drugs such as tranquillizers, hypotensives and antihistamines will also be slower in their reactions and may be quite unsafe in operating a machine or driving a vehicle. Hearing and visual deficiencies will render the individual more accident prone if suitable precautions are not adopted.

OCCUPATIONAL ILL-HEALTH

Ill-health and disease can be caused or influenced by life-style, environment and internal factors, and people who work in a similar environment and are exposed to the same agents are each likely to respond differently. The extent of any adverse reactions will vary with their age, sex, and general constitution and fitness, and will be influenced by previous or coexisting disease, and unsuitable diet, excess alcohol or smoking, fatigue, genetic factors and their endocrine and immunological status. In the work place unusual work practices, idiosyncratic behaviour and inadequate standards of personal hygiene may also prove significant in the development of occupational ill-health or disease.

Increasingly jobs and processes must be designed to suit people of all ages, sizes and states of health taking into account all the above factors to eliminate the possibility of ill effects. The able and disabled must both be considered. More studies are required to evaluate the physical demands which work makes upon fit and healthy people especially affecting their hands, feet, limbs and eyes. Fortunately, many engineers, ergonomists, occupational psychologists and others are now applying their minds to designing and adapting processes, equipment and machinery to fit the capabilities and limitations of human beings. We now have the technical knowledge available to reduce dramatically the stresses to which workers have been exposed in the past. People are less accustomed today to hard physical labour than formerly and lifting and handling devices now available enable backbreaking work to be carried out without risking hernias, prolapsed intervertebral discs and torn muscles.

For many years the various Factories Acts have contained a list of 'Notifiable Diseases'. On receipt of notification of such a condition from a doctor or an employer the Health and Safety Inspectors have the power to investigate the cause and will also request the advice and assistance of the local Employment Medical Adviser (see Table 19.2). The development of Industrial Injuries and Occupational disease compensation legislation over the years has resulted in an increasingly lengthy list of 'Prescribed Diseases' (see Table 19.3). Workmen's compensation is paid to victims of such conditions providing certain criteria are met. Benefits are also paid for certain diseases where the employment which caused the disease was before the establishment of the industrial injuries scheme in July 1948.

The exposure of employed people to toxic substances and other hazards is the

Table 19.2 Notifiable diseases (Fife & Machin, 1976)

Acute, subacute or chronic disease of any organ due to:	
Aniline	
Arsenic	
Benzene	
Beryllium	
Cadmium	Or any of their compounds
Carbon bisulphide	
Lead	
Manganese	
Mercury	
Phosphorous	
Anthrax	
Chrome ulceration due to chromic acid, or bichromate of potassium, sodium or ammonium	
Compressed air illness	
Epitheliomatous ulceration due to tar, pitch, bitumen, mineral oil or paraffin	
Occupational cancer	
Toxic anaemia	
Toxic jaundice due to tetrachloroethane or nitro- or amido-derivatives of benzene	

concern not only of the workers themselves but also of employers, health professionals, trades unions, university departments of occupational health and many others. Mechanical, physical, chemical, biological and psychosocial hazards are being identified in many work places as vigilance and awareness are increased (see Table 19.4). During the decade 1970 to 1980 several hundreds of new chemicals have appeared annually increasing the potential hazards to health. The World Health Organisation has set up a central unit to coordinate international work in assessing their effects on health.

The ill effects of certain hazards may necessitate early retirement on grounds of ill-health. In some circumstances an employee may be dismissed since the employer feels unable to keep him or her on in a state of chronic ill-health or inefficiency despite the fact that his work place may have caused the health problem. The Employment Protection (Consolidation) Act 1975 gives some help to employees in these circumstances but may subsequently result in ill will and poor relationships at work.

Historically the worker himself has been the gauge of working conditions and of atmospheric contamination, reacting and responding according to his general state of health, his knowledge and personality, and the pressures of others as discomfort or irritation develop and as signs and symptoms of mental or physical ill-health appear. He or his representatives have made it quite clear when conditions were no longer fit for work. However, for many years, the law and concerned employers have seen that workers in specific hazardous occupations have been monitored in various ways to assess the effects upon them of exposure to the hazard.

Fortunately health and safety legislation has caused a significant fall in the numbers of occupational diseases diagnosed since the early 1970s. There are, however, still large numbers of people being affected in many occupations by non-fatal but nevertheless incapacitating conditions such as dermatitis, tenosynovitis or periten-

Table 19.3 Prescribed diseases (HMSO, London, 1979)

Disease number
1. Lead or a compound of lead
2. Manganese or a compound of manganese
3. Phosphorus or phosphine or poisoning due to the anticholinesterase action of organic phosphorus compounds
4. Arsenic or a compound of arsenic
5. Mercury or a compound of mercury
6. Carbon bisulphide
7. Benzene or a homologue
8. A nitro- or amino- or chloro-derivative of benzene or of a homologue of benzene or poisoning by nitro-chlorbenzene
9. Dinitrophenol or a homologue or by substituted dinitrophenols or by the salts of such substances
10. Tetrachloroethane
11. Tri-cresyl phosphate
12. Tri-phenyl phosphate
13. Diethylene dioxide (dioxan)
14. Methyl bromide
15. Chlorinated naphthalene
16. Nickel carbonyl
17. Nitrous fumes
18. Gonioma kamassi (African boxwood)
19. Anthrax
20. Glanders
21. (a) Infection by leptospira icterohaemorrhagica
(b) Infection by leptospira canicola
22. Ankylostomiasis
23. (a) Dystrophy of the cornea (including ulceration of the corneal surface) of the eye
(b) Localized new growth of the skin, papillomatous or keratotic
(c) Squamous-celled carcinoma of the skin
24. Now covered by diseases numbered 41 & 42
25. Inflammation, ulceration or malignant disease of the skin or subcutaneous tissue or of the bones, or blood dyscrasia, or cataract, due to electro-magnetic radiations (other than radiant heat), or to ionising particles
26. Heat cataract
27. Decompression sickness
28. Cramp of the hand or forearm due to repetitive movements
29. & 30. Now included in 28
31. Subcutaneous cellulitis of the hand (Beat hand)
32. Bursitis or subcutaneous cellulitis arising at or about the knee due to severe or prolonged external friction or pressure at or about the knee (Beat knee)
33. Bursitis or subcutaneous cellulitis arising at or about the elbow due to severe or prolonged external friction or pressure at or about the elbow (Beat elbow)
34. Traumatic inflammation of the tendons of the hand or forearm or the associated tendon sheaths.
35. Miner's nystagmus
36. Poisoning by beryllium or a compound of beryllium
37. (a) Carcinoma of the mucous membrane of the nose or associated air sinuses
(b) Primary carcinoma of a bronchus or of a lung
38. Tuberculosis
39. Primary neoplasm of the epithelial lining of the urinary bladder (Papilloma of the bladder), or of the renal pelvis or of the ureter or of the urethra
40. Poisoning by cadmium
41. Inflammation or ulceration of the mucous membrane of the upper respiratory passages or mouth produced by dust, liquid or vapour
42. Non-infective dermatitis of external origin (including chrome ulceration of the skin but excluding dermatitis due to ionising particles or electro-magnetic radiations other than radiant heat
43. Pulmonary disease due to the inhalation of the dust of mouldy hay or other mouldy vegetable produce and characterised by symptoms and signs attributable to a reaction in the peripheral part of the bronchopulmonary system, and giving rise to a defect in gas exchange (Farmer's lung)
44. Primary malignant neoplasm of the mesothelium (diffuse mesothelioma) of the pleura or of the peritoneum
45. Adeno-carcinoma of the nasal cavity or associated air sinuses
46. Infection by brucella abortus
47. Poisoning by acrylamide monomer
48. Occupational deafness
49. Viral hepatitis
50a. Angiosarcoma of the Liver
50b. Osteolysis of the terminal phalanges of the fingers
51. Carcinoma of the nasal cavity or associated air sinuses

Source: DHSS notes on the diagnosis of occupational diseases prescribed under the Industrial Injuries Provisions of the Social Security Act 1975. HMSO, London 1979.

Table 19.4 Hazards

Mechanical	*Biological*	
Falls of people } from heights / on the flat	Bacteria	
Falls of materials } from heights / on the flat	Viruses	
Stepping on } objects	Spores	
Striking against } objects		
Struck by a falling object	Fungi	
Use of hand tools	Moulds	
Lifting and handling of	Enzymes	
goods	Parasites	
materials	Insects	
equipment	Animals	
Excavations and tunnelling } (burial entombment, asphyxiation)	Reptiles	
Struck by falls of materials } (burial entombment, asphyxiation)		
Machinery		
power		
non-power		
Transport		
rail		
non-rail		
Use of lifting equipment including hoists & cranes		
Physical	*Chemical*	
Heat	Solids	
Cold	e.g. metals	particles
Humidity	wood	grit
Pressure	rock	dust
high	coal	powders
low	fibres	
Noise	natural	
Vibration	manmade	
Ultrasonics	Liquids	
Electricity	e.g. acids	
Fire	alkalis	
Explosions	oils	
Microwaves	solvents	
Radiation	Fumes	
ionising	Gases	
non-ionising	Vapours	
lasers	Mists	
infra-red		
ultra-violet		
Friction		
Repetitive movements		

donitis crepitans, and the 'beat' conditions mainly a affecting the knees, hands or elbows of those in the mining industry (Health and Safety Executive, 1979). Back pain and back injury cause many lost days from work as well as considerable discomfort and incapacity.

FIRST AID SERVICES

First aid provision in the work place extends beyond the provision of first aid boxes with specific contents required by the law, and trained first-aiders. Depending upon the hazards, various other measures need to be installed or readily available to ensure speedy attention at times of crisis.

For years First Aid legislation in Britain was embodied in numerous Acts, Regulations and Orders. However, the law on first aid has now changed as a result of the new Health and Safety (First Aid) Regulations 1981 (Health and Safety Commission, 1981). This has replaced the existing legislation by across-the-board regulations, a code of practice and guidance notes affecting all employers, workers and self employed people, and certain people working 'off shore'. Certain emergencies, including coronary thrombosis and cerebrovascular accidents, necessitate rescue and transportation of injured, ill and possibly unconscious people from awkward and difficult situations and away from dangers such as electricity and heights. Regular practice sessions should be carried out to ensure that occupational health, safety and rescue staff as well as first aiders have a slick routine and that each is familiar with his or her rôle in such a crisis.

OCCUPATIONAL HEALTH SERVICES

Occupational health services are not required by law in Britain, but many employers are now recognising the value of employing trained occupational nurses, physicians and other specialists, in addition to safety experts and the statutory 'first aiders', in order to provide a comprehensive programme of prevention and care for employees.

The provision of occupational health services varies according to the concern of employers, the resources allocated and to geographical factors. The decision to establish such a service will depend upon the numbers employed, the nature of the hazards in the working environment, management policies, the pressures of safety committees and employee representatives, and legislation.

Many companies and organisations now employ their own occupational health staff ranging from part-time trained nurses without additional occupational health training to a full team of appropriately qualified doctors, nurses, occupational hygienists, technicians and safety advisers. In some cases they may also retain the services of a physiotherapist, chiropodist and dentist. Other firms elect to subscribe to one of the group occupational health services which offers a service to people in factories and other work places nearby. The staff of group services are invariably peripatetic and will visit work places to see employees, to study the working environment and to give advice.

In a discussion document entitled 'Occupational Health Services: The Way Ahead' (Health and Safety Commission, 1977) revealed that only about 2.5% of the firms surveyed, employing 31% of the workforce had both medical and nursing staff.

It is estimated that there are about 9000 nurses in Britain providing some sort of occupational health care for employees of whom about 2000 State Registered Nurses hold the Occupational Health Nursing Certificate.

Occupational health services and advice should now be made available to as many people at work as possible to assist in the appropriate placement of employees, to promote, maintain and restore physical and mental health and to ensure that workers are free from risk.

The activities of an occupational health services are likely to include:

1. pre-employment health screening and recommendations regarding placement
2. regular health supervision, statutory and voluntary, including physiological monitoring when necessary
3. general health advice and referrals when appropriate
4. assessment following sickness absence and advice to employees and management
5. rehabilitation and resettlement following accidents, illness and surgery
6. counselling and referral to appropriate agencies
7. health promotion by means of:
   a. identifying individual employees in need of help, advice and referral, including food handlers
   b. identifying those 'at risk' in their work and recommending appropriate action
   c. health education
8. identification and monitoring of health risks in the working environment
9. supervision of, or treatment of accidents and illness occurring at work
10. Supervision and in-service training of first aiders
11. accident prevention in collaboration with safety officers, safety committees and safety representatives
12. the establishment of contingency plans for major disasters with management and external agencies such as police and ambulance services.
13. advice and recommendations to management, employees and their representatives on health, safety and welfare matters, including the planning and design of new processes or departments, and the appropriateness of protective clothing and devices
14. maintenance of confidential health records and statutory records
15. liaison and cooperation with management, safety advisers, employee representatives, personnel and welfare staff, other health care practitioners and social/welfare agencies, as appropriate.

Ideally the occupational health programme should include the early identification of employees who are at risk not only as a result of work with known or suspected hazards but also those at risks as a result of their own imperfect health. Work in specified processes or with certain chemicals is subject to statutory health surveillance to ensure that early signs of over exposure or ill effects are identified as soon as possible.

Employees who are suffering from chronic ill-health, or are recovering from injury or illness should be able to obtain help from occupational health staff with rehabilitation and resettlement into their old job, or to a new position.

Occupational health staff should work closely with management, personnel staff, safety advisers, committees, representatives and first aiders, as well as other staff representatives. At the same time as maintaining strict confidentiality regarding the affairs and health status of individual employees they should make relevant recommendations to help improve the health and well-being of the workforce. Thus it is essential that they should make regular visits to every department and work place, seeing and talking to staff at all levels in order to identify problems and the causes of ill-health, including inadquate hygiene, and to identify those suffering from deteriorating health.

Occupational health staff can contribute to induction courses, education and training programmes for new employees and those changing to work with new hazards. In describing their service and giving formal and informal advice and demonstrations on health, hygiene and preventive measures, they can encourage new attitudes towards health and the development of personal responsibility and self care. They can also contribute to accident prevention programmes and participate in plans for action in the event of major disaster. They will be expected to provide some form of counselling service, to support people who are emotionally upset, those suffering from mental ill-health, and to give general and specific health advice on a wide range of personal and group problems which may extend beyond the work place. Their links with other health, safety and welfare practitioners and experts will prove invaluable. where food handlers are employed they will be expected to provide particularly close health supervision and appropriate health education in order to protect the consumer.

If the employer has no member of staff who has specialised in occupational health he can call upon the Health and Safety Executive for help and advice and guidance through the Employment Medical and Nursing Advisers. Independent occupational physicians and nurses, hygienists, ergonomists, occupational psychologists, safety consultants and others are also increasingly available to assess problems, give advice and suggest remedies.

Although most employers try to create a safe working environment, the pressures for productivity or the provision of a good service often taken precedence over the need to spend time and money considering ways and means of creating a safer, healthier and more comfortable work place for emplyees. Sometimes, despite legislation, considerable pressure may have to be applied by the workers themselves or by their representatives, in order to persuade the employer or departmental manager to take action to improve unsatisfactory working conditions. Occasionally they may even call in outside experts to confirm that their concern is justified. The well-informed employee, such as a trained safety representative or shop steward, may have to draw the employer's attention to the law and its requirements (see Table 19.1) as the only way of getting an unsatisfactory situation rectified.

An employer is normally in business not only to provide a product or service but to make money. However, it is not possible to run a company, organisation or service satisfactorily without fit and healthy employees who are well trained, motivated and capable of carrying out the work to be done, and appearing at work when expected. It is obvious that the absence of one or more workers as a result of sickness, domestic crisis or other reason is going to prove disruptive.

Occupational health care for workers is now essential. Although working people spend only a part of their life at work, many may spend years in the same hazardous environment. Occupational health staff must now be extremely well informed to keep up with new developments, legislation and the many hazards around. Training is essential. Health workers of all disciplines must meet together regularly, communicate often and cooperate with each other in order to identify the causes of ill-health, ensure that steps are taken wherever possible to alleviate adverse conditions and to promote, restore and maintain those standards of good health to which all people aspire.

REFERENCES

Fife I, Machin E A 1976 Redgraves health and safety in factories. Butterworth, London

Health and Safety Legislation. Should we distinguish between men and women? Equal Opportunities Commission 1979

Health and Safety at Work Act 1974 HMSO, London, ch 37

Health and Safety at Work 1977 Safety Representatives and Safety Committees. Regulations, Code of Practice and Guidance Notes. Health and Safety Commission 1977. HMSO, London

Health and Safety at Work Survey. Financial Times April 18th 1980

Health and Safety Executive 1980 Notification of accidents and dangerous occurrences. Health and Safety Series Booklet HS(R)S. HMSO, London

Health and Safety Executive 1979 Health and Safety statistics, 1976. HMSO, London

Health and Safety Executive 1981 First aid at work. Health and Safety Series Booklet HS(R)11. HMSO, London

Health and Safety Commission 1977 Prevention and health. Occupational health services: The way ahead. Discussion document. HMSO, London

FURTHER READING

Gardner W, Taylor P 1975 Health at work. Associated Business Programmes, London

Tyrer F H, Lees K 1979 A synopsis of occupational medicine. Wright, Bristol

Waldron H A 1976 Lecture notes on occupational medicine. Blackwell Scientific, London

20

Promise to care — The single woman caring for elderly dependants

Sheila Quinn

Thirty years after the foundation of the welfare state it is easy to pretend that statutory services have replaced the family. It is often lamented that the family is a vanishing institution; that the changing roles of women are making it increasingly difficult to provide the tender, loving care for the old that was supposedly characteristic of earlier times in history, in short that the modern family no longer provides the care needed by the elderly sick. It is also postulated that value patterns are shifting away from the virtues of 'duty', 'service' and 'sacrifice' and that personal service is now regarded as demeaning. As a result the remaining solution is 'the warehousing of old sick people in nursing and old age homes.'

It is true with regard to the 'vanishing' family that divorce rates are on the increase, and that increasing numbers of children are being raised in one-parent households and that there are other signs of fragmentation of the family with regard to marital and child rearing roles. However, according to one prominent American psychologist, Neugarten:

> It remains to be seen if the same fragmentation will become true of the parent-caring role. Middle-aged children may continue to come to the aid of their aged parents in the future just as they are still doing in 1976.

Community Care of the elderly can be a very emotive subject, especially as the proportion of the elderly in the population increases every year. The needs of the individual and his family must be balanced against those of society as a whole. Often lip service is paid to the idea of caring for the aged in a non-institutional setting without provision of any extra resources to this end. Contrary to popular myth, the vast majority of old people are still looked after by relatives and friends. The proportion in residential institutions is no higher today than it was 50 years ago. Only about 5% of the elderly population are cared for outside of some type of family situation.

One often forgotten group when one refers to the family, is the large number of single women who devote a long period of their life to an elderly infirm relative, but whose situation is often neglected and whose contributions of care are often taken for granted. There are an estimated 310 000 single women involved in caring for elderly relatives and they have been credited with saving the welfare state large sums of money, when one considers the increase in various statutory services like meals-on-wheels, home helps and sheltered accommodation that would be needed if their services were withdrawn. Few of this group avail themselves of these services and with the growing pressure on resources they are increasingly encouraged to manage on their own.

Little financial aid is specifically available to help this group apart from the Attendance Allowance and the Invalid Care Allowance. The Attendance Allowance is paid tax free, without test of means, and in addition to any other income or benefits being received, if the patients require either constant attention in respect of body functions or constant supervision to prevent danger to themselves or others. There are two rates, the higher one for those needing attention or supervision by day and night, the lower one for those needing attention day or night. It is not necessary for anyone to give up work before the Attendance Allowance can be claimed, but the current rate would not go very far to meeting the cost of help in the home in order that the carer can continue on working. Anyone under pensionable age (except married women under certain circumstances) who does give up work to look after a relative, who receives the Attendance Allowance, may be able to claim the Invalid Care Allowance. This seems small compensation for the financial, social and emotional problems that can develop. It is only since 1978 when the Home Responsibilities Protection Regulations were introduced that state pension rights for those who give up work for home caring have been protected.

How does this caring situation of single woman caring for aging patient arise? It is related to the kinship ties which are still very much in evidence today especially among the working class community. It is still common to find the family rallying round to look after parents as they grow older.

In *Family and Kinship in East London*, a study of Bethnal Green in 1955 Young and Wilmott, illustrated this local kinship system of the ties between mother and daughter which help to form the extended family.

In contrast, Fletcher in *The Family and Marriage in Britain*, refutes the argument about the family of the past being more caring: 'The modern family fulfils more functions than did the family before or during the 19th century development of industrialisation.'

In the general conclusion of Townsend's survey of old people also in Bethnal Green, a working class area of London, he states

> If many of the processes and problems of ageing are to be understood old people must be studied as members of families (which usually means extended families of three generations); and if this is true, those concerned with social and health administration must at every stage, treat the old as an inseperable part of a family group, which is more than just a residential unit.

Studies have shown that it is rare for a working class child to leave home before marriage, and the sense of duty and attachment to the home are particularly strong if one parent dies. Townsend's survey of old people in Bethnal Green shows that in such a situation the child may delay marriage, sometimes indefinitely, in order to stay with the remaining parent. Children appear to substitute as fathers and occasionally as mothers, and this seems to be the way the family adjusts to the loss of a member. As time passes, the older children feel they can move away from the home district leaving other siblings there. Thus emerges a close tie between the parent and the youngest children and one child usually remains near-at-hand.

Studies have found that the most frequent type of household in terms of siblings and relatives is that of daughters caring for aged parents. Brockington & Lampert

(1966) in their studies of a group of Stockport's over-80s found that 26.7% of the men and 31.7% of the women were cared for by daughters.

In the Townsend Bethnal Green investigation, 24% of the old people lived with an unmarried child and the cross-national study by Shamus et al, (1968) of old people who were living with other relatives, over half were with an unmarried child.

The situation is universal. Bernice Neugarten sums it up in *Care of The Elderly*:

> In 1970, it was clear that the older the individual and the sicker, the more likely he or she would be living with a child. It often goes unnoticed that at present, in the United States, for every older person living in an institution, there are some 2.5 others living with a child.

Evidence indicates that without the aid of relatives the welfare services in relation to the elderly would need to be extended considerably. Brockington & Lampert (1966) found that:

> Old people living with their children, and particularly those living with daughters and single sons, inspite of the greater amount of disability suffered by them, had made the least calls on the welfare state.
>
> There are a significant excess of persons who had been living alone among the institutional population, whereas those who had been living with the younger generation or with other persons were under represented.

The strain on the carer can result in a heavy burden, especially when other responsibilities are involved. Trevor Howell (1970) points out in his survey of 500 patients about to be admitted to a geriatric unit:

> Sometimes the son or daughter happened to be the breadwinner of the home as well as the attendant. In such circumstances continued absence from work often jeopardized the latter's career. It was noted that very old parents in particular readily wore out elderly daughters.

Shenfield (1957) points out:

> Some daughters looking after parents may suffer ill-health and strain themselves, and are frequently prevented from enjoying activities outside the home or taking regular holidays. Sometimes the strain created leads to reproaches and unhappy relationships and increases the feelings of hopelessness and dependance experienced by an infirm old person.

Little research has been done specifically into the plight of single women involved in this caring situation. However, The National Council for the Single Woman and her Dependants formed specifically with the needs of this group in mind, has piloted an investigation of the problems encountered by its members. A postal survey of 360 women was carried out in 1977. Low income was found to be the main problem with 50% of all respondents having no paid employment and a large number were in receipt of benefits like the Attendance Allowance. It was found that many women devoted a great deal of time to caring, both in terms of actual hours spent daily and the number of years they had been involved in this role. 40% of the respondents had been involved in caring for a period of 3–15 years with 25% involved in this activity on a 24 hour basis.

Loneliness was a frequent complaint as so much time had to be given up to caring that it was often impossible to maintain personal friendships. The longer the time spent in caring, the more acute the loneliness became. A significant number, 18% of dependants showed some form of mental incapacity. Another problem encountered concerned mother/daughter domination in the relationship. This is an important factor that can be overlooked when counselling this group. One of the main conclusions reached by the report, that is significant to health workers involved in community care, was the areas in which it was felt they needed counselling, e.g. decisions concerning giving up work, the possible implications of the caring role extending over one or two decades, benefits and help they were entitled to, help with planning a caring routine, and the psychological implications that may arise out of the situation.

These conclusions formed the basis for a survey undertaken by the author, looking at the attitudes of health visitors towards this group, and their knowledge of problems experienced as a result of the situation. Health visitors were chosen for a number of reasons. Previous studies (Whitfield, 1972) have shown that the main professional workers, if any, that these carers came into contact with were district nurses, general practitioners and, occasionally, the clergy. Rarely did the health visitor become involved.

However, using the definitions of the role of health visiting in relation to health and the individual put forward by various authors, the potential for providing the professional help needed by this group, becomes evident.

In 1956 the Jamieson Report on Health Visiting stated:

> In association with the general practitioner the health visitor will be concerned with a wider range of families than any other comparable worker. She thus has the opportunity to act as a common point of reference and source of standard information, a common advisor on health teaching, a 'common factor' in family welfare.

This viewpoint was emphasised more recently in a report commissioned by The Council for the Education and Training of Health Visitors, (1977) An Investigation into the Principles of Health Visiting, which defined the unique position the health visitor was in which could help her when working with this group; as she could 'identify emerging problems as needs before there is a general awareness, "expert" agreement or societal willingness to admit the need.'

Also conducive to the needs of this group, who are often housebound by their duties, is the major setting of the health visitor's work, the home. Most of the carers interviewed by Whitfield wanted occasionally to be able to talk the problem over with someone with a nursing background who would be able to discuss the question of bodily functions.

It was considered that the health visitor, with her nursing background, knowledge and awareness of the sociological and psychological problems that can affect an individual, and 'licence' to visit all families, healthy as well as ill, in the home environment, has a lot of scope to provide assistance to this group.

The research was undertaken in one inner London area which was judged to have an average social class mixture, ratio of elderly in the population and in relation to health visitors, a reasonable number working in general practice attachment. Out of a total of 30 health visitors, six of whom were general practice attached, 20 returned a questionnaire formulated to find out the extent, if any, and nature of their involvement with single carers and finally what potential role they saw for themselves when working with this group.

The respondents were divided into two groups, those that had had contact with a single woman caring for an elderly dependant (Group A) and those who had had no contact (Group B.) Group A, consisting of six health visitors, two of whom were general practice attached, gives weight to Whitfield's findings that the majority of these carers are often only in contact with the general practitioner out of all the professionals in the primary health care team. The majority of referrals had been through the general practitioner, however, an increasing number are being received from hospitals on discharge of an elderly relative.

The majority of health visitors saw the potential for the development of social, emotional and financial problems. Alcoholism and psychiatric problems as a result of this situation were also highlighted.

The majority also saw the need for professional support, e.g. counselling, as well as more practical help, i.e. sorting out entitlement to benefits. Both groups agreed with the idea that the health visitor has the potential ability to develop a central role with this group. Various suggestions as to the future role of the health visitor included mobilising resources, i.e. home helps and aids for the disabled, regular home visits to monitor and reassess home situations as to the needs of both the elderly dependant and carer, referral to an other agency, counselling, organizing voluntary sitters who generally build up a supportive relationship with the carer in order that she will have someone to turn to in times of stress. It was also felt that the social services should take a more active part in assisting this group.

The fact that the sample who had been in contact with this group of carers was small, indicates perhaps how neglected this group is. Whitfield in her study had to canvas a number of inner London Boroughs to construct her sample of 20 carers actually known to the social services.

Sadly, with the recent expenditure cuts to the social services and the possibility of more to follow and the rallying call for a return to 'the caring family' and more voluntary services, it is easy to overlook this group who take so little from the social services, while devoting often a large part of their adult life to fulfilling a 'promise to care.'

It is to be hoped that health visitors will take the lead in pointing the way for all health workers engaged in primary health care and committed to preventative medicine, in providing professional support and counselling to this group.

FURTHER READING

Brockington F, Lampert S M 1966 The social needs of the over 80s. Manchester University Press, Manchester
Exon-Smith A N, Grimley-Evans J 1977 Care of the elderly. Academic Press, London
Fletcher R 1966 The family and marriage in Britain. Penguin, London
Howell T H 1970 A students' guide to geriatrics. Staples Press, London
Jack S A (Chairman) 1977 An investigation into the principles of health visiting. CETHV, London
Land H 1977 Who cares for the family? Journal of Social Policy 7 (3)
Shamus E et al 1968 Old people in three industrial societies. Routledge and Kegan Paul, London
Shenfield B E 1957 Social policies for old age. Routledge and Kegan Paul, London
Townsend P 1963 The family life of old people. Penguin, London
Whitfield S 1972 The burden of caring. Unpublished Social Sciences Project, submitted to City University
Young M, Willmott P 1957 Family and kinship in East London. Penguin, London

21

Alcoholism in the community

Keith J. B. Rix and Elizabeth M. Lumsden Rix

In the United Kingdom the prevalence of alcoholism is increasing at an alarming rate. While a small proportion of alcoholics are to be found in prisons and hospitals, the vast majority are in the community. However, only the tip of the iceberg is recognised by community agencies (Table 21.1). The overall prevalence varies from one part of the country to another but the high proportion of undetected alcoholism is a consistent finding. What is more, the actual prevalence of alcoholism itself underestimates the magnitude of the problem. For every alcoholic there is usually a spouse and children whose health, well-being and, sometimes, lives are endangered. The government has not been unaware of this serious problem and within the last few years its Advisory Committee on Alcoholism has reported.

Table 21.1 Alcoholics known or unknown to agencies in Camberwell, London (based on Edwards et al, 1973, with the permission of the Royal College of Psychiatrists).

Sex	Prevalence rates	
	Alcoholics known to agencies*	Alcoholics identified by house-to-house survey†
Males	8.6	61.3
Females	1.3	7.7

* Per 1000 aged 16 years or over
† Per 1000 aged 18 years or over

A ROLE FOR COMMUNITY HEALTH WORKERS

The Advisory Committee on Alcoholism (1978) identified the primary health care team as one of several groups which should be able to provide treatment and care for the majority of alcoholics at what is called 'the primary level', the level at which the alcoholic makes contact with the services and where the problem is recognised. It is distinguished from 'the secondary level' whose workers have had special training relevant to alcoholism.

The report states that the main tasks of primary level workers should be:

1. to recognise problem drinking and its causes and effects
2. to have an adequate knowledge of the help required by the problem drinker and the family
3. to give help as far as it lies within their scope

4. to know when and where to seek more expert help
5. to provide continuing care and support before, during and after any period of specialist treatment
6. to provide adequate follow-up.

In relation to the primary health care team in particular it is stated that the team has considerable opportunity to identify problem drinkers but its aim should also be to provide treatment and care.

Four basic elements of care are delineated as the responsibility of secondary level workers:

1. specialised knowledge, advice and support to primary level agencies
2. 'second opinion' interviews of clients and families
3. depending on the outcome of the assessment in (1)and (2), acceptance to secondary care. This is a shared responsibility between primary and secondary levels. The emphasis must be on teamwork
4. specialist forms of treatment — general medical, psychiatric and counselling.

HOW COMMUNITY HEALTH WORKERS VIEW ALCOHOLISM

The advisory committee's recommendations have to be placed in the context of community health workers' knowledge and perceived capabilities in relation to alcohol problems. A Scottish study in the Lothians found that staff in non-specialist agencies were 'noticeably lacking in confidence with regard not only to dealing with alcoholics, but in identifying the problem and treating clients in the early stages' (Bell & Rae, 1978).

Detailed study of a variety of professionals has revealed that they feel insecure in responding to patients with alcohol problems because: (a) they lack appropriate knowledge; (b) they lack techniques in the special area of counselling the person with alcohol problems; (c) they are pessimistic about the likely outcome of their intervention in relation to the drinker or his family; and (d) they lack confidence in their own abilities in this field and often appear anxious at the thought of working with problem drinkers (Cartwright et al, 1975). Nurses specifically lack appropriate knowledge of alcohol problems and may have negative attitudes towards alcoholics. Wilkins (1972) surveyed student health visitors before they were given a lecture on alcoholism and concluded that they lacked sufficient knowledge of alcoholism to enable them to perform their work adequately. Rotheram (1980) examined male student and qualified psychiatric nurses and found that even 'qualified nurses could benefit from basic information about alcohol'. More alarming was his finding that the qualified nurses had less positive attitudes towards alcoholics than the student nurses.

PREPARING COMMUNITY HEALTH WORKERS FOR THEIR RECOMMENDED ROLES

Cartwright et al (1978) have suggested that certain requirements must be met before community workers can function effectively with alcoholics:

1. information about alcohol problems;
2. techniques for working with drinkers;
3. support and supervision;
4. clear definition of their role and contribution to the management of a case.

This chapter is intended to provide some of the information which community health workers will need to meet these requirements for participation in the recognition, treatment and care of alcoholics. In addition, the role of the community health worker in prevention will be discussed.

THE RECOGNITION, TREATMENT AND CARE OF PROBLEM DRINKERS

Information about alcohol problems

Current concepts

The World Health Organisation (Edwards et al, 1977a) has defined an *alcohol related disability* as: 'An impairment in the physical, mental or social functioning of an individual of such nature that it may be reasonably inferred that alcohol is part of the causal nexus determining that disability'. The definition is a broad one since it covers impairments which may be caused by a single episode of alcohol intoxication as well as those related to the repeated drinking of alcohol. Table 21.2 shows some alcohol-related disabilities commonly encountered in the community.

Table 21.2 Some common alcohol-related disabilities

Physical	Gastritis
	Peptic ulceration
	Pancreatitis (acute and chronic)
	Accidents (road, industrial, home)
Mental	Anxiety states
	Depression
	Morbid jealousy
	Parasuicide
	Dementia
Social	Loss of friends
	Debts
	Monday morning absenteeism
	Lost job
	Marital breakdown
	Driving offences
	Criminal offences

The World Health Organisation has identified one particular variety of alcohol-related disability for special attention and this is the *alcohol dependence syndrome*. Its leading symptom is regarded as an impaired control over intake of alcohol and it has a number of 'essential elements' (Edwards & Gross, 1976). These are (a) an increasingly stereotyped pattern of drinking in which the normal variability according to social situation or mood is lost, (b) a progressive increase in the importance of obtaining alcohol so that it climbs higher and higher on the drinker's list of priorities with increasing costs in the context of health, family and work, (c) an increased tolerance to alcohol so that more alcohol is needed for the desired effect, (d) the development of withdrawal symptoms ranging from tenseness, apprehension, restlessness and tremor with nausea or vomiting to soaking sweats and occasionally even seizures or hallucinations, (e) the relief or avoidance of withdrawal symptoms by further drinking, (f) the subjective awareness of a compulsion to drink and (g) reinstatement of the syndrome after abstinence. It is important to realise that disabilities can occur without dependence on alcohol and sometimes a mild or even moderate degree of dependence may not be accompanied by significant disabilities. Enquiry about both disabilities and dependence is part of the assessment of the alcoholic.

The detection of hidden alcoholism

The community health worker who sets out to detect the hidden alcoholics in the community can now take advantage of the findings of recent epidemiological and clinical studies which have allowed the definition of various groups at high risk of being alcoholic. Some of these are listed in Table 21.3.

These 'at risk' factors can be used to compile an 'At Risk Register' for an individual general practice or health centre. The idea originates from the pioneering work of Wilkins (1974) who identified a number of the groups listed in Table 21.3. In its simplest form the register has two components. First, the records of patients regarded as 'at risk' can be tagged to indicate to the next person using

Table 21.3 Factors indicating increased risk of alcoholism

Occupational	Alcohol beverage trade
	Hotel, restaurant, and catering staff
	Fishermen, seamen, boatmen and bargemen
	Financiers, insurance brokers and financial agents
	Lorry drivers' mates and van guards
	Railway workers
	Electrical engineers, winders and reelers
	Authors, journalists and related workers
	Medical practitioners
Family history	First degree relative alcoholic
	Behaviour problems in children
	Anxiety or depression in spouse
Medical history	Any of the conditions listed in Table 21.2
	Plus: epilepsy (onset after 25 years)
	tuberculosis
Social history	Child neglect
	Family disharmony
	Suspected abuse of self certification of incapacity to work
	Three or more spells of absence from work in previous year for 3 days or less
	Three or more jobs in previous year
	Record of criminal convictions
	Financial or accommodation problems
Home conditions	Cigarette burns on carpets, furniture or bedclothes
	Alcohol in bedroom
	Large quantities of 'empties'
Physical appearance	Obesity (if male)
	Smell of alcohol on breath
	Hoarse voice
	Oedematous facies
	Dilatation of facial or conjunctival vessels
	Cigarette burns on hands or chest
	Multiple bruises, abrasions or lacerations
	Signs of liver disease

them that alcoholism is under suspicion or that evidence for it should be sought. Secondly, each time a case record is tagged, a card bearing the name of the patient goes into a card index. When the diagnosis has been either confirmed or refuted the card can be removed. At regular intervals someone should go through the card index and make up a list of those patients who have not subsequently been seen. Discussion can then take place concerning the possibility of a special review for some or all of them.

Techniques for working with problem drinkers

The acquisition of technical skills depends rather more on demonstration and supervised practice than theoretical accounts so this section is scarcely even an introduction to the methods which are employed in assisting alcoholics to change their pattern of drinking or reduce the causative factors or remedy the various problems which have resulted from their drinking.

Broaching the subject

Having once decided that alcohol is almost certainly causing dependence or harm, someone will need to broach the subject with tact and care to avoid alienating the patient. What needs to be avoided is what Edwards (1968) has called 'the careless frontal attack' and likened to the caption from an old-fashioned *Punch* joke:

Doctor (not knowing what he means by the term): Do you admit you're an alcoholic?

Patient (not understanding the term any more than the doctor but sensing it's an insult): Certainly not!

Edwards' paper still bears reading for its masterly account of how to approach a patient with a suspected drinking problem.

It may be useful to note that it is often possible to talk to a patient without using the words 'alcoholic' and 'alcoholism'. It is often possible to talk about alcohol-related disabilities as 'problems related to drink' and dependence as 'depending too much on alcohol' or 'relying too much on the drink'.

Taking a drinking history and setting goals

Before any help can be offered to the problem drinker it is necessary to understand how the person comes to be in the situation he is and what the dimensions of the problems are. Attention must be given to the various constitutional, personality, interpersonal, social, occupational and cultural determinants of the drinking habits (Rix & Lumsden Rix, in press). The degree and extent of alcohol dependence have to be established as these will have implications for the choice of treatment goal (abstinence or harm-free drinking) and also for the likely need of drug or hospital treatment during the initial period of alcohol withdrawal. Asking in detail about consumption over the previous week and about episodes of drinking not only gives information about the extent of dependence and disabilities and the current determinants of the drinking but it may reveal strengths and assets already being utilised to prevent the problem getting worse. The more detailed the inventory of the disabilities, as also the analysis of the causal factors, the more detailed will be the set of goals which the community health worker and patient will set. The application of the Nursing Process will assist greatly in providing a framework for this aspect of intervention in alcohol problems.

Giving advice

For male alcoholics with an intact marriage a single concentrated package of well-considered and individually tailored advice given to the alcoholic and his wife together and based on a thorough analysis of the alcoholism and all its antecedents and maintaining factors can be as effective as a standard treatment programme with the usual blend of inpatient and outpatient psychiatric treatment (Edwards, et al, 1977b). This research has led to an increasing optimism in alcoholism treatment and a shift towards simpler and less costly types of intervention.

The nature of the advice will, of course, depend on the nature of the problems and related targets. Unlike the research study where the whole process of assessment and advice was carried out in a single morning in an outpatient clinic, it will often be necessary or appropriate in the community to spread these over a number of contacts with the alcoholic and his family.

Counselling alcoholics and their families

Some community health workers will find themselves going further than simply giving advice. They will counsel alcoholics and their families using methods which will vary according to their training and experience. It is not intended that community health workers should necessarily be psychotherapists but since they are increasingly drawn into the psychosocial aspects of family life, most are already involved in counselling and the use of psychological skills in their daily work. Ford (in preparation) found that in his provision of an alcoholism advisory service to a primary health care team 'the primary care staff (had) sound counselling ability' without having had formal training.

Regardless of the choice of technique the health worker has to assist the alcoholic, and the family if one exists, to take over full responsibility for what happens about the alcoholism. One of the unwanted side-effects of the disease concept of alcoholism has been the view that the responsibility for the outcome of the condition lies not with the alcoholic or family but with the therapist in line with the traditional model of disease in which the patient is the passive recipient of the therapist's treatment. This is particularly a problem with inadequate or dependent personality types.

Knowing when to refer

There exists a range of non-specialist and specialist services which may make important contributions to the treatment of individual patients. How far a community health worker needs to refer to such services will depend on both the nature of the individual's problems and the experience and skills of the worker. A health worker who can provide advice but not counselling may need to refer a patient or family when it becomes apparent that advice is not enough. The counselling may be provided by someone else in the primary health care team, a specialist agency such as a local council on alcoholism, a local authority social worker, or the local psychiatric service. When psychiatric referral is needed (Rix, 1981) referral should, as a rule, be to a general psychiatry service in the first instance unless the regional alcoholism treatment unit is geographically accessible and within the health district or health authority. When peer support seems of likely value the patient and family may be referred to the local branches of Alcoholics Anonymous and Al-Anon or Ala-Teen respectively.

Support and supervision

The when and where of referral become less problematic if adequate support and supervision are available. These may take different forms depending on local circumstances.

The Advisory Committee on Alcoholism has envisaged that community health workers should have access to a local community-based team from which to seek help in the treatment of more difficult cases. It has envisaged that such a team should comprise 'as a minimum, a psychiatrist — perhaps part-time — a nurse, social worker and voluntary counsellor, all with specialist skills'. The Lothian Liaison Committee on Alcohol-Related Problems (1978) has produced detailed proposals for a 'community alcohol team' and its tasks are shown in Table 21.4.

Table 21.4 Tasks of a community alcohol team (adapted, with permission, from a report of the Lothian Committee on Alcohol-Related Problems, 1978)

Provision of information to primary level workers concerning alcohol problems and their recognition
Provision of information about available help in the area
Support and consultation to primary level workers
Acceptance of some referrals for treatment or supervision of primary level workers on specific cases
Coordination of alcohol-related services in the area
Demonstration of new ways of tackling alcohol-related problems

There are some other approaches which could be regarded either as alternatives to or forerunners of the community alcohol team. Clarke (1980) has described a method by which a psychiatrist has provided supervision through case discussions for those health visitors involved with families with psychosocial problems. Ford (in preparation) has described how a community psychiatric nurse has provided education, training and supervision for general practitioners and health visitors working with problem drinkers and their families. Ford's model differs from that of Clarke in that the specialist often sees the problem drinker or spouse with the member of the primary health care team.

Role definitions and contributions to the management of cases

A discussion of the role which a particular community health worker adopts in relation to a particular patient brings into focus the issue of professional boundaries. Potential conflicts may arise between health visitor, community nurse and social worker when boundaries overlap (Sladden, 1979) and health visitors, for a variety of reasons, may find themselves doing 'social work' (Clark, 1974). It has been commented that there is a danger that 'by trying to avoid mutual encroachment, social workers and nurses may leave untilled a vast and potentially fertile tract of territory' (Sladden, 1979). Many alcoholics are to be found in this territory so some attempt at a definition of the roles of community health workers in relation to alcoholism is vitally important.

All community health workers are in a position to recognise alcoholics but who broaches the subject depends both on the confidence and competence of the health worker and on who knows the patient best. Whoever broaches the subject is probably the person best placed to begin an evaluation of the patient's problems. Without exception the general practitioner should be involved in this process and he will, in any case, have to examine the alcoholic at an early stage and investigate medical problems. The definition of problems and the setting of targets will, in most cases, be a joint exercise undertaken by the general practitioner and another member of the primary health care team.

Although the nature of the problems may call for the involvement of various members of the primary health care team, it is important that one member of the team, not necessarily the general practitioner, should have oversight of the patient and seek to assist the patient in changing his or her pattern of alcohol consumption and reducing the factors which have caused the drinking problem.

The general practitioner will plan and supervise domiciliary withdrawal from alcohol (Ritson, 1979) and arrange for a district nurse (Rix, 1979) or health visitor to monitor the progress of withdrawal. The district nurse may have a special role in relation to the traumatic and medical or surgical complications of alcoholism (Rix, 1979) but the health visitor will probably have much more to do with families in which child abuse or the foetal alcohol syndrome exist. An attached social worker will probably be the person of choice when marital or other interpersonal difficulties figure prominently but some health visitors and district nurses find themselves providing some limited advice in this area. Community psychiatric nurses usually limit themselves to the aftercare of alcoholics discharged from hospital treatment programmes but where they have an attachment to a particular practice or health centre, they may take responsibility for cases where a greater experience of psychotherapeutic or behavioural techniques is indicated but in which hospital treatment is not necessarily indicated or feasible.

There are few rigidly defined roles for the various members of the primary health care team. Flexibility and an awareness of one's own and one's colleagues' limitations are all important.

THE PREVENTION OF ALCOHOLISM

Although the prevention of alcoholism is probably to a large extent a matter for politicians, there are some important roles for the primary health care team (Scottish Council on Alcoholism, 1978; Rix and Lumsden Rix, in press). These include the provision of alcohol education to children and to people who have an increased risk of alcoholism.

The Scottish Council on Alcoholism (1978) has recommended that alcohol education should be a continuing process from mid-primary school onwards. Parents provide the first learning experiences for most children and community health workers, in particular health visitors, have the opportunity to discuss alcohol education with the parents of young families. Sometimes the opportunities arise in families where there are problems but they may also arise with normal families seen in the context, for example, of a 'well baby clinic'. Health visitors who are attached to schools may be able to assist in organising a programme of alcohol education which is integrated with the rest of the school curriculum (Scottish Council on Alcoholism, 1978). Community health workers themselves should probably avoid talking to school children collectively about alcohol since there is a risk that as 'experts from outside' they may add to the mystique of alcohol which could be counter-productive.

Health visitors may not have the time to give individual advice on alcohol education to all the parents of young families but the families of alcoholics deserve special attention. The children of both sexes have an increased risk of alcoholism themselves and yet they are less likely than most children to be exposed to an example of responsible drinking.

The next best predictor of alcoholism is probably occupation. The occupational groups listed in Table 21.3 constitute appropriate targets for health education and any community health worker who has contact with people in these groups should be able to offer appropriate education and advice. The occupational health service nurse may have particular opportunities both at the individual level and through organised courses to bring information to the attention of employees.

In addition to these and other groups specifically at risk there are those people who are at risk merely by virtue of their excessive consumption of alcohol. Here prevention is particularly appropriate for males who drink more than the equivalent of about four pints of ordinary strength beer or eight standard measures of spirits daily and for females who drink more than the equivalent of between two and three pints of beer daily or more than five measures of spirits daily.

An important female target group is pregnant women since the foetus appears especially sensitive to alcohol. A foetal alcohol syndrome has been described which comprises a growth deficiency persisting from before birth, facial, cardiac and limb defects and mental deficiency. There are other non-specific abnormalities which also appear to be related to maternal heavy drinking and what is encouraging is

Table 21.5 Some rules for safe drinking (adapted from Rix K J B 1979 Alcohol: Questions and Answers, with the permission of the Scottish Council on Alcoholism)

1. Set yourself a limit and do not exceed it
2. Know how much over how long a time makes you drunk — drink less over a longer time
3. Measure your drink carefully
4. Dilute spirits with at least as much water or something non-fizzy to slow absorption
5. Avoid 'topping up' — wait until your glass is empty
6. Avoid drinking on an empty stomach — if possible, restrict drinking to meal times or when food is available
7. Sip your drink — don't gulp it
8. Break the 'rounds' system — drink at your own speed
9. Avoid making lunch-time drinking a habit
10. Learn to enjoy a non-alcoholic drink
11. Provide food and non-alcoholic drinks for your guests as well as alcoholic drinks
12. Do not force an alcoholic drink on someone who declines it
13. If you go to a party, take a taxi or select a non-drinker to do the driving
14. Do not laugh at the drunk
15. Do not use alcohol to solve emotional problems
16. Avoid drinking as a means of 'unwinding'
17. Avoid alcohol as a night-cap
18. Do not drink to intoxication
19. Remember that alcohol and drugs may not mix
20. Examine your drinking habits each year and be alert to signs of a developing alcohol problem

that these, at least, appear preventable through the encouragement of the expectant mother to reduce her alcohol consumption during pregnancy (Rosett et al, 1977).

Central to much of alcohol education is the concept of healthy, safe or responsible drinking. Table 21.5 lists some of the rules by which safe drinking is usually governed. Immunity from alcohol problems is not guaranteed to those who observe these rules but, in view of the importance which remitted problem drinkers and alcoholics attach to such simple measures as advice from health professionals (Saunders and Kershaw, 1979), it would be foolish for community health workers not to offer the simple guidance which could be all important in stopping or reversing the development of a problem which has been correctly identified as having reached epidemic proportions.

REFERENCES

Advisory Committee on Alcoholism 1978 The pattern and range of services for problem drinkers. Department of Health and Social Security and the Welsh Office. HMSO, London

Bell E, Rae E 1978 Responding to alcohol-related problems in the Lothians. Scottish Council on Alcoholism (unpublished)

Cartwright A K J, Shaw S J, Spratley T A 1975 Designing a community response to problems of alcohol abuse. Report to the Department of Health and Social Security by the Maudsley Alcohol Pilot Project

Cartwright A K J, Harwin J E, Shaw S J, Spratley T A 1978 Implementing a community-based response to problems of alcohol abuse. Report to the Department of Health and Social Security by the Maudsley Alcohol Pilot Project

Clark J 1974 The health team in action. British Broadcasting Corporation, London

Clarke M G 1980 Psychiatric liaison with health visitors. Health Trends 12: 98–100

Edwards G 1968 Patients with drinking problems. British Medical Journal 4: 435–437

Edwards G, Gross M M 1976 The alcohol dependence syndrome: provisional description of a clinical syndrome. British Medical Journal 1: 1058–1061.

Edwards G, Gross M M, Keller M, Moser J, Room R 1977a Alcohol related disabilities. WHO Offset Publication No 32. World Health Organisation, Geneva.

Edwards G, Hawker A, Hensman C, Peto J, Williamson V 1973 Alcoholics known or unknown to agencies: epidemiological studies in a London suburb, British Journal of Psychiatry 123: 169–183.

Edwards G, Orford J et al 1977b Alcoholism: a controlled trial of 'treatment' and 'advice'. Journal of Studies on Alcohol 38: 1004–1031.

Ford T An alcohol advisory service for a health centre. (in preparation)

Lothian Liaison Committee on Alcohol-Related Problems 1978 Alcohol-related problems: a shared response in the Lothians. Edinburgh.

Ritson B 1979 Detoxification — and who needs it? Update 20: 607–612.

Rix K J B 1979 Alcoholism and the district nurse. Nursing Times Community Outlook 75: 275–280.

Rix K J B A 1981 strategy for intervention in alcohol problems. Update 23: 1057–1063

Rix K J B, Lumsden Rix E M Alcohol problems: A guide for nurses and other health professionals. Wright, Bristol (in press)

Rosett H L, Ouellette E, Weiner L, Owens E 1977 The prenatal clinic: a site for alcoholism prevention and treatment. In: Seixas F A (ed) Currents in alcoholism, vol. 1. Grune & Stratton, New York

Rotheram F 1980 Nurses and alcohol-related problems. Nursing Times 76: 2197–2198

Saunders W M, Kershaw P W 1979 Spontaneous remission from alcoholism — a community study. British Journal of Addiction 74: 251–265

Scottish Council on Alcoholism 1978 Report on health education and prevention.

Sladden S 1979 Psychiatric nursing in the community: a study of a working situation. University of Edinburgh Department of Nursing Studies Monograph No. 6. Churchill Livingstone, Edinburgh

Wilkins R H 1972 The health visitor and the alcoholic. Journal of Alcoholism 7: 92–97

Wilkins R H 1974 The hidden alcoholic in general practice. Elek Science, London

FURTHER READING

Edwards G 1968 Patients with drinking problems. British Medical Journal 4: 435–437

Edwards G, Gross M M 1976 The alcohol dependence syndrome: provisional description of a clinical syndrome. British Medical Journal 1: 1058–1061

Rix K J B 1979 Alcoholism and the district nurse. Nursing Times, Community Outlook 75: 275–280

Rix K J B, Lumsden Rix E M Alcohol problems: A guide for nurses and other health professionals. Wright, Bristol (in press)

Shaw S, Cartwright A, Spratley T, Harwin J 1978 Responding to drinking problems. Croom Helm, London

Wilkins R H 1974 The hidden alcoholic in general practice. Elek Science, London.

22

Mental handicap in the family

Cynthia Finlayson

INTRODUCTION

> The mother of a handicapped child soon becomes a complete slave to his dependency. As a result, she devotes all her time to his necessary care, neglecting her other household duties, her other children, if there are such, and inevitably, her husband . . . there is only one way to lessen all this grief . . . and that is immediate commitment to an institution at the time of diagnosis.
>
> Aldrich (1947) in The American Journal of Mental Deficiency.

> The mentally retarded person has the right to live with his own family or with foster parents; to participate in all aspects of community life, and to be provided with appropriate leisure time activities. If care in an institution becomes necessary, it should be in circumstances as close to normal living as possible.
>
> Article 4 of the Declaration of Rights of Mentally Retarded Persons, United Nations General Assembly 1971.

In recent decades there has been a remarkable change in attitude towards dependent members of society reflected in the move away from institutionalisation towards community care. Ideally, families that look after a dependent relative at home are supported in their task by a variety of community services. Community care should not mean that society unburdens its responsibilities on to the shoulders of the family. In practice, however, there may be little effective support. This is especially likely in the case of mental handicap, for the principle of institutional care has always been best accepted for the mentally subnormal and the mentally ill, with the consequence that community services are often poorly developed and the needs of families in this situation are not always well understood.

Clearly, people experience different problems in caring for a mentally handicapped child at home. The disabilities of subnormal children are variable and every family of a subnormal child is unique in its access to personal, social and material resources. Thus, although it is possible to describe the consequences of a child's specific impairments in terms of nursing and educational demands made on the family, it is less easy to describe how the presence of a subnormal child affects the functioning of the family as a whole. Despite the wide variety of difficulties that may arise, personal accounts of life with a subnormal child do seem to reveal a central core of experience, relating not so much to individual circumstances as to the problems of adjustment to stresses inherent in the situation.

The pattern of experience begins with learning about the existence of handicap, an unavoidably traumatic event. The shock is numbing. In retrospect, little can be remembered of the period following discovery, including medical explanations and advice so often given along with the diagnosis. Gradually the numbness wears off and the mind struggles to overcome the unacceptable by rejecting the truth of diagnosis, the existence of the child and offers of help. There frequently is tremendous anger, a need to attack, to attach blame, to relieve feelings of guilt and fear. Anger and denial belie a natural anguish which may take days or even months to work through. Members of the health team may be involved with counselling, but it is far more likely that they become convenient targets for frustration and bitterness. These feelings are probably never fully resolved, even after handicap is accepted.

Case history

The process of acceptance

The birth of a female infant with Down's Syndrome to Julia B was notified to the health visitor in the usual way. At the primary visit she spent some time with the mother discussing feeding difficulties, but in the course of an hour Miss B made no mention of the child's appearance, behaviour or diagnosis. The health visitor thought that perhaps her client had not been informed of the problem. She contacted the paediatrician concerned, to learn that Julia had been told and, indeed, had taken part in a long interview with the doctor and had seemed to take the bad news very well. At her next visit the health visitor eventually broached the subject. Whilst not denying knowledge directly, Miss B changed the subject and began to show hostility to her previously welcome caller. On another occasion she became very angry when the health visitor offered to introduce her to another mother in a similar situation and, on subsequent occasions, she refused to answer the door to her. A different health visitor who called some months later was allowed to examine the child and the mother spontaneously provided information about delayed milestones, although she did not mention Down's Syndrome until the end of the visit '. . . because I wanted to see if you'd notice'.

Recalling the incidents over a year later Julia said: 'I suppose they did tell me in the hospital, I really don't remember very well. It was all a bad dream. I don't think I believed it really. It seemed right when the visitor came and didn't say anything, nice and normal, but then she came back and started probing and I just froze inside. It was like learning it all over again. Then she tried to be "understanding". God, I resented that! How could she possibly know what it was like? I was sorry when she stopped coming though, because I did have a lot of problems, especially with feeding. It was awful, sitting at home with an unresponsive baby who wouldn't suck. I thought I'd go mad, stuck with a baby who couldn't even *use* me. The clinic was no good either. I only went once because I couldn't stand the waiting room with all those normal women with their normal babies. Funnily enough, though, I think it's easier in some ways to cope with a handicapped baby, all wrapped in a shawl and dependent, you can pretend it's like any other; but when the baby's bigger and should be doing things, it's obscene to have a drooling infant then. That was the worst time, when I couldn't pretend any longer and realized I had a lifetime of responsibility ahead of me.'

Of course handicap is not always diagnosed so early in life. It is rarely possible to say at the time of birth that a child will be mentally subnormal, for only a few children are born with a characteristic physical appearance or signs suggestive of mental deficiency. In most cases diagnosis is made after a long period of observation and investigation, so that even if deficiency is severe and suspected early, it may not be confirmed for many months, sometimes longer.

Case history

Anger and isolation
Mrs G is the mother of Michael, a shy, severely subnormal nine-year-old. He was her first child and she had no reason to suspect that he was mentally subnormal when he was a baby. However, she did wonder whether something was physically wrong when he was still not walking at 19 months and so she took him to an infant welfare clinic from which he was duly referred to hospital. At the hospital she was told not to worry because he was just a late developer and they made a follow-up appointment to see him in a year. By that time he was walking, and she had expectations of a fully normal child. When she was then told that her son would never get beyond the mental age of a three-year-old, she was completely stunned. She still feels bitter, believing that the hospital allowed her to nurture unrealistic expectations for a year longer than necessary.

At about this time she had a second son, and it eventually became apparent that he was deaf. As soon as this was discovered, peripatetic teaching, playgroups, special schooling and plans for the future were organized. There had been no such help for Michael and she still marvels at the comparison, especially as the task of caring for him has always been the greater one. Even whilst her younger son was being helped, she was still harbouring a hundred unanswered worries about the older child's future.

She and her husband desperately wanted to overcome the uncertainty they felt about the future and to understand what had gone wrong for their child. Even now they are confused about the diagnosis, unsure about the terminology they have heard applied to Michael, not even sure whether the handicaps of their two children might somehow be linked by a genetic factor. Having come to terms with the problem they naturally wanted answers to the many questions that came to mind. One social worker speaks of how parents in this situation need 'someone to prepare them for the future and *to dare to look ahead with them*. To talk about what will happen when they can no longer cope, and when they die . . . . They also want the social worker or health worker to withstand their expressions of fear or panic'. (Wallace, 1978).

Mrs G remembers her worst days as those before she found a place in a playgroup for Michael. She had few neighbours or friends with whom she felt able to leave the little boy. Everyday tasks such as shopping and visiting the launderette had to be planned as though they were major expeditions if she were to take both children with her, one a baby in the pram and the other mobile but wayward and unresponsive. Her husband assumed responsibility more and more for the jobs which took her out of the house, a necessary step but one which served to isolate her at home. The feeling of isolation became especially unbearable when the second baby needed frequent hospital visits and was then found to be deaf; it all seemed too much. Loneliness and depression overwhelmed her and for several months she was a frequent visitor to her general practitioner, 'begging for tablets to sleep and forget'. Looking back, she feels that she coped over this period by holding very low expectations of Michael's behaviour and concentrating on his physical care only, a personal defence she now regrets, believing she may have held him back. Eventually she succeeded in getting a playgroup place and this helped considerably. Later still, Michael's admission to school marked a turning-point, relieving her of the day-long burden of responsibility, and also bringing her into contact with services and facilities she had not known existed. She also became involved in a local self-help group, and suddenly found tremendous practical and social support within her own community.

Mrs G is now involved in running a playgroup in her area for mentally handicapped children knowing how little help she received with Michael until he started school. As leader of this group, she sees her role as helping mothers in the same situation by not only caring for their children for part of the day, but also acting as adviser and liaison officer; sharing her hard-won knowledge about services and facilities.

Michael's problems came to light in the second year of life, the stage that Julia felt that her daughter's handicap began to show to the world. There is little doubt that the second year of life marks a new phase in the life of a subnormal child and his family. The extent of handicap becomes obvious and there is a period of learning and adjustment as the parents realize the nature of the child's difficulties and their implications for the future.

Mental handicap is associated with impairment of intellectual, physical and social function. Intellectually there are three main areas of difficulty: poor reasoning ability giving rise to difficulty with generalization and the capacity to learn from experience; a poor attention span which means that one-to-one learning is usually required; and a learning deficit, which means that the retarded child will take longer to learn than a normal child of the same mental age. It follows that teaching the subnormal child is a lengthy, dispiriting task. It is necessary to wait longer for certain capacities to appear, and then to work longer and harder for abilities to be acquired through learning. Toilet training, for example, may take five years or more of determined and disciplined teaching with cooperation from all the family. Months or even years may pass without any apparent progress, yet over the same period other basic skills are likely to be taught, equally unrewarding and fraught with social implications if learning fails to take place. In time, day to day routines in potting, feeding and hygiene become emotionally charged events, coloured by a history of failure and by the thought that the alternative to reform is to be reconciled to socially unacceptable behaviour.

Mastery of basic social skills is obviously important if the child is to take his place within the family and wider community, and what limited ability there is will be directed towards this goal. Some unfortunate children are, however, further handicapped by behavioural disorders which are largely independent of learning experience and which may be intolerable to live with, even in the absence of subnormality. How does a family relate positively to a child who screams for hours on end, or to a child who mutilates himself? Temper tantrums, unusual sleeping patterns, hyperkinesis and ritualistic behaviour are but a few of the behavioural abnormalities that may be associated with mental subnormality.

The task of caring is usually complicated further by the presence of physical disability. Mental handicap and physical handicap are strongly correlated, and it is relatively rare for subnormality to exist alone. It is not intended to discuss physical disabilities at any length here. It suffices to say that mentally subnormal children may suffer from a range of coexistent physical problems, commonly epilepsy, sensory defects and orthopaedic disorders, all with obvious direct implications for care.

The child's handicap, therefore, affects the family on two levels. The need for social training associated with the difficulties of teaching generates a background of stress; a constant striving for minimal achievement in the face of high levels of frustration. Against this background are difficulties arising from the child's other needs, the physical demands of routine care on a day-long, life-long basis; extra laundry if he is incontinent, extra lifting if he is physically disabled, extra time and emotional energy if there are difficulties with washing and feeding, constant alertness if he is a danger to himself or to others. Some severely handicapped children will tend to die young, and for the rest there will be the gradual acquisition of a level of social competence. Inevitably, the burden of caring is greatest for the family of a young subnormal person (Table 22.1).

Table 22.1 Incapacity amongst mentally handicapped people

Incapacity	Age		
	Under 15	15 and over	Total
	%	%	%
non ambulant	24.06	6.23	11.25
behaviour difficulties requiring constant supervision	14.06	11.23	12.06
severely incontinent	12.55	5.20	7.54
needing assistance to feed, wash and dress	28.33	15.49	19.25
no physical handicap or severe behaviour difficulties	21.00	61.85	49.90

Source: Cmnd 4683

Case history

Physical and social adjustment

The H family live in a council maisonette in an inner city area. There are two sons: Alan, who is a sixth-former at the local comprehensive school and Alex, who attends a special school. Alex is severely subnormal, hyperkinetic and epileptic.

For years Mrs H has managed to care for Alex without any outside help. He requires constant attention and almost total nursing care in routines such as washing, dressing and toiletting. Recently he has achieved a degree of bladder control but as he frequently has epileptic fits, it is still necessary to change his clothing at least once a day. The fits continue during the night and as there is a danger that he might injure himself, Mr and Mrs H and Alan maintain an all-night vigil, taking four-hourly turns to watch over him.

The physical demands on Mrs H are quite overwhelming. When she becomes too exhausted to carry on, her husband takes days off work to relieve her. In this way he uses up his annual leave, and the family have not had a holiday since Alex was born.

The long nights take their toll and Mr H is very worried that he may soon be sacked as his attendance at work is unreliable and he feels that, through being tired, he does not give satisfactory service. This job is particularly important to him because it operates flexi-time and so enables him to help out at home more easily. His wife has taken a part-time job since Alex started school and she feels that it is keeping her sane, but she too fears that she may lose the life-line of an outside interest.

Alan has recently performed poorly in his 'O' Levels and now has to drop back a year at school. This is probably due to the stresses involved in looking after Alex, but he resists any suggestions that his brother should leave the family, even for a temporary break. He has, in fact, declared that he will not marry and plans to look after Alex until he dies.

The family have reached the end of their tether. In writing for help on their behalf, the consultant paediatrician said:

> This continues to be an immensely difficult problem where medical help has been only marginal and sometimes damaging, and where community facilities provided have really been limited to . . . school with little more than good intentions in addition.

Their story illustrates the sheer physical grind of caring for a severely subnormal child and the emotional cost that this care extracts. All things considered, they are a remarkably cohesive family and the marriage even seems to have strengthened under stress that would make many a partnership founder.

Tension is beginning to show, however. Mrs H is physically drained and she realizes that, as Alex gets bigger, she will be less able to cope. She and her husband share fears for the future. What will happen to Alex when they are old or if Mr H loses his job, or if Alan cannot care for him? It seems inevitable that they must accept periodic short-term admissions for Alex to a specialized unit, yet they fear and resist this, believing it to be a first step in the direction of sending him to an institution. To complicate matters, their feelings of failure are aggravated by Alan, who bitterly opposes the idea and accuses them of being hard and uncaring. His declared intention never to marry and to care for Alex until he dies is a prospect they view with mixed feelings, for if he does not, then what will become of Alex? If he does, then what will his life be like?

Every family finds the best way of meeting the needs of its members between them, and it is not unexpected to find that the siblings of mentally handicapped children will often assume heavy responsibilities in their care. It appears that the needs of mentally normal children in the family are increased. Small children may be frightened of the handicapped child if he is aggressive; older ones may suffer feelings of shame and embarassment. They may well receive less attention than the handicapped child, causing feelings of resentment and insecurity. As adulthood approaches, a life-time of caring cannot be easily set aside. It may be very difficult, or impossible, to persuade the young person of the moral limit of his or her responsibilities if they do not see a viable community alternative to care in the home.

Looking ahead takes courage. Ahead of Julia, Mrs G and the H family is the day when their mentally subnormal children leave school, a day normally associated with a child's full acceptance into the adult community and the end of parental duties. For these families, the day will probably mark the child's return to them; not for them the prospect of light relief or time alone.

Thus the family is caught, emotionally, physically and socially, in a long-term commitment to the child's needs. Society shares that commitment in its support of community care and may significantly affect the quality of the experience through provision of appropriate community services.

REFERENCES

Wallace E 1970 Mental handicap: meeting the real needs of families. Social Work Today 9: 33

23

The position of old people in the community

Marie Wragg

Old age is not regarded as something to look forward to. When we are children, we often wish we were grown up or had a job or place of our own. The future looks rosy and we feel confident we can cope with anything that comes along. As life goes by and inevitably brings some disappointments in its train, we begin to have a more realistic view of old age and its problems. Our society does not appear to value old people. There are very many of them, however, not always enjoying life, sometimes desperately lonely. This should be very much the concern of the community. Community health is very much the concern of administrators and politicians but it should also be the concern of all who care about their fellow men. Much has been done for the physical welfare of the old. In this chapter, the focus will be on some psychological aspects of ageing which have been largely ignored but which should be appreciated by those whose work gives them first hand experience of old people whether they are professionals or voluntary workers.

A story was going the rounds recently of an elderly man who said 'I belong to the unfortunate generation. When I was young, I was taught to look up to my elders, but now I am old, I have to look up to the young.' On the whole, it is true that the old are not revered today and the young are accorded great importance. Because of their spending power, young people are wooed and flattered by those advertising consumer goods. At times, one is aware of the 'tyranny of the cult of young' (Jonas, 1973). Many old people go out of their way to ape the young in clothes or language, often with disastrous results. One wonders how it has come about that old people are not respected. After all, it is not so long since the old were revered and the commandment 'Honour thy father and thy mother' strictly observed. Of course, countries vary a great deal in this respect. Even today, in country areas in China, children go to the family temple to light joss sticks and burn paper money for a grandmother who has gone to the spirit world. In India too, and among Jewish communities, the old have a valued place.

Not so in the Western World! There are many reasons for this. It has become a truism to say that in the last 50 years we have been passing through a time of the most rapid social changes in history. There has been an explosion of technological knowledge. It is not so long ago that we saw on colour television the first man stepping on to the moon and later, returning safely through space to the earth. The kind of research which led to this tremendous achievement is almost impossible for the layman to understand. Much of what the old learned as children is now out of date (as their grandchildren are quick to point out!) So the old are not now revered for their knowledge and wisdom. Furthermore, the attitudes and values and standards the old of today were taught in their youth are no longer generally accepted. Emphasis is placed on productivity. There are elderly musicians, artists, politicians and film stars who are seen to make a contribution to society but most people over 60 or 65 are regarded as almost useless in the community. Again, the emphasis today is on the latest fashion and on novelty. Advertisers sell their products by calling out: 'New! New! New!' The expression 'planned obsolescence' has entered our language. It seems that things should not be built to last.

As a result of these changes, today old people tend to be ignored or undervalued, unappreciated, barely tolerated. Nor have these changes come to an end. It is quite possible that many people alive today will see the introduction of a shorter working day, a four-day week and retirement at 50 so the proportion of old people not working will tend to increase. As it is, there is a much longer expectancy of life than in earlier times owing to better health services and medical care. In other words, the proportion of old people in the community is increasing steadily. Hilgard's research (1953) shows that on average, the happiest years are between 25 and 45 but from the age of 60 onwards, people are less happy. It should be noted that early old is usually taken to begin with retirement, 60 for a woman and 65 for a man to 75. Then the years 75–85 are very old and extreme old age 85 onwards.

THE PSYCHOLOGICAL NEEDS OF THE OLD

From the above comments, it is clear that anything like a ccomprehensive approach to old age would need to look at many sociological, historical and medical considerations as well as the psychological factors to be examined here. Two fields are particularly relevant, the psychology of needs (or drives or motives as they are sometimes called) and also that of character and personality, bearing in mind the practical applications involved. When psychologists have been trying to discover what makes people tick, they have frequently listed various needs that seem to be universal in human beings and, indeed, at times in animals too. The number of these drives has proliferated. One research worker, Murray (1938) named 28. A helpful classification is that of Morgan (1961) and this will be followed here. He first mentions basic, inborn. biogenic, physiological needs, formerly called 'instincts'. These are clearly linked with the body, such as the need for food, drink, sleep, sex, excretion and maternal care. Some, like sex are partly inborn and partly affected by learning. On the whole, the physical care of old people is well catered for by the National Health and Social Services plus the contribution of various charitable organisations.

There are other needs not so clearly linked with the body. These are sometimes called 'general drives'. Activity is one that can be clearly observed in animals, children and young people. Old people too are healthy if they keep going and should be encouraged to take whatever exercise they can according to their age and ability. Curiosity or exploration is another general drive. It is the base of all our knowledge and can act as a spur. Curiosity in the elderly can be gratified at several different levels. There are adult education courses in archaeology, painting, yoga, local history and many more. Townswomen's Guilds, clubs for the old and similar organisations offer stimulating talks. Elderly people with little previous education have followed their chosen subject up to degree level through the Open University. Success is richly rewarding and gives a feeling of great satisfaction.

Another general drive Morgan calls 'affectional' — the need for love and warmth and appreciation. The place of this need in the early formative years is well known. Bowlby (1961) has shown that a child who is not given affection then may be unable later to show affection to others and may become an 'affectionless character.' Many an elderly person who has been starved of love in early life will blossom like a flower when meeting a doctor or nurse or social worker who is really concerned. Now that so many families are separated by distance or divorce or work, warmth and affection are more and more necessary for healthy old age. Morgan then turns to more complex drives varying very much in different cultures. Affiliation is a need. We all want to belong to a group. The lonely old lady or gentleman with no relatives or friends nearby can feel very deprived. Even casual acquaintances who may become friends, are valued. A report by Thomson (1981), tells how useful for the elderly and others has been a free minibus service for patients in Croydon. It was found that elderly people improve greatly if kept out and about: 'the old people look forward to their minibus trip. They put on their best clothes and regard it as a special day out.' Many needs are satisfied here: activity, affiliation, curiosity, affection. Status is a need linked with affiliation and social approval. The loss of previous status when retirement comes can raise problems. By the time a man reaches 65 he is often a 'somebody' at the top of his profession or trade then suddenly he becomes a 'nobody'. A single woman or a widow who has been enjoying work outside the home may find a similar frustration. This can be very hard to take.

Security is another need not always satisfied, not surprisingly considering the violence shown in lurid detail on our television screens and described in newspapers. Many old people have to live in huge blocks of flats with younger ones out at work and no one to call on for help. Such people need a great deal of reassurance and encouragement if they are to get rid of their fears. Another complex need is achievement. We all like a pat on the back. Men and women are urged to get to the top, regardless of the fact that only a very few can do so. There are not many plums after all, so there is inevitably disappointment and disillusion among many. This may lead to bitterness in old age. One hears the phrase 'I never had a chance'. Horney (1937) reported a 'need to be needed'. This is most noticeable in elderly people who may feel they are only fit for the scrap heap yet with a little trouble from friends, relations and professionals their gifts and experience can be used. This will give them enormous satisfaction.

Independence is another need met so often in the elderly who, when they become ill, may be afraid of being 'put away' or having to live with a daughter-in-law who does not relish the prospect either. This is one reason why, whenever possible, old people should be encouraged to keep their own homes. Self-esteem and dignity are linked with independence. Freedom is valued so it is a good thing to do away with pointless rules and regulations in Homes for the Aged. Sadly, they are often still treated as children. When someone says to an old person 'Oh you naughty girl! Look what you've done' this can be very wounding. Another need is for some kind of religious dimension that can be of great value, particularly when grief and bereavement and eventually death are inevitable.

Some needs or motives we may not even be aware of as they are part of our unconscious. A habit of rejecting all offers of help may rise from a chip on the shoulder going right back to early childhood. Through life we form our own special goals and motives or needs which is why one man likes Beethoven, another, jazz. During our youth and middle age, we have not always had the time to devote to our goals but in old age they can be rediscovered and developed. A good listener can soon discover what they are.

In concluding this section on the psychology of needs, there is a very simple piece of research that can be undertaken. Ask any group of elderly people this question: 'What do you think will give you the greatest happiness when you are old?' The answers obtained illustrate very clearly the drives that have been described. 'To be able to be independent to the end' (independence). 'To remain active' (activity). 'To see my children and grandchildren frequently' (affection). 'Some congenial companionship' (social contacts). 'Security' 'Peace of mind' 'A secure faith' 'Interests of one's own choosing'.

A good nurse or social worker therefore will realise how important certain needs are and, where possible, take steps to satisfy them.

PERSONALITY AND THE OLD

We are dealing with individual people so the temptation to generalise must be resisted. So often one hears people say that old people are so forgetful or tiresome or obstinate. Some are but by no means all. There is also the danger of thinking in terms of stereotypes, that is, fixed sets of over-simplified beliefs such as 'Italians are always emotional.' Some are, some are not. We should pay more attention to individual differences. This is where the fascinating study of personality comes in. It is a study which is essential to all those whose work involves people whether they are doctors, health visitors, nurses, teachers, advertisers, policemen, industrialists. In many cases, they have to sum people up rapidly before they can establish rapport and decide how to organise their work. No two people, not even identical twins reared together, can be exactly alike. Each person has his or her unique set of abilities and habits and, except for identical twins, his unique hereditary endowment. Personality formation begins from the moment of conception when a specific combination of genes and chromosomes, the bearers of heredity, takes place. Over the years, a pattern develops, a style of life, a way of reacting to the family and later to the outside world. It is well known that the early years are very influential. It is thought that the ductless glands influence mood and temperament. Other aspects of the total personality such as attitudes, beliefs and prejudices are not inborn but acquired during life from parents, relatives, friends, teachers, colleagues. We tend to conform to the standards and ideas of our social group. There is a concept called 'role expectancy' which indicates the tendency to behave in the way in which we are expected to do by the social group. We adapt to different roles in different situations. The blustering foreman on the workshop floor may be a different person altogether in his own home. Role conflict may occur when a person has to switch roles or is not sure which role he is supposed to adopt. However straightforward old people can appear on the surface they are individualists trying to come to terms with a rapidly changing world, their own personal world and the confusing and complicated physical world around them. This can be a distressing process.

One question that is often asked is: can personality change? Personality does have a basic continuity. Habits and motives learnt over the years are not easily forgotten. The aggressive old lady who has tyrannised her family for many years does not become an angel of sweetness and light when she fractures a hip and has to depend on others. A person does not change very quickly or very greatly. But there *are* changes brought about by marriage, a new job, an intense religious experience, success or failure. Psychotherapy and counselling techniques can help people to get rid of bad habits and form new ones. A person's weaknessess can be minimised and neutralised. Take aggression, for example. The wise mother encourages her boisterous son to let off steam by kicking a ball rather than his little brother. Instead of fighting one another in riots and wars, we adults might instead fight disease, injustice and ignorance.

When studying the psychology of personality, many have tried to classify people as particular types such as extrovert and introvert, aggressive or submissive. Referring to individuals who frequent the Corbett Senior Centre, Fontana (1977) divides the elderly into four types: the relaxers, the waiters, the joiners and the do-gooders. This is misleading and oversimplifying. So much depends on the situation. Personality is not simple enough to be described in this way except loosely in casual conversation. Many psychologists, for example Allport (1937) prefer to describe the collection of traits that characterize a particular person. A trait is 'an aspect of personality that is reasonably characteristic of a person and distinguishes him in some way from many other people.' Morgan (1961) for example, mentions cheerful, sociable, reserved, over-anxious. Several of these traits can be seen in old people. Danger signals are depression and moodiness and feelings of persecution. The good companion will reassure her patient when necessary, offer encouragement and praise his or her efforts to cope with any negative feelings.

In any work with old people, personal relationships are of paramount importance. For these to be successful, every effort should be made to understand oneself. This can be even more difficult! Eysenck & Wilson (1975) tried to increase the insight of the reader. They said: 'lack of insight is unfortunately very common: it is one of the things your best friend will not tell you'.

CONCLUSION

Any approach to old age should consider both the community and the individual for they are closely linked. Old people are increasing in number. It is only right that they should be cared for. In most cases, they have made a useful contribution to the community for many years. The community has shouldered its responsibility to some extent. Medical and social services in the United Kingdom are better than they have ever been although there are still gaps and much room for improvement. For example, more home helps and meals-on-wheels are needed everywhere, particularly now when hospitals are so short of staff they have to send patients home before they are well enough to look after themselves. It is possible, however, that too much attention is paid to the physical needs of old people, important though they may be and not enough to their psychological needs. The community might do more to prepare people for retirement to ensure that these needs are satisfied. Ideally this preparation should begin when people are in their forties or fifties. Many firms have started pre-retirement schemes and others are offered by bodies responsible for adult education. Part-time work after 60 or 65 might be encouraged and could give a great feeling of achievement to the pensioner. Research in industrial psychology has shown that old people can acquire new skills if they are prepared to change their attitudes and if they are highly motivated. They can then feel they are of some value to society. Of course, in an age of high unemployment there would have to be preparatory talks with the government and unions on the practicalities involved. If old people were able to work regularly on a paid or unpaid basis, there would be far fewer complaints of fatigue. So often, fatigue is brought on by psychological factors such as boredom and a feeling of uselessness.

However good the facilities provided by the community are, it is the pensioner who has to make use of them. From the point of view of the individual, these are broadly two ways of adjusting to old age, disengagement or activity (Cumming & Henry, 1961).

Disengagement or withdrawal is the method used for centuries by the Great Christian Mystics or hermits or elderly Hindus. It would appeal to reserved, introverted people with inner resources. In old age and, indeed, through life, it is good to consider the spiritual side of life. By the seventies, a personal philosophy of life should have been evolved. 'Disengagement' might also signify detachment and acceptance. One has to come to terms with one's disabilities, bereavements and thoughts of one's own death. Some societies, however, in particular the United States tend to set a premium on outward looking extroverted people, the kind who are the life and soul of the party. This view takes the line that having a full and varied life of activities is the better preparation for ageing. As we have seen, individual differences should be borne in mind.

There are differences of sex, age, region, social group, education, experience. A person can find it as rewarding to cultivate a small allotment as to listen to a symphony concert. There are innumerable hobbies and interests from which to choose. After 60 or 65 for the first time there may be leisure to devote to travel, art, bowls, the local school or hospital. More opportunities could be created for voluntary service to the community. In U.S.A. Jonas (1973) refers to some of these schemes, for example counselling and tutoring children, school dinner supervision, foster grandparents. A remark often heard is 'It's good to be needed again.' In New York, there is an organisation called SERVE (Serve and enrich retirement by volunteer experience). Members spend three days a week visiting mentally retarded children. Recently, in England Jolly (1981) a nurse, has written a book describing a scheme for 'ward grannies' for children whose parents cannot visit the hospital. She claims this has proved a source of confidence and help for the patient. One can imagine how rewarding this work must be to all concerned.

There should be a new look at the years of retirement. It should be possible to enjoy:

> that which should accompany old age
> As honour, love, obedience, troops of friends
>
> Shakespeare

Instead of adopting a negative attitude to old age, both the community and the individual should cultivate positive feelings. We should remember the wise words of Montaigne: 'The value of life lies not in the length of days but in the use we make of them: a man may live long yet live very little.' Old age, like every other, has its problems but it can be a time of happiness and fulfillment. Life can begin at 60.

REFERENCES

Allport G W 1937 Personality. Holt, Rinehart and Winston, New York
Bowlby J 1961 Child care and the growth of love. Pelican, London
Cumming E, Henry W E 1961 Growing old in the process of disengagement. Basic Books, New York
Eysenck H, Wilson G 1975 Know your own personality. M Temple Smith, London
Fontana A 1977 The last frontier. The social meaning of growing old. Sage Publications London
Hilgard et al 1953 Introduction to psychology. Harcourt Brace Johanovich, New York
Horney K 1937 The neurotic personality of our time. Norton, New York
Jolly J 1981 The other side of paediatrics. Macmillan, London
McCllelland D C, Atkinson J W, Clark R A, Lowell E L 1953 The achievement motive. Appleton-Century-Crofts, New York
Montaigne Michel de 1533–1592 Essays I ix
Murray H A 1938 Explorations in personality. Oxford University Press, New York
Shakespeare 1564–1616 Macbeth V iii 22 1606
Thompson W R 1981 All to the good. Readers Digest April, p 78

FURTHER READING

Vida Carver 1978 The ageing population. Open University, London
Jonas Doris, Jonas David 1973 Young till we die. Hodder and Stoughton, London
Morgan L T 1961 Introduction to psychology, 2nd edn. McGraw Hill, New York
Tournier 1972 Learning to grow old. S.C.M. Press, London

24

The family role in care

Elizabeth Raymond

Who should care?

A nine-year-old boy, only son of elderly parents, lay dying in hospital. Day and night his parents took turns to stay with him on the ward. Day and night a team of three student nurses took turns to give him 'special' attention. When he died, the students shared their grief with the parents, for they cared.

An elderly, emaciated lady lay dying alone at home. The relief nurse paid an evening visit, handling the patient roughly, almost violently, as she attended perfunctorily to her presure areas. The nurse did not really care.

Another lady lay dying at home, on a mattress on the living-room floor of one of the most expensive flats in London. The nurse visited regularly, seeking to bring what relief she could. She was bewildered and distressed by the patient's adamant refusal to accept any help or treatment whatsoever. This nurse cared for her patient, yet the patient had lost the will to live, and did not care any more.

Another lady lay helpless in her own excreta for many months, known only to her neighbour. who collected her pension and gave her food. How much did that neighbour care?

A middle-aged nurse looked after her handicapped mother for three years after the old lady had a stroke. The friend who helped her, a non-nurse, had taken responsibility alone for her own mother for twenty years. Two more friends shared the burden in the last weeks, and the old lady died peacefully, in her own home, surrounded by those who cared.

The word care may be interpreted in a number of ways. The brief accounts just given have been chosen to highlight the aspect of caring which has to do with the extent to which the patient matters to someone. The family history of the lady who had lost the will to live suggested that life experiences had taught her that she did not matter to anybody.

In exploring the family role in care, the premise underlying this chapter is that people matter more than theories or systems. The patient cannot be cared for effectively alone. The family matters, and each individual has his or her own need for care. The professionals matter too, and if they are to play their part effectively, their individual needs must be taken into account.

Definitions of the word care in the Concise Oxford Oictionary centre on three themes. There is the theme of *responsibility*, both in terms of taking charge of someone, and also in the sense of giving heed or serious attention to what the carer is doing. There is the theme of *providing* for someone's needs, for example for food or nursing attention. Finally there is the theme of *feeling* for the one cared for, for example feeling concern, interest, regard, or affection.

It should already be apparent that the author's view is that there is no single blueprint for the role of the family in caring for a sick member. Rather there is a need for a partnership between family, friends, and professionals present in any given situation, and within this partnership there is the need to identify the role of the particular family in its particular context.

Similarly, the role of the family in relation to the terminal illness of a member cannot be laid down arbitrarily. The response of family members to a dying relative will necessarily arise out of the attitudes to that relative, to disease and to death which have been developed over the preceding years. In part, the attitudes of individuals to disease and death will have been influenced by prevailing attitudes of society. Many commentators have suggested that there have been two clear trends in recent decades, and that these attitude trends have been related to the breakdown of the extended family structure and to the better health and increased longevity of the population. It has been suggested that there has been a move away from a kind of group mentality, where the whole family regards itself as involved in the misfortunes and sicknesses of the individual members, and towards the attitude that each must fend for himself, as others are subject to their own pressures too great for them to assume the added burden of caring for another. It has also been suggested that whereas at the turn of the century sickness and death were regarded as a familiar part of everyday life, constantly to be reckoned with, today there is a kind of collective denial of reality and an attempt to avoid accepting mortality as inevitable. Elisabeth Kubler-Ross (1973) expresses a relationship between these two trends when she comments:

> I think there are many reasons for this flight from facing death calmly. One of the most important facts is that dying nowadays is in many ways more gruesome, more lonely, mechanical and dehumanized . . . Dying becomes lonely and impersonal because the patient is often taken out of his familiar environment and rushed to an emergency ward.

The word lonely is repeated in consecutive sentences and will find an echo in the minds of nurse readers who recall the dying patient on the ward, curtains drawn round the bed, alone in a crowd. E. Mansell Pattison (1977) completes the circle by suggesting that the lonely, mechanical, dehumanizing aspects of death in hospital are the consequence of the death-denying attitudes of the hospital staff. He says: 'The denial of death is seen in hospitals — in the apprehension and avoidance of the dying patient.' and he quotes Feifel (1965) as saying that: 'Physicians deny death more vigorously than the general populace.' In justifying his concern with attitudes to death and dying, Mansell Pattison makes it very clear that, in his own words: 'In dismissing death as 'taboo' — we dismiss the dying as well.' Attitudes to death and dying have recently received considerable attention in health professional circles, and it is not proposed to discuss the topic further here, except to reiterate the significance of these attitudes for the level of care which the dying patient may expect to receive. The remaining part of this chapter is concerned with the factors which influence the family role in care generally.

FACTORS AFFECTING THE FAMILY ROLE IN CARE

Social expectations

The relative significance of social expectations is very variable. They constitute a group pressure on the individual, the intensity of which will depend on the importance of the group to him. In close-knit communities, such as rural communities and immigrant groups, expectations have changed little over the years, and the community generally expects the family to take responsibility for the sick, the handicapped, and the elderly. In the urban situation there is more ambivalence. On the surface, practical difficulties such as distance between the homes of children and their elderly parents, are recognised. However, when the need for care arises, the true expectations of society appear to have changed less than might have been expected. In particular, society still appears to place heavy burdens of expectation on the single daughter. The attitude continues to prevail widely that she should give up whatever she may be doing, and go even hundreds of miles in order to care for a parent. Further ambivalence in society's attitude is apparent in the continuing campaign for voluntary euthanasia, when, as Cardinal Heenan observes in his preface to *The Hour of our Death* (Lack & Lamberton, 1975) modern medicine is such that: 'with remarkably few exceptions, patients even in the last stages of a ravaging disease can be kept comfortable and happy.'

There is ambivalence too in society's expectations of the family when confronted by mental illness and mental or physical handicap. Ambivalence is expressed in social policies, housing design, and economic resources. Since the 1959 Mental Health Act (Ministry of Health, 1959) reports and legislation have increasingly tended to put pressure on the community and families to retain the elderly and the mentally ill and handicapped in their care. Recently financial allocations to health and social services have been progressively reduced, and state provision for the elderly and the mentally disordered has always had a low priority relative to acute services. In 1976, 17.1% of the population were over pensionable age, and the proportion is still rising. It is projected that by the turn of the century, one-third of this group will be 75 and over (Office of Population Censuses & Surveys, 1976). There will never be enough homes for the elderly to meet the need, yet how many houses are built with 'granny-flat' accommodation? On the whole, housing design seems to have reflected two other factors which may have a bearing on the family role in care. These are:

Population mobility and family size

Society's attitude to the family role in care is rooted in the centuries old pattern of village life in which the extended family members lived in close proximity, and were so interdependent on one another that there was no question but that they cared for one another, especially as resources for care outside the family were scant. With larger families, more individuals were available to share the load. In the 20th century, there has been a dramatic shrinkage in family size with falling birth rates. At the same time, mechanisation, faster transport, and the growth of the cities, with changing patterns of employment, have all contributed to the splitting up of the extended family. Consequently, today the burden of care is often inordinately heavy for just one or two relatives. Contrary to popular opinion, the majority of families will still go to tremendous lengths to provide care. Considering the frail elderly, for example, Hunt (1978) showed that 41.5% of old people receive help from their relatives. According to Isaacs et al (1972) many adult children make efforts to care for their frail, failing parents at what is sometimes overwhelming cost to themselves. The cost involved begins to become apparent when account is taken of the age and state of health of the care-giver.

Age of the care-giver

When considering the need of the elderly for care, it needs to be borne in mind that the decline in health, mobility, and ability to manage independently, which is associated with ageing, usually begins after the age of 75 years. This means that the care-giver may be an elderly spouse, also in need of support, or a child reaching middle age. The latter may be a single daughter needing to go to work and coping with the emotional and physical difficulties which may be associated with the menopause. As the years pass, the middle-aged care-giver approaches her own retirement, fall in income, and the needs of old age.

State of health of the care-giver

In 1971, 54% of men aged 75 years and over, and 22.7% of similarly aged women lived alone with their spouses. (Age Concern Research Unit, 1977). Within this age group the care-givers themselves constitute a group with a disproportionately high incidence of disabling conditions, cardiovascular and respiratory disease, rheumatoid arthritis, osteoarthritis, and so on, quite apart from problems associated with ageing such as dulling of the special senses. A so-called 'social admission' to hospital of an elderly person may be the result of the failing health of the spouse, who can no longer manage broken nights, incontinence, and the strain of carrying the burden alone.

Other health problems may be manifest in the family caring for a handicapped member over many years, particularly where there is some form of mental handicap. It needs to be remembered that the parents of a handicapped child have been bereaved of the normal child they anticipated. As with any loss experience, they will have needed to mourn the loss, but this grieving process is not always satisfactorily accomplished. Feelings of guilt, a sense of being punished, and a feeling that the child demonstrates a defectiveness present in a parent are all feelings which, unless resolved, may not only result in mistreatment of the child, but also in abnormal patterns of behaviour governing the whole family. Families may refuse to acknowledge the handicap and not allow the child appropriate assessment and help, or may become totally preoccupied with the needs of the handicapped child to the exclusion of the needs of the rest of the family. The family caring for a handicapped member tends to become isolated anyway. The family feels that others do not understand or want to become involved, and in many instances this assessment is correct. Years later an ageing parent or a sibling may be found still caring for the handicapped individual who has dominated the development of the carer's whole social life and relationships. The carer's feelings can be a mixture of guilt, anger, resentment, and helplessness, and the assumption that people learn to live with such things is often false.

Even in the most normal of care-giving situations, the birth of a healthy baby, the family role in care and the health of the care-giver are intertwined. As a district midwife, the author often had cause to ponder the apparent inconsistency in nature which requires the utmost attention to the newborn child precisely at the moment when the mother is most drained of resources, with her hormonal balance in a state of change, and with all the other physiological changes of pregnancy needing to be reversed, not to mention the need for rest and recuperation after the exertion of labour. Where other members of the family are not present to share the load, postnatal depression is hardly a surprising consequence. In the past, grannies and aunts were the accepted helpers, as well as older sisters of the new baby. Today, where the nuclear family is isolated and left to fend for itself, the father has had to take on the role of helper almost perforce. For this to happen there has to have been some change in attitude as to what is regarded as manly, and obviously tensions arise in families where husband and wife are not agreed in this respect.

The quality of relationships within the family.

Where the care of handicapped or elderly members of a family is concerned, it is the experience of the author that onlookers are often prone to make very superficial judgements. The middle-aged daughter who takes on the care of her elderly parent is invariably credited with commendable devotion, whilst the daughter who does not is labelled uncaring. Remarks are made such as 'She's got three children, but they never visit her, poor old soul!' Undoubtedly there *are* devoted daughters and uncaring children too. However, each human relationship is complex and unique, and much may be hidden behind the apparent attitude of the would-be care-giver. A child may grow up in a home where parents have been dominating and have made heavy demands, both emotionally and practically, on the child. If, as is the case for one person known to the author, those parents have also verbalised their view of their child as a 'nasty piece of work', it is hardly surprising that the child has become an adult suffering from an intensity of anger, guilt feelings, and depression. The adult is still a child tied emotionally to mother's apron strings, but when care is given it is not given out of devotion, but because the child feels emotionally blackmailed into doing so. The quality of such care appears to be rather suspect. Another example is of a child growing up in a home where an alcoholic father constantly made promises he failed to keep, in addition to the violent abuse he meted out to wife and children. One adult child of this family despises the father and feels no sense of responsibility for him whatsoever. Since most families prefer not to wash their dirty linen in public, it is unlikely that the casual observer would be aware of the true nature of relationships in either of these families.

During the routine family visiting undertaken by health visitors, they are in a good position to observe the quality of mothering which a mother gives to her child. Again and again they see the profound effect which the mother's own relationship with her mother has on the way she learns to care for her child. In the first place, th strongest influence on her concept of normal mothering must be that which she has herself experienced, and even when the experience has been unsatisfactory, it all too often provides the model which the new mother imitates. There seems to be much justification for the argument that unless individuals have received love, they will find themselves unable to give love, or at least severely limited in their ability to do so. There is ample evidence that many who have been abused in childhood abuse in turn when they become parents.

The way in which parents relate to their children, and the quality of care they give, is also related to the interaction between themselves and other individuals. A distressed baby may be the clue to an unhappy marital relationship. Indeed, as a health visitor, the author only finally solved the problem of an incessantly crying child when the parents separated. It subsequently emerged that the marriage had been almost at the point of breakdown long before the baby was born, despite the united front presented by the couple. In another family, a five-year-old boy was referred to the child guidance clinic at the end of his first term at school with major communication difficulties and unable to behave in a socially acceptable way in class. This family had been unknown to the health visitor, but, since a second baby was on the way, relationships with the parents were gradually established. Both parents had extreme difficulty in demonstrating love and affection, and with a wide age gap between husband and wife, their relationship was more that of a Victorian military father with a frightened and conforming child. An extreme example of the effect of such problems in parents on their children is recorded in the book by Virginia Axline, *Dibs: In Search Of Self* (1976). After Dibs had been at school for two years the following description is recorded:

> The teachers had tried their best to establish a relationship with him, to get a response from him. But it had been touch and go. Dibs seemed determined to keep all people at bay . . . When he started school, he did not talk and he never ventured off his chair. He sat there mute and unmoving all morning. After many weeks he began to leave his chair and to crawl around the room, seeming to look at some of the things about him. When anyone approached him, he would huddle up in a ball on the floor and not move. He never looked directly into anyone's eyes. He never answered when anyone spoke to him.

Yet the same child, who was regarded by his parents as mentally defective, scored an I. Q. of 168 when tested one week after play therapy sessions ended!

Perhaps enough has been said to establish the major importance of relationships within the family with respect to the nature of care which the members are capable of giving to each other.

Emotional maturity

The ability of each individual to form relationships is very dependent on emotional maturity. We live in a society in the West which still tends to seek explanations for human behaviour on a rational basis. Yet the motive force comes from our emotions, which are basically operating at a level deeper than conscious rational thought. If we are honest, we are often forced to admit that the so-called reasons we give for our actions are in fact explanations we have to produce in order to satisfy a need for structure and predictability, without which the world inside ourselves would be an unknown and frightening place. British society in particular is suspicious of emotion, except perhaps on the football pitch! Yet emotional maturity comes as we learn to recognise and make friends with our emotions, including such emotions as anger, fear, and grief.

The quality of care family members give may be greatly enhanced or damaged depending on the emotional maturity of the care-giver. Indeed, whether or not a particular member accepts a caring role may be determined predominantly by their emotional response to the situation. Nursing a sick relative may require actions which cause some physical pain, and the thought of causing pain to the loved one may cause real emotional turmoil in the care-giver. Particularly where terminal care is required, the care-giver may be very frightened, frightened of the dying process itself, or afraid of seeing the loved one dead. In situations such as these, the nature of the support which health professionals provide becomes very important.

The attitudes of health professionals

Since the health professionals are those in whom society has vested authority when it comes to matters of health, their attitudes can carry considerable weight in influencing the family role in care. The two main areas in which their attitudes are significant are with respect to who should provide the necessary care, and where the care should be provided. If a patient is cared for at home, and family members are present, then the most usual state of affairs is for shared care to be negotiated between the family and the professionals. The district nurse traditionally recognises her status as a guest in the home of the patient. Even so, she has a responsibility to ensure that family members are helped to participate as fully as they are able, while ensuring that they are not carrying a burden which is excessive either physically or emotionally. When terminal care is involved, the family members who are left at the death of the patient will need to grieve. It can be very important to those close to the deceased to feel that they have done all that they could, and on occasion health professionals are guilty of depriving them of the opportunity to do so instead of making efforts to ensure adequate support whilst enabling them to share in the process of dying. Like birth, death is an event which properly belongs to the family. The author has a vivid recollection of wishing to be alone with her dying mother, a patient in an intensive therapy unit, and of finding a student nurse doggedly remaining in attendance, anxious lest her patient should have a cardiac arrest. It felt like an eternity before a perceptive staff nurse asked the student to leave. The following few minutes, which were a final leave-taking between mother and daughter, subsequently proved to be important for the author in accepting the finality of death, and knowing that nothing was left unresolved to give cause for guilt feelings or added distress. Even when patients have been admitted to hospital they remain part of the family and there is still a need for negotiation between staff and relatives concerning the family role in care, bearing in mind that the visitor by the bed may be the person who until now has fed, washed, and changed the patient for many months. While they may be in desperate need of relief, what they do not need is to be given the impression that they are of no further use, and possibly even that their loved one's admission to hospital is the consequence of their failure to cope.

Professional qualifications do not render a human individual invulnerable, and all that has been said about the needs, feelings, and attitudes of family members will apply to doctors, nurses, and all other health professionals. It needs to be recognised that nurses in particular need to develop coping mechanisms to protect them from the full force of the emotional impact of some of the situations in which they have to provide care. Even though this may be necessary to a degree for the nurse, it cannot be totally in the patients' interests, since it will lessen the feeling component of the care given. Ideally, the subjective caring of family and the objective caring of health professionals operating in partnership, can complement and balance one another to the benefit of all concerned. Even this partnership may experience considerable pressure without the existence of community support, which is expressed in the form of agencies such as voluntary car drivers, night sitters, home helps, and a host of others. Not only the professionals, but the community, where it exists, has a part to play in supporting the family which seeks to fulfil its caring role.

This chapter began with the question: 'Who should care?' Despite all the changes in social structure, family size, and life-styles during this century, it is hardly possible to escape the fact that the family still plays a central role in care. Care begins with the family, and ideally it also ends there. The human individual who has no family is deprived indeed. However, if a family is to fulfil this role at birth, through the vicissitudes of life, and at death, then that family needs to receive care also, in the form of support from the professionals and support from the community. The individuals comprising the latter two groups themselves need care and so the process of caring becomes one in which all the participants, lay and professional, are mutually interdependent. It has been said that, as the human individual grows to maturity, he passes from the stage of dependence, through the stage of independence, to an acceptance of the need for interdependence, for both giving and receiving. Perhaps, our national health care system will have reached maturity when this interdependence of family, community, and professionals is fully recognised and expressed in all our health care policies and practice.

REFERENCES

Age Concern Research Unit 1977 Profiles of the elderly, vol 1. Age Concern Publications, Mitcham
Axline V 1976 Dibs: In search of self. Pelican, London
Feifel H 1965 Death and dying: attitudes of patient and doctor. Group for the Advancement of Psychiatry, New York
Hunt A 1978 The elderly at home. OPCS, HMSO, London
Isaacs B, Livingstone M, Neville Y 1972 Survival of the unfittest. Routledge & Kegan Paul, London
Kubler-Ross E 1973 On death and dying. Tavistock Publications, London
Lack S, Lamberton R (eds) 1975 The hour of our death — a record of a conference on the care of the dying. Geoffrey Chapman, London
Mansell Pattison E 1977 The experience of dying. Prentice-Hall, New Jersey, USA
Ministry of Health 1959 Mental Health Act. HMSO, London
Office of Population Censuses & Surveys 1976 Population estimates series PP1 no 1. HMSO, London
The Concise Oxford Dictionary 1964 Oxford University Press

[illegible] V 1979 [illegible]. Pelican, London

[illegible] 1969 Health and [illegible] doctor. [illegible] Foundation of [illegible], New York

Professional approaches

The concept of 'helping' those in need is inherent in the concept of man as a social animal, and has for generations provided the main motivation of those who choose to work in the field of health care. But what do we mean by help? Who can best help whom, and how? The help provided by families for their own members and for members of other families within small interdependent communities has been supplemented at various times and in various cultures by religious orders and by various institutions of the state. In our own society, helping people with health problems came, as the result of the growth of scientific knowledge, to be regarded as a job for 'experts' and this has led to the specific occupational groups which are sometimes referred to collectively as 'the health professions'. The notion of professional help, based on the possession of esoteric knowledge which the client does not have, has been criticised by writers such as George Bernard Shaw, who described the professions as conspiracies against the laity, and Ivan Illich, who accuses the medical profession in particular of causing not only 'clinical iatrogenesis' (the physical damage caused by doctors in their attempts to cure people) but also 'social iatrogenesis', by which he means the destruction of the patient's autonomy, and the expropriation of his or her own responsibility for individual health care.

Members of the health professions themselves are now questionning their roles and their relationships with patients and looking for new ways of offering 'help'. This section describes just some of the differing, even competing, approaches which professional carers have used. A particular problem for members of the health professions is sharing care both with members of other professions and with the patient and his family. The complexity of people's problems often requires different kinds of expertise which are not likely to be found in one person, but without collaboration and cooperation between the various people involved there will be duplication and gaps in the care provided. The concept of teamwork in primary health care has been much debated, as has the need for continuity of care between the primary and secondary care sectors. Another concept which is the source of much debate is evaluation; in this case also the controversy is not about its desirability. but about how best it can be achieved. The contributions presented here do not pretend to provide solutions, but we hope they will provide stimulation for further debate.

Finally, Barry Reedy reminds us that our own system of delivering health care is not the only possible one, and may not even be the best one. At a time when resources for health care are very scarce and the structure of the health care system is undergoing rapid change, it is particularly important that we benefit wherever possible from the experiences of others in determining what will best suit our own needs.

25

Professions and professionalism

Monica Baly

The Victorians, who were brought up to accept that people were divided into the ruling class, the middling sort, the industrious labouring classes, and paupers, would have been less confused than we are about what constitutes professionalism. The professions were primarily middle class occupations which needed a long training and in which practitioners controlled their own standards and either worked independently for a fee, or, if they were not independent, were paid on a different basis from those who merely sold their labour for a wage. The other criterion which distinguished professions from other occupations was that the professions provided services which the public needed which could not be equated with the profit and loss account of the market system.

In the 18th century and before, there had been the learned professions of divinity, physic and law; these were the services that once were the prerogative of the early Church but whose practitioners now trained in the universities. In the census of 1841 these were the only professions listed though there were recorded 'other educated persons' whose occupations some 40 years later were generally to be found under the heading of 'the professions'. By the middle of the 19th century the growing complexity of industrial society, the new style of management of landed estates, and the demands of possessions overseas enlarged the need for professional services of all kinds — a need that was largely met by the thrusting aspirations of the growing middle classes whose sons were being educated in the public schools on the pattern set up by Dr Thomas Arnold. Nor was the social mobility always upwards, for younger sons of the aristocracy often found it necessary, and at times preferable, to earn a living in a profession or in business, the law being a particularly lucrative passport to the reformed parliament.

In 1858 the Medical Act laid down the procedures by which a physician or surgeon might qualify, and this in turn led to the creation of professional bodies to control the standard of registration and the discipline and conduct of their members. This pattern was followed by other professions who were usually granted charters, such as the Institute of Chartered Accountants and the Royal Institute of British Architects, and this was the model that nurses hoped to follow when the College of Nursing was established in 1916.

With increasing legislation to protect trade and property, and the growing, if unwilling, state intervention in public health and social policy, the attorney, once the standard butt of comic opera, joined the ranks of the respectable. When Lady Bracknell said, 'Markby, Markby and Markby, a firm of the highest repute in their profession, indeed I am told one of the Mr Markbys is occasionally seen at dinner parties' (Wilde, 1895) she was making a social comment on the changing status of occupations in the late 19th century; the solicitor had arrived. So too had accountants, architects, engineers and surveyors — all so necessary to the growing Victorian cities — occupations which organized themselves with long periods of articles, qualifying examinations and professional bodies to control admission and conduct. Teaching, on the other hand, was more diffuse, and it was some time before the training colleges inaugurated by Sir James Kay-Shuttleworth (1804–1877) produced recruits who were classified as 'professional'.

There was of course no equivalent outlet for middle-class women, in spite of the fact that in 1841 the proportion of unmarried women was the highest it has ever been. However, even if there had been no Nightingale reforms, the advent of anaesthesia and Listerian asepsis would soon have demanded a different type of nurse; indeed there is evidence that before 1860 the better hospitals were attracting women capable of helping the doctors and learning from them. The significance of the Nightingale reforms was that the training was taken out of the hands of the doctors, and, by making nurses accountable to nurses, one condition of being a profession was fulfilled. The emphasis on high standards of personal conduct met another; nurses, like solicitors, became respectable.

Miss Nightingale has been blamed because, 'although she gave women a role outside the home and elevated nursing to a profession she shaped nursing in the traditional role and did not disturb the interaction of the sexes' (Johnson, 1978). This conclusion by Malcolm Johnson is not entirely supported by the contumacious relationships of some of the early new matrons who eventually ruled where men had once done, but in any event Miss Nightingale's mission was to the sick and not to the emancipation of women, to such a role she did not aspire. Nevertheless it is paradoxical that nursing was accepted as a profession just at the time when hospital nursing was less about organising care and more about being an adjunct to the new hospital doctor and using technical instruments. Therefore, in hospitals at least, the reforms produced two conflicting roles for nurses: the managerial role which tended to destroy the concept of professional independence for those below; and ironically, the role that gave most kudos, the technical role, in which the nurse was, she felt, responsible to the doctor. It is not Miss Nightingale's fault that the main professions that women were able to carve for themselves were concerned with the tasks that had been traditionally theirs in pre-industrial times — the care of the sick, the teaching of small children and social welfare. James Stuart Mill (1869) wrote: 'occupations the law and usage make accessible to women are comparatively few and the field of their employment is overcrowded.' Small wonder that these occupations could get good recruits for low pay; men, in their more profitable occupations, saw no reason to change the balance.

PROFESSIONALISM IN THE 20TH CENTURY

During this century occupations have become more complex and society more egalitarian. On the one hand the division of labour, mechanization and automation have made many tasks boring and meaningless so that those with varied or creative jobs are regarded as lucky; on the other hand, until comparatively recently, education in England was such that only a minority attained the training necessary for such jobs, a situation that was socially divisive. However the inter-war concept of a profession typified by Carr-Saunders definition of a profession as 'a distinctive occupation, orientated more towards service to the client than earning salaries and maximizing profit' is now outdated because more and more professionals, including doctors and lawyers, are paid employees and collective bargaining has in many cases become a function of professional organizations, although payments may be clothed in such euphemisms as 'per capita fees for a contract *for* service'. Moreover, the special status of the older professions has been eroded by the emergence of new groups such as social workers and the paramedical professions whose work may be unsupervised, who equally affect the quality of people's lives, and whose negligence can cause great harm for which they are answerable at law. The confusion has been confounded by the change in the legal definition of a Trades Union. Before the Industrial Relations Act of 1972 unions were registered with the Registrar of Friendly Societies and their principal purpose had to be 'the regulation of relations between employers and employees or their associations.' The new Act allowed registration to *bona fide* negotiating bodies who had this clause as *one* of their objectives, and although the Trade Union and Labour Relations Act 1974 restored union rights to the *status quo ante*, it is still possible for an organisation in which this purpose is not the principal article to register as an independent union. Furthermore, because of the peculiar diverse growth of unions from the shop floor upwards in the U.K., as opposed to the Continent, there are unions with articles more akin to professional associations; some white collar unions are affiliated to the Trades Union Congress, some are not; some pay a political levy, some do not. There are many confusing variations on the theme.

THE HALLMARKS OF A PROFESSION

Since there are now no precise definitions of a profession does it make sense to talk about professionalism, and would the country be poorer if there were no groups for whom such concepts as health, education and justice were good ends in themselves pursued not primarily for gain? If professionalism is a goal still worthwhile what are its hallmarks? Many sociologists have written about the professions in the shifting class structure but few people have attempted to set down the modern acceptable determinants. In her book *The Professional Ethic*, Norah Mackenzie tried to bring together the ethical and other distinguishing characteristics of the professional, and in one chapter she lists 15 of which perhaps the most succinct was written over 2000 years ago; it is Plato's account of the Socratic teaching, that, 'medicine looks not to the interest of medicine but of the body' — the professional, says Plato, pursues excellence for its own sake. Nearer our own time Sir Harold Himsworth (1953) in a well-known lecture gave two characteristics which subsume many offered by other authors and which are worth looking at in detail as they relate, — or fail to relate, — to nursing. Sir Harold said that for a profession to exist there had to be a tacit social contract between the profession and society where society allowed the professional 'status, authority and privilege as shall be required for him to discharge his professional duty.' Thus, society allows the professional to be above the law in some respects for example, the doctor and nurse are allowed to possess dangerous drugs and the doctor to make incisions in the body, the lawyer to possess information not disclosed elsewhere, but in return society requires certain undertakings. Sir Harold sees these as being 'a special competence — the technical skill to meet, to an ever increasing extent the needs that called the particular profession into existence . . . unless society has the requisite degree of confidence in the competence of its professions they are helpless.' But he says this degree is 'never ordinary, the needs to be met are too vital to survive the suspicion that the best has not been available. It is this that makes the continual prosecution of research an essential factor in maintaining confidence, it is this that makes the striving after excellence, rather than mere competence, the criterion of professional endeavour.'

But it is not just skill and length of training that distinguishes the professional in the eyes of the man in the street, there is something more, and that something must be trust. Bernard Shaw said 'all professions are a conspiracy against the laity' and in a world of increasing specialisation many would be inclined to agree, for with every step towards more esoteric knowledge the ordinary citizen is more vulnerable. How can clients be sure that their individual good is not being sacrificed to the general social interest? How can clients, blinded by science, trust their professional advisers? There is only one way, and that is that professional men and women must submit themselves 'to a standard of morality more exacting than required by the community in general'. The watchword to all professions therefore must be, 'Act always so as to increase trust.'

IS NURSING A PROFESSION?

In his book *Professional Men* Reader, commenting on the attempts of women at the end of the 19th century to break into the professional world, concentrates on women in medicine saying, 'of course there was nursing but this was not comparable with medicine because nurses were not expected to exercise independent judgement' — a good reason, he concludes, why people thought it a suitable occupation for women. This is not a view shared by Miss Nightingale. The picture may have been partly true of nurses in hospital as they worked more closely with the increasing number of doctors, but there was a world elsewhere where district nurses, health visitors and the early industrial nurses were on their own and did exercise independent judgement, although admittedly their decisions did not deal with needs 'as vital' as those often dealt with by medicine and the law.

The next area of doubt is 'the special competence that called it into being'. Many would argue that nursing has no special competence other than that derived from past empiricism and eclectic borrowings from other sciences. There is nothing wrong about borrowings — most of the new sciences are eclectic as is much of medicine itself. What, until recently, gave pause for thought was the lack of a body of knowledge about nursing, and even where research had been carried out the findings were either not known or not heeded. Until nursing is genuinely research based its claim to professionalism will be weak. However, now that in so many respects the wheel has gone almost full circle and what can be cured has been cured, we are back to the importance of *care*, and here nurses should come into their own as independent practitioners prescribing regimes of care as the religious sisters so often did before the doctors invaded the hospitals. Knowledge is being built up in areas where care is paramount, such as stoma therapy and terminal care; and the nursing process, in which care plans are written down, should help with the compilation of nursing knowledge in such fundamental areas as nutrition, elimination, mobility and the care of the unconscious patient.

Perhaps nowhere is the confusion about nursing as a profession greater than in the area of professional responsibility. The quintessential professional is the unsupervised private practitioner working for a fee. No one doubts that such a person is legally responsible for his professional actions; the difficulty seems to arise when a person is employed. However, doctors in hospital are employed, albeit by a higher tier of management, and they are often seen to be held responsible, so why not nurses? Nurses are sometimes confused because they are accountable to another nurse, but this makes no difference, and the truth is that every professional person is responsible for his or her professional acts. A district nurse who administers the wrong drug, correctly prescribed by another professional, accountable to another nurse and the servant of an employing authority, is still negligent, and, depending on the circumstances, may be held liable in a court of law. This responsibility implies obligations. First, there is a professional and legal duty to keep up-to-date with new developments and to be and remain a safe practitioner. Second, as a duty to oneself and the profession to ensure that legal liability is covered in such a way that the best advice and defence is available if necessary.

Finally, if nursing is to meet all these obligations, the recruits to the profession and those who qualify must be capable of meeting them and it is this need that should be pre-eminent in recruitment and educational policies.

THE PROFESSIONAL ETHIC

Professions organize themselves in different ways but most have some method of disciplining their members. In medicine it is the General Medical Council; in nursing it has been the General Nursing Councils until their functions are taken over by the Central Council of Nursing Midwifery and Health Visiting; in other cases it may be the professional institute itself that acts as the disciplinary court. Although this seems harsh it acknowledges the ineluctable truth of Sir Harold Himsworth's point about the need for a 'code of morality more exacting than that set for ordinary men'. When personal conduct is such that it reflects on the profession then action may be taken by the disciplinary court, although in practice de-registration usually only occurs when conduct, such as drug addiction or alcoholism, renders the practitioner unsafe, or when the scandal involves patients or clients. Nevertheless, conviction in the civil court, however apparently unconnected, will be reported to the professional body.

But apart from the exhortation to be a safe practitioner and to obey the law, what guidelines can professionals use when confronted by the minefields of ethical issues now associated with many health problems and techniques? Should, for example, all life be saved and prolonged? If not, what are the criteria for not striving to keep alive? Should the suspected malformed embryo be aborted? Should the spina bifida victim be saved for a life of paralysis? Is it ever right to betray a patient's or a client's confidence? Can duty as a nurse ever conflict with duty as a citizen? Less dramatically, but now a moral problem, how should scarce resources be allocated? And of course, can members of the caring professions ever be justified in withdrawing their labour as a means of industrial protest?

Depending on a person's own ethical code or religious beliefs, not all these questions pose a dilemma. Some are certain about the sanctity of all life, others are equally sure that life in this world is but transitory. But even for the devout follower of any religion, not all the answers are given and each age throws up its own ethical issues; it was not for nothing in another time of great intellectual upheaval that Cranmer prayed that 'we might both know and perceive what things we ought to do.'

Some of these questions have always troubled men and for over 2000 years men have tried to find principles on which to base moral action. The notion of justice is fundamental and was discussed by Socrates; to some it means 'to every man his rights or his merits', but Socrates came up with the challenge that in pursuing justice for merit it was never right to harm anyone. We can equally argue that justice means 'everyone according to his needs', and this second meaning must affect our attitudes to the need for subsistence wages. The main guide given by Socrates in the end was that justice must be disinterested, a thought to be borne in mind when supporting a 'just wage claim'.

On the other hand we may take our moral stand from Hume (1711–1776) who, taking his cue from Locke, said that man starts with a natural goodness and in weighing our actions we ought to take into consideration the happiness or misery of others. The idea that moral good could be measured by utility and pleasure was taken up by Jeremy Bentham (1748–1832) and enunciated in his principle of 'the greatest happiness for the greatest number' which was the underlying principle of much mid–Victorian legislation and is still used, often loosely, to justify short-term suffering in the interests of long-term greater good — a theory that can be used to justify strike action that inflicts harm on innocent people. The difficulty here clearly is 'whose greater good is the harm to be suffered for, and who decides what is 'good' and who will suffer?'

However, perhaps the greatest of the modern moral philosophers was the man who refuted Hume and the thinkers of the Enlightenment, Immanuel Kant, (1724–1804); Kant held that all moral concepts had their seat in reason and were not an inborn characteristic, that feelings, including sympathy, could be wrong and that there was only one unconditioned good, — the good will — a 'will' that is good not because of what it does but because of its intention: that is, a human action is morally good when it is done for the sake of duty, although Kant never suggested that duty had to be disagreeable — simply disinterested. To find a governing principle, Kant posited two imperatives: the hypothetical and the categorical, and it is the second that has come down to us as Kant's categorical imperative. 'Act only on that maxim through which at the same time you can will it should become universal law.' In other words should I prescribe the other person to act towards me as I am intending to act towards him were our positions changed? Although this provides a work-a-day maxim it does not cover all conduct; Kant himself had a very convoluted argument to show that suicide was morally wrong but his argument was logically unconvincing; nor can it answer our questions about such things as cloning or test-tube babies. No philosophy can, although since so many problems in health care now centre on ethical issues, perhaps ethics and philosophy should be restored to the syllabus for doctors and nurses.

The Rcn Code of Professional Conduct covers many of the points made by the International Council of Nurses in their Code of Nursing Ethics both of which are in accord with the general ethical principles that have come down through the Christian ethic and the major moral philosophers. Emphasis is placed on the responsibility of nurses to protect the well being and dignity of each individual person in their care which is in no way affected by 'the type of origin of the person's needs or illness or by his age, sex, mental status, social class, ethnic origins, nationality or personal beliefs' which means that the Kantian question must be applied to every patient. From this it follows that 'measures that jeopardize the safety of patients, such as unnecessary treatment, hazardous experimental procedures and the withdrawal of professional services during employment disputes' should be opposed by all professional people. In other words, the Benthamite, utilitarian view that good ends can justify bad means is not acceptable. And why is this view not acceptable? It is because the betrayal of the confidence of people in the integrity of the professional destroys their trust and without trust the professions are helpless. Apart from the Christian and Socratic injunction not to inflict harm there is a practical question; if members of the caring profession do inflict harm, who in the future will come to them for care? This is not to say that there are no circumstances in which a profession should take industrial action; such circumstances are conceivable, but before embarking on such action much thought needs to be given to whether the long-term loss of confidence is worth the short-term gain, and whether the proposed action is 'just' that is, disinterested.

Finally, there is the intriguing question of whether it is right to follow truth wherever it leads. In the first Bronowski lecture Dr George Steiner (1978) reminded us that Thales (c.b.624 B.C.) the celebrated Greek mathematician and philosopher fell down a well while looking at an eclipse; studying the stars he could not see the ground beneath his feet; similarly, Archimedes, (c.287–212) whose clever devices had for so long kept armies at bay, was murdered in his garden while studying a problem of geometry. Human progress has always depended on men who ignored the ground beneath their feet — Copernicus, Galileo, Newton and Darwin each in their turn upset preconceived notions about the world — and life would have been more comfortable if they had suppressed their findings. In the last resort we are back to Plato and to the truth as the ultimate aim — more important than man, and, even if we wished, it is impractical to try to turn our backs on the search because, whatever the prohibition, men will always seek what is hidden. The difference now is that the new scientific, and particularly the biomedical, discoveries may open up doors that disturb our ideas of justice and decency, indeed our very ethical codes. We already have life on the machine and the conspicuous consumption of economic resource to push back death or to produce new life, or to invade the mathematics of the genetic code, or to destroy all life — what if findings on the intelligence quotient of one race or group as against another lead away from our ideas of the equal value of all men? Kant went to great pains to show that man's moral behaviour rested not only on his good will, but on his free will, and in the end we are still free to choose how scientific truth shall be used. No man is an island, and nurses, who may well be the patient's best advocate and protector in these matters, cannot stand aside from the great ethical debate.

REFERENCES

Carr–Saunders, Wilson C 1933 The professions. Oxford University Press, London
Himsworth H 1953 Change and permanence in education for medicine. The Lancet 17 October: 789
Johnson M 1978 Nursing auxiliaries and nursing professionalization. Nursing Times February 23: 313
Kant I 1785 The critique of pure reason (trans. Paton H) As groundwork of the metaphysic of morals under the title of The moral law 1948 p 84. See also p 421 of the second edition of The Critique. Hutchinson and Co., London
Mackenzie N 1971 The professional ethic. English University Press, London, ch 7, p 41
Mill J S 1869 The subjection of women. Everyman Library 1970, London
Plato c356 BC The republic. Trans. Lee Desmond, 2nd edn. 1974, p 73. Penguin, London
Reader W J 1966 Professional men. Weidenfeld & Nicholson, London
Royal College of Nursing 1976 A code of professional conduct — A discussion document. London
Shaw G B 1905 The doctor's dilemma. Act 1. Odham's Press, London
Steiner G 1978 Has truth a future? BBC Publications, London
Wilde O 1895 The importance of being earnest. Act III sci. 1974 edn. Penguin, London

FURTHER READING

Baly M E 1975 Professional responsibility. Wiley, London
Baly M E 1980 Nursing and social change, 2nd edn. Heinemann, London
Mackenzie N 1971 The professional ethic. English University Press, London
Paton H J 1948 The moral law. Hutchinson, London
Peters R S 1981 Moral development and moral education. Unwin Education Books, London.
Reader W J 1966 Professional men. Weidenfeld & Nicholson, London

26

Possibilities and problems of interdisciplinary teamwork

Maura Hunt

The need to yoke together separate but interlinked professional skills has arisen over the past 20 years in response to the growth in the complexity of services, the expansion of knowledge and the subsequent increase in specialization. One person may suffer from limitations of knowledge or experience, a team of different but inter-related workers can wipe out these deficiencies. In 1959 the Younghusband Report on social work services made the point that 'In view of the fast growing complexity and scope of modern knowledge no one profession dealing with a range of human needs can make exclusive claim in relation to the others, each has its essential function as well as its necessary overlap with others. This overlap is required for intelligent cooperation and teamwork. It should also enable a holistic approach to be made to the multiple needs of man.' Experience of teamwork methods of working has produced mixed reactions and results which have been mainly negative. Most studies of interdisciplinary teamwork have concluded that the majority of teams are working at levels well below that which is considered potentially possible. Critics of a team approach use this data as 'proof' that teamwork is ineffective and inefficient. The data may be correct but the conclusion reached from it is open to question. The question is not 'team versus no teams' but for the achievement of certain health and social services' goals a team approach is required. The interdependence of health and social service personnel in coping with some problems, such as non-accidental injuries to children, makes them a team by definition whether or not they formally call themselves a team. A team situation exists if a task to be done requires the interdependent efforts of two or more people. Interdependent means that workers involved must work together and coordinate their activities since the job cannot be done by one person alone. This does not imply that members of a team do everything together in a face-to-face interactive manner. It does imply that at various points in time the nature of the task will require coordinating to schedule work, allocate priorities and share information as a basis for problem-solving and decision-making.

Problems related to teamwork do not appear to be inherent in all such methods of working but seem to be associated with the extent to which team members' roles and functions are clearly defined and complement each other. In a study (Wilson 1958) of a surgical team in an operating unit it was found that the roles of each member were so well-defined and each member was so interdependent in the execution of the task, that even individuals who were personally antagonistic to each other could act in accord during the course of the operation. Since verbal communication was often unnecessary if each member knew his job and carried it out competently, unacceptable personal characteristics could be overlooked. An orchestra and a football team can work in similar ways. Legend has it that in the U.S.A a famous double-play combination in a baseball team did not speak to each other off the field for years. In contrast, teamwork can involve considerable communication problems when members' contributions are overlapping or ambiguous or when the degree of interdependence is limited. As a result of a study of relationships between different occupational groups in an American psychiatric hospital it was concluded that:

> Once you gather under the same roof a number of different occupational groups with overlapping skills you may invite problems of competition for prestige and salary, conflicting conceptions of role duties, desires and demands for greater autonomy and independence and other problems which create conflict among personnel and add problems for the administrator. Rushing, 1964.

At a conference of psychiatrists, social scientists and nurses who were engaged in interdisciplinary mental health research, it was found that communication problems were so widespread among them that anyone claiming to have experienced no difficulties in teamwork must be 'in a delusional state' (Luszki, 1958).

BARRIERS TO INTERDISCIPLINARY TEAM FUNCTIONING

Ideally, teamwork involves the definition of common goals and the development of a plan of action to which each member makes a different but complementary contribution towards the achievement of the team's aims. This is not easy to attain and there are some common barriers which stand in the way of effective teamwork functioning. These barriers are:

1. Educational preparation of team members
2. Role ambiguity and incongruent expectations
3. Status differentials
4. Authority and power structures
5. Leadership styles.

Educational preperation

A professional role is learned as an individual goes through a specific educational programme that is designed to teach these skills and knowledge essential to carrying out the work associated with the role. The segregated nature of the educational preparation of the various professionals providing the health and social services can hinder teamwork. Professional educations can provide a limited perspective with jargon, ideologies and values which different professions regard as unique and which are not understood by outsiders. This can present problems of communication in interdisciplinary situations for as Strauss (1962) has remarked 'professionalism complicates the task of developing teamwork between occupations. Each profession tends to develop a parochial specialised point of view. As a result, jurisdictional disputes become common and the overall system starts to break down into a number of semi-autonomous departments.'

Role ambiguity and incongruent expectations

There are many and varied definitions of role but it seems generally accepted that it constitutes the behaviour expected of an individual by virtue of his occupying a specified position in a social situation (Biddle & Thomas, 1966). Role expectations for a certain office and its occupants exist in the minds of members of groups to which they belong, thereby representing standards in terms of which they evaluate performances of their fellows. The context of these expectations includes preferences with respect to what a person should do, what he should think, how he should act and relate to others. These role expectations are perceptual, they exist in the minds of the occupant of a specified position and in the minds of those he associates with in carrying out his work. But expectations do not remain in their minds, they tend to be communicated in many ways, sometimes as direct instructions, sometimes less directly as when a colleague refers a task or expresses admiration or disapproval towards some exhibited behaviour. If team members' expectations of each others' roles are in accord few problems may occur, but if there are serious perceptual discrepancies considerable difficulties may arise.

In a study of teamwork in general practice professional stereotypes and role ambiguities were found to abound (Gilmore et al, 1974; Hunt, 1974). Doctors and nurses often described social workers as 'long-haired trendies' who were unrealistic about problems and lacked 'commonsense'. In turn social workers seem to have images of doctors and nurses which presents them as authoritarian with limited psychological and sociological insights.

Status differentials

Difficulty in integrating members of different status has been identified frequently as a major stumbling block in many interdisciplinary team efforts. Status involves the ranking of an individual by his fellows on the basis of socially acknowledged qualifications which are ascribed to him (Vollmer & Mills, 1951). Explicit status distinctions in a group tend to reduce interaction and social support among members. A study of personnel in a large general hospital found that social interaction typically followed status lines and was inhibited by status boundaries (Wiessen, 1958). Most social contacts of doctors were with other doctors, nurses primarily associated with other nurses and the same was true for other kinds of ward personnel. The results of another study (Candhill, 1958) demonstrated that formal and informal rank were related to participation in staff conferences in a psychiatric hospital. With regard to formal position, senior doctors tended to participate most in discussions concerning patients, residents were next highest in participation and nurses and other workers, like occupational therapists, participated least. Informal status ranking had a similar effect on communication in that the amount of participation of various residents was directly associated with their competence as evaluated by their seniors and with the respect they enjoyed among their colleagues. Moreover, the outcome of a discussion varied according to the status of the individual raising the topic. On topics introduced by a senior doctor only 8% of the discussions were inconclusive, whereas 14% of the topics raised by residents and 21% of topics raised by nurses resulted in inconclusive discussions. This trend tended to evoke frustrations among lower status personnel. Similar communication patterns were identified in teamwork studies in general practices (Gilmour et al, 1974). Analysis of tape recorded team meetings revealed that GPs tended to initiate most of the topics discussed and made the majority of the interventions. Deferential behaviour was exhibited by district nurses and health visitors as reflected in their lack of disagreement with doctors on issues discussed and their apparent inability to initiate debates with doctors on problems within the team which they found frustrating.

Authority and power

Authority has been described as a position that secures acceptance of decision made, enforces performances of roles and ensures coordination of team members' activities (Given et al, 1977). Authority derives from the mandate of an organisation and is associated with specific positions not persons. Power is not inherent in a position, as authority is, but resides in a person and is bestowed by a group. Power relates to the degree of control one member has over the performance and functions of others in the group and influences the organisation of relationships. In health care settings the doctor is traditionally accorded the highest power and authority which enables him to influence others and provides little motivation for him to work with others unless he needs their skills to facilitate his own which he can usually 'order' rather than negotiate.

Leadership styles

Status, authority and power are closely linked and interrelated with the assumption of leadership roles. Democratic societies seem to be fascinated by ways in which groups may be led, by qualities of leadership and by kinds of situations from which leaders arise (Douglas, 1976). Primary health care teams display these tendencies but discussion mainly focuses on the 'natural' right of the doctor to assume leadership as is usual in hospital. Nurses and other health care personnel are referred to as 'ancilliary', 'supplementary' to medicine and 'paramedicals' implying that they are extensions of the doctors and therefore work under their supervision. A writer on 'the changing scene' in general practice presents a commonly held medical view when he states 'increasingly the concept of the family doctor as one in constant attendance is being diluted, albeit necessarily, to his being just one of the people giving care. The general practitioner sees himself and, in perorations, is seen by others as the leader of the team' (Dopson, 1971).

In relation to social workers it would appear as if doctors are seen as occupying a position of higher social and professional status giving them greater power and influence. Tibbitt (1975) in analysing medical and social work relationships points out the inequalities existing between them by stating that:

> The medical profession has a long history, enjoys high social prestige and has developed a large body of specialist knowledge.... These factors have placed it in a favourable position to attract further resources and to extend its domain. Social work, on the other hand, is a new profession still aspiring to full professional recognition. It does not enjoy high social prestige, it has no widely accepted specialist knowledge base . . .

In studies of general practice teamwork (Gilmore et al, 1974; Hunt, 1974) there was a reluctance on the part of doctors, district nurses and health visitors to admit that any formal leadership operated in their groups or that any leader was required. It was noticeable that groups which had regular team meetings and whose members developed some coherent goals and policies had identifiable and dynamic leadership which gave impetus to the groups and coordinated their activities. In all cases such leadership was provided by doctors with the exception of an experimental one set up as part of the study (Gilmore et al, 1974) in which a health visitor acted as 'coordinator', a title that was more acceptable to the team than 'leader'. Provided with some preparation and external guidance and support, the coordinator developed the role sucessfully.

With reference to primary health care teams a nursing writer recently stated that 'teams of unequals don't work' (Kratz, 1978). While lip service is sometimes paid by doctors to the idea that nurses and social workers are 'equal' professionals, in terms of salary, status and power, the scales are heavily weighted in favour of the doctor. It is summed up by Mills (1951) who writes: 'The power position of groups and of individuals depends upon factors of class, status, and occupation, often in intricate interrelation. Given occupations involve specific powers over others in the actual course of work; but also outside the job area, by virtue of their relations to institutions of property as well as the typical income they afford, occupations lend power'. In view of this it seems unrealistic to envisage teams of 'equals' developing in a multidisciplinary sense in the health and social services which will have any real meaning.

Since leadership is essentially a relationship in which one person uses his power and influence in getting a number of people to work together and accomplish a common task (Gibb, 1969) any form of leadership will work if it is acceptable to most of the group members and meets their needs. There are signs that some factions among nurses are questioning the traditionally undisputed relationship between doctors and nurses which has been described as the nurse doing 'the doctor's bidding with unquestioning, unknowledgeable, but — always — reliable dispatch' (Etzioni, 1969). This development is potentially a source of conflict in teamwork and it is suggested by American nurses that 'the general status disparity' and the growing unacceptance of it by nurses is producing a 'structured-in conflict' between doctors and nurses (Dachelet, 1978).

MANAGEMENT OF TEAMWORK PROBLEMS

In studies of general practice teamwork (Gilmore et al, 1974) the most commonly adopted method of dealing with problems and communication difficulties was to reduce communication between team members. Difficulties in most teams tended to be avoided rather than faced and dealt with. In only a minority of teams studies were any regular meetings of all members held which provided opportunities for policy making and the resolutions of difficulties. On this basis most did not merit the title of 'team' since a basic requirement for such a distinction is that all members should engage in fact-to-face interactions and engage in cooperative and coordinating activities.

This evasion of any attempts to engage in problem solving and conflict resolution appeared to be related to (1) ambiguity about the differences between interpersonal and interprofessional relations; (2) high priority on the maintenance of harmonious relations and a negative view of conflicts; (3) deferential attitudes associated with the predominately female composition of nursing.

The lack of distinction between interpersonal and interprofessional relationships tended to inhibit attempts to deal openly with conflicts and to pursue working goals. Evidence of 'successful' teamwork was often presented as the use of first names by team members, their participation in social activities and the maintenance of pleasant, unruffled contacts. These norms tended to place constraints on any open expression of conflicts, of interests, or disagreements over goals and methods. The result was that decisions were sometimes subverted by a process of tacit agreement or problems were repressed and never solved. These tactics did not necessarily correlate with teamwork developments as reflected in innovative or coordinated services to the public. It seemed to suggest that maintaining harmonious relationships became and end in itself rather than being regarded as a means of achieving better quality services for the public which constitutes the *raison d'; etre* of multi-disciplinary groupings.

Conflict was mainly regarded as evidence of teamwork failure while it is suggested that absence of conflict cannot be taken as an index of the strength and stability of relationships. It is considered impossible for any group to be entirely harmonious because it would be devoid of any process, structure or change. Stable relationships may be characterised by conflicting behaviour because it is argued that it is only when relationships have reached a level of stability that frequent conflicts can be engaged in (Coser, 1956). When conflicts cannot be openly tolerated there is likely to be an accumulation of hostile and ambivalent feelings between individuals who interact regularly which has been termed 'unfinished business' (Golembiewski, 1970). A distinction needs to be drawn between realistic and unrealistic conflict which has been differentiated as 'realistic conflict is tied to a rational goal and conflict concerns the means of achieving the goal. In unrealistic conflict the conflict becomes the end in itself' (Norther, 1969).

The fact that nurses are still predominantly female would seem to be related to their tendencies to adopt submissive roles and to attempt to maintain harmony at all costs. The status of nursing is a reflection of the status of women when the skills and qualities required are regarded as extensions of the 'natural' roles of wife and mother epitomising stereotyped feminine attributes. An American nurse has recently stated 'Take away sexism and you take away one of the mainstays of the health hierarchy' (Dachelet, 1978). An indication that doctors are unused to nurses openly engaging in critical debate about their relationships with each other is provided by some published medical responses. A doctor writing in the British Medical Journal spoke approvingly of a nursing speaker's critical comments on aspects of the National Health Service at a recent conference. He was less approving when a critical view of doctors was presented by the same speaker for he observed 'and then, sadly, came the "doctor bashing" ' (Scrutator, 1978). This suggests that there is never any validity in criticisms made of doctors which creates barriers in communication, for by suggesting that the sender of the message is prejudiced the contents of the message can be ignored.

TEAMWORK DEVELOPMENT AND POSSIBILITIES

It appears that teams have problems related to the following:

a. setting goals and identifying priorities

b. analysing and allocating role responsibilities
c. examining and developing teamwork processes
d. managing interpersonal and interprofessional relationships
e. evaluating outcomes of their teamwork endeavours.

It is now being suggested that these concerns are not, as is often assumed, merely the results of individuals' personality defects. Rather, their existence is an indication that a team has not developed the means of dealing with the problems which are inherent in trying to accomplish tasks which require interdependence. There are indications that problems will not disappear of their own accord nor can most interdisciplinary teams innately know how, or learn solely through work experience, how to deal more effectively with these issues. Ideas are being presented which suggest that the knowledge and skills needed to manage inherent teamwork problems can and must be learned through an explicit educational process aiming at team development based on an action-research approach (Rubin, 1971). This involves activities which help teams to solve their own actual problems that result from the interdependent nature of their work. The team is helped initially by outside research consultants to collect data from team members about particular obstacles to team development, reach decisions about solving the problems, implement the problem solving decisions and re-evaluate the outcomes. This action research approach, it is suggested, helps teams to solve their immediate problems and go on to develop ways of maintaining this problem solving means of working. These methods try to deal with the following fundamental questions arising in teams:

1. What are we supposed to be doing?
2. Who is doing what?
3. How do we accomplish our work?
4. How does it feel to work in this setting?

The investment in time to do this is not insignificant in that several of these action research efforts have estimated that for any team to 'get into shape' would require a commitment, for an initial programme, of a minimum of 3–3½ hours per week over a period of 8 weeks to team development activities. Few health teams in Britain appear to engage in this kind of effort, either in setting up teams, or in the preparation of students during professional courses. A great deal of lip service is paid to the need for interprofessional education as part of professional courses for workers in education, social and health services but very little is done to translate these ideologies into practice. Such a commitment would require statutory bodies controlling professional education to jointly plan their respective syllabi with this in view and for curriculum planners to incorporate such learning experiences into their courses rather than have interdisciplinary education produced as activities to fill odd spaces in programmes. Bringing together different disciplines, either at training or practice levels, for a few one-off sessions is only of benefit in initiating these activities. It will have limited effects if it continues in this form and merely gives the impression that this constitutes teamwork development.

Spatial proximity. Even if teams are adequately prepared for working in interdependent ways they may experience difficulties in implementing their ideas if they are hampered by environmental or administrative factors. Dewey (1935) has pointed out that 'the educational task cannot be accomplished merely by working on men's minds without action that effects actual changes in institutions'. Spatial location of group members relative to each other and the probability of contact in the course of daily activity limit in a very tangible way who is likely to interact with whom. It was found in a study (Gilmore et al, 1974) that in moving into a shared office a team of health visitors and district nurses gave fewer 'don't know' responses to questions about the roles of members of the other group. It was also reported that where doctors shared a staff room with the nursing team status differences were reduced and informal communication was facilitated. Another study indicated (Stevenson & Parsloe, 1978) that better relationships developed between social workers and health visitors when they shared the same premises. Proximity facilitates regular meetings and sharing of information though it does not guarantee cooperation (Bruce, 1978).

Administration. Both nursing and social work occupations are administrated by hierachial structures while medicine has a more autonomous organisation. Promotion in nursing and social work requires the surrendering of professional service skills and the assumption of full-time administrative or teaching tasks. In contrast, the most eminent doctor can still practise his basic professional skills. Administrative constraints can cause problems in teams by restricting innovation and enforcing rigid professional boundaries. Since not even established professions can lay claim to a unitary or exclusive body of knowledge to which other professions have no access there needs to be an acceptance of overlap and blurred boundaries between allied occupations. On the other hand, teamwork requires a recognition by members of each other's differences as well as similarities. If all members share the same knowledge and skills there is no need for a multidisciplinary team. Yet in teamwork studies (Gilmore et al, 1974) there was often a reluctance among doctors and nurses to admit that other professionals had knowledge and skills dissimilar to theirs. Some doctors went so far as to state that they possessed all the knowledge and skills that social workers, district nurses and health visitors had but that these occupations did not have the level of medical expertise used by doctors.

Interdisciplinary consultation. If differences were recognised each member of the team could act as a consultant to his colleagues in his particular sphere of special interest. In this way each team member could keep himself and his colleagues up to date in a specific field of interest thereby making use of the main benefits of teamwork by creating a pool of interrelated knowledge and skills within the team. Caplan (1959) has described this kind of consultation as 'an interaction process taking place between two professional workers, the consultant and the consultee. In the interaction the consultant attempts to help the consultee solve a problem of his clients within the framework of his usual professional functioning. The process is designed so that while help is being given to the consultee in dealing with the presenting problem, he is also being educated in order that he will be able in the future to handle similar problems in the same way with other clients in a more effective manner than in the past.' For such a consultation scheme to develop in interdisciplinary teams it would be necessary for members to develop confident occupational identities, to be able to recognise and admit professional limitations and to ask colleagues for help without suffering loss of self-esteem.

THE FUTURE OF THE TEAMWORK

Manifestations of some disillusionment with the progress made in primary health care teamwork seems to be emerging in recent times. Very obvious disenchantment with general practice teamwork is being expressed by health visitors. In a report of the Health Visitors Association's Annual General Meeting in Scarborough in 1977 it was recorded that no one at the meeting 'could have failed to notice the rapturous applause every time a speaker expressed the profession's frustration with working alongside general practitioners' (Clode, 1978). This disillusionment seems to reflect real difficulties in integrating curative and preventive orientations. It may also be presenting a more realistic approach to teamwork in that, over the last decade, general practitioners, health visitors and district nurses have been hastily thrown together without any preparation or help in developing teamwork in the hope that some unspecified 'good' results would emerge from these haphazard tactics. This more realistic view of the problems and complexities of teamwork may represent a healthier approach than the past, rather euphoric, views that existed and may lead to more focused attempts to promote effective teamwork endeavours.

In spite of the communication problems which interprofessional work presents it looks as if it will continue to form the working system within which health and social services will be provided for some time. The trend towards finer divisions of labour and specialisations carries built in contradictions in relation to theories which focus attention on the 'whole' person. Yet, the quest for this approach simultaneously fosters a theory of integration with the practice of fragmentation (Wilson, 1970). The only response to this dilemma that seems feasible is for allied health and social service personnel to continue their efforts to coordinate their activities. The preparation of health and social service personnel for working in teamwork settings is an educational task of great importance for the future and merits more attention than it is currently getting in Britain in terms of research and experimentation. The emphasis on attaining professional status can be achieved at the expense of meeting the community's needs. Rose (1975) claims that: 'To put the client into a central position we need de-professionalisation. With a critical awareness of all the forces that oppose us, we have to make the myth of a service ethic a reality.' Another critic (Webb, 1975) of professionalism as a superordinate goal considers that: 'The greatest barriers to teamwork are not merely ignorance, role uncertainty and confusion, but also those of modifying professional constructions and perceptions of the world, the balance of power which exists between one profession and another, and that which exists between professions and clients.'

Acknowledgement

This chapter is reprinted from 'Teamwork: For and Against: an appraisal of multi-disciplinary practice', 1979, BASW Publications, Birmingham.

REFERENCES

Biddle B J, Thomas E J (eds) (1966) Role theory — concepts and research. Wiley, Chichester
Bruce N 1978 The social work/medicine interface. University of Edinburgh (unpublished)
Caplan G 1959 Concepts of mental health and consultation, US Department of Health, Education and Welfare, p 119
Candhill W A 1958 The psychiatric hospital as a small society. Harvard University Press p 295–296
Clode D 1978 'Of primary concern . . .' Health and Social Service Journal 12 May p 539
Coser L A 1956 The function of social conflict. Routledge and Kegan Paul, London, p 85
Dachelet C Z 1978 'Nursing's bid for increased status'. Nursing Forum XVII (1): 18–43
Dewey J 1935 Liberation and social action. Putnam, London p 4
Dopson L 1971 The changing scene in general practice. Johnson Publications, Surrey, p 47
Douglas T (1976) Group work practice. Tavistock, London, p 68
Etzioni A 1969 The semi-professions and their organisation. Collier-MacMillan, West Drayton, p 59
Gibb C A (Ed) 1969) Leadership. Penguin, Harmondsworth, p 231
Gilmore M, Bruce N, Hunt M 1974 The work of the nursing team in general practice. Council for the Education and Training of Health Visitors, London
Given B, Simmons S 1977 The interdisciplinary health care team — fact or fiction?, Nursing Forum XVI (2): 165–184
Golembiewski R T, Blumberg A eds 1970 Sensitivity training and the laboratory approach. Itasca III, I E Peacock
Hunt M W 1974 An analysis of factors influencing teamwork in general medical practice. M Phil Thesis, Faculty of Social Sciences, University of Edinburgh
Kratz C 1978 Letter in Nursing Times 15 June p 1011
Medalie J 1978 Family medicine — principles and applications. Williams and Wilkins, Baltimore
Mills, C W 1951 White collar. Oxford University Press, London
Northern H (1969) Social work with groups. Boulder Col. U. P.
Report of the working party on social workers in Local Authority Health and Welfare Services 1959 HMSO, London
Rose H 1975 Socialisation and professional ideologies as obstacles to cooperation. European Centre for Social Welfare Training and Research
Rubin I M, Beckhard M 1971 Factors influencing the effectiveness of health teams. M.I.T. Working Paper 561–571 p 20.
Stevenson D, Parsloe P 1977 Social Work Research Project. Universities of Aberdeen, Bristol and Keele
Strauss G (1962) Tactics of lateral relationships: the purchasing agent. The Administrative Science Quarterly Sept 7: 161–186
Tibbitt J E 1975 The social work/medicine interface, a review of research. Central Research Unit, Scottish Development Department
Webb A L 1975 Coordination between health and social services, a question of quality. Eurosocial Report No 4, European Centre for Social Welfare Training and Research
Wiessen A T 1958 Hospital ideology and communication between ward personnel. In: Jaco E G ed Patients physicians and illness. Free Press pp 453–458
Wilson R N 1970 The sociology of health. Random House

27

Continuity of care

Muriel Skeet

You ask me what it is I do. Well actually you know, I'm partly a liaison man and partly PRO
from '*Executive*' by Sir John Betjeman

In its time, liaison has meant 'illicit amour'; the sounding of 'mute final consonant before a following vowel'; and, preceding the title of officer, a 'go-between for allied troops'. More recently in the health and social service field it has come to mean a person who provides, for patients, a connection between home and hospital by way of services and support systems.

In this context, the liaison officer is usually a nurse and more often than not, responsible for patients of either one specialty, e.g. ophthalmology or geriatric medicine, one disease, e.g. diabetes or cancer, or one technique or procedure, e.g. mastectomy or stoma. Someone who integrates care and services for all those patients who form the 'current export' from hospital is, unfortunately, a rare animal and represents one of the more regrettable omissions from our health service.

To a greater or lesser degree, every patient who returns home from hospital has to make a major adjustment and remains vulnerable until rehabilitated to his normal life-style. This applies especially to the patient of advancing years, yet it is these patients who most often suffer physical, mental and emotional distress, much of which could be avoided. Early assessment and competent planning could have prevented many of the horror stories which have illustrated reports on the subject (Skeet, 1970; Roberts, 1975; Age Concern, 1975; Pitkeathley, 1978; Continuing Care Project, 1979; National Corporation for the Care of Old People, 1979).

This chapter, therefore, is concerned with the quality of those arrangements which are made for the continuing care of aged patients discharged from acute hospital wards. Its framework is based on the 'six honest serving men' of Rudyard Kipling.

WHAT

Before we plan its continuation, it is necessary to consider of what the initial care, as opposed to treatment, of these people consists. It is a subject which has attracted a fair amount of attention in recent years but much of the literature relates to either long-term care or to short-term care in geriatric units. The little that has been published on the care of old people in acute wards and departments has been sharply critical. It has even been said that 'the aura of the workhouse lingers on' and that we are trying to run our health and social services for elderly people in ways that 'stem from compulsion and custody as in the past' (Norman, 1980). Another report points out that we 'admit patients to hospital and we discharge them: we may even order (old people) to hospital and there we hold or detain them. We also release them from hospital.' This, the writer suggests, is 'the language of prison, of the police and of criminal law. It is not the language of hospitality' (Binks, 1978).

Of course for everyone, entry into hospital implies a surrender of some autonomy, mainly for the sake of the services which the institution can render. But the maintenance, or regaining, of an identity is vital to every patient if he is to re-establish himself in the community. Because of his disorientation when moved away from familiar surroundings and support systems, the elderly patient needs especial help in this respect. Some certainly receive outstanding kindness and respect from hospital staff, but many are labelled like pieces of luggage and even then incorrectly addressed by name or title. As one observer has said, 'from the point of view of maintaining one's identity it cannot help a grandmother to be consistently addressed as "Miss" nor for a venerable maiden lady to be called "Granny".' It would seem superfluous to say that old people are as much individuals as any other group, but if they are not seen to be so in hospital, it is not surprising that they are not planned for as such on discharge.

This anonymous grouping of the aged manifests itself in other practices. In her excellent discussion paper 'Rights and risks', Alison Norman points out:

> Choice in what we eat is a basic exercise in autonomy, energetically exercised even by two-year-olds. But one senior nurse states that, in his experience, breakfast for the elderly patient is almost always tea, toast and porridge. Lunch, instead of being the high point in a patient's day, is often his most boring . . . . In one ward I observed that these patients had minced beef for dinner and scrambled egg for tea every day for their six-week stay . . . surely the diet could be more varied and include, for example, diced chicken, creamed fish, braised meat and other soft foods . . . Even when menus giving a choice of food are provided, they are often filled in by ward clerks who do not consult elderly patients. Yet helping old people to complete these forms provides an opportunity for daily one-to-one contact in which a volunteer could be effectively used.

This example shows both the lack of recognition of the importance of meals to old people and also the lack of imagination in the use of volunteers. Both can be, and are, reflected in subsequent arrangements for the provision of community services or continuity of care.

A choice of time to sleep is refused only to the very young, to prisoners and to people in institutional care. A normal pattern for most elderly people would be late rising, a nap after lunch, and bed when they feel tired. Such a regime often produces a natural sleep pattern with little need for sedation. Because this is not achieved in hospital, the old, and the very old, person is often sent home with sedatives which only increase his confusion and apathy. Until we get right the 'what' of care for old people in hospital we are unlikely to get right the 'what' of care requested on their discharge. Members of the community team therefore have additional responsibilities to discover and assess as well as to care.

WHY

It has also been reported that some hospital staff see their job as being completed when their patient is 'better' having had his lesion or disease dealt with (CCP, 1974). In the case of young adults they may indeed quickly learn how to fend for themselves, but this attitude can result in the readmission of those patients who are aged (Skeet, 1970).

We no longer live in the days when a few old people are being cared for by many middle-aged relations. The reverse is true. Consequently old people are often caring for each other. When the situation seems to be well managed we may comment to each other and marvel that people in their seventies and eighties are coping so well. But often it is happenning at great cost (Skeet, 1970; Skeet, 1977). Carers need care and supporters need support. Scarce resources must be used discriminately if only in our own interest as taxpayers. Help from the welfare state for these people is vitally needed and often is not forthcoming. In some instances this has resulted in the admission to hospital of the carers themselves, 9% in a survey undertaken by the Continuing Care Project (1979). We can also be misled when told that there is a son or daughter at home. There are now some *very* old patients being discharged from hospital and their sons and daughters are themselves in their sixties or seventies. Particularly tragic is the plight of parents with a physically or mentally handicapped son or daughter living with them. The offspring is also ageing and probably needing more, not less, help.

The modern dilemma of the diminishing family is probably one of the most serious aspects of the lack of continuity of care. The reasons why this should be are likely to remain for a considerable time and, if anything, become greater. Society itself must help and work in partnership with those providing professional support. First, the needs must be assessed locally and made known locally. People forming the local community can then be mobilised and given relevant briefing, knowledge and skills. This is an outstandingly appropriate task for the Voluntary Aid Societies in the form of St John's, St Andrew's and the Red Cross.

If this does not happen, the lives of old people will deteriorate into existences and hospital waiting lists will grow even longer than they are now.

WHEN

Writing on social vulnerability, Williams (1979) noted:

> Two types of situation can arise which cause a change in the social equilibrium of an old person. Both produce domestic deterioration — one insidiously and the other dramatically. The first is where — although basic care is being given — a time arrives when certain tasks, necessary activities and even hobbies, become too demanding and there is a slow but steady lowering of the quality of living. The second is when a crisis occurs because there is a sudden breakdown in the provision of basic care.

Isaacs & Neville (1972) in their study of the Scottish health services, detail in their report three categories of old persons. The first is the *protected*, where the old person being in an institution is protected from social problems (of some kinds). The second is the *defended*, where the old person is cared for by relatives and, being in a state of social equilibrium, is defended from social problems (again of some kinds). The third is the *defeated*, where the old person fails to receive basic care or where relatives are suffering an intolerable strain in providing it. It is important, Isaacs says, to recognise that if an old person is having difficulty with one task, he may also be having difficulty with others. The full extent of the problem may remain unperceived unless this is recognised. For instance, it may become impossible to continue to walk the dog. Then the garden becomes too difficult to manage. Slowly household maintenance may suffer and then care of shoes and clothes becomes overlooked. If this is the state of affairs before illness, how is the old person going to cope after surgery or after his spouse has had a stroke? It is when such things as these are known that better or wiser planning can be undertaken.

Some problems, of course, are more subtle and therefore the 'when' may not be so obvious. Many old people, for example, fail to keep up with changing economic circumstances and do not easily assimilate new information. Pension rates change, licensing fees for television are raised and these facts have to be understood. Poverty is often seen as a problem of old age and while it may be due to a lack of money, sometimes it is due to having an expenditure out of all proportion to today's values and needs (Williams, 1979). Today's old people come from a thrifty generation which has been taught to save for a rainy day, and although now is the rainy day, and they are unlikely to live to see a rainier one, they still feel the necessity to save, or at least not to spend. It is a habit. They are therefore reluctant to buy food, clothes and fuel, even when having the resources for doing so. Their savings preclude state help and so the lowering of standards continues.

There are other problems and difficulties of course — mental, sexual and spiritual. There is also the phenomenon of the 'captive spouse'. Because of the disability or frailty of a husband or wife, the patient may be going home to work harder than at any other time. Only when such facts are known and communicated can plans for continuity of care be made and timed to meet the greatest needs of discharged old people.

HOW

It cannot be over-emphasised that continuity of care can only be achieved by careful planning and that careful planning can only take place after careful assessment. This should take place as soon as the transfer, from home to hospital or hospital to home, is known. the former cannot always be anticipated, but discharge from hospital should never come unexpectedly to a patient nor to those attending him.

The decision to discharge should be based on accurate, relevant and up-to-date information concerning each patient. Those involved must build up a picture of him in his normal situation, psychological, social and domestic. Only in this way can potential needs be identified and plans made to meet them. The newly admitted elderly patient may be an unknown quantity to those working in hospital, but it is likely that he is well known to a number of people in the community. In an era of scarce resources, it is important to look at information already available and those who hold it should communicate with members of the hospital staff. This can help to identify at an early stage, not only potential problems but also potential support.

If, on the other hand, no attempt is made to pass on to hospital staff the relevant facts, a false picture of the patient may be drawn up by them, having regard to the patient's ability within hospital where he is dependent upon others. It is not reasonable to expect the patient himself to anticipate how he will feel and manage when he returns home. Whilst in hospital, he may be lulled into a sense of unreal optimism about his capabilities. Constant attendants will give him confidence and his very surroundings will often enable him to get about more easily than he would at home.

It is appreciated that the question of confidentiality arises. All professionals have the right to keep confidential notes, but surely basic information should always be shared with colleagues. If there is any doubt, the patient's permission to do this should be requested. This permission is rarely refused, especially when a patient understands that the information will be passed on to colleagues better able to help with his particular anxieties or difficulties. In this way, information on home circumstances, support available, and services already being received or likely to be required, can be recorded and made available to all who should be concerned. Because conditions and situations change rapidly, frequent reviews may be necessary.

Equally severe difficulties have been reported in communication from hospital to community when a patient is discharged. One notorious subject of complaint is the delay in notifying the patient's general practitioner. Even when a communication is received it may contain sparse and inadequate information and not stimulate the doctor to give visiting the priority it deserves.

Sometimes, although a wide variety of services and support systems exists in the community, they are not mobilised. This may be because no-one has realised the services are needed, or because the service-providers have not been informed soon enough, or because the patient, when he does realise that he needs help, does not know where, how or whom to ask for it.

Communication, collaboration, cooperation and coordination between and amongst all members of the health and social teams as well as patients and their families are vital to the 'how'.

WHERE

If communication, collaboration, cooperation and coordination actually take place accurate assessment, efficient planning and effective care can result. The latter may be totally in the patient's own home or it may include visits to day centres, clinics, clubs or therapy groups. For the assessment and planning stages, it has been discovered that, at the present time, there are considerable differences, mostly dependent upon whether the old person is in a geriatric unit or in an acute unit. In the former, there seems to be general agreement that the concept of geriatric care presupposes some kind of multi-disciplinary approach, a goal of rehabilitation, and a positive approach to the patient's health and welfare in the community.

In these units the responsibility for identifying needs is seen as shared and never as falling to one person. The key is seen to be 'coordination', not 'domination' by one person. The method and place may vary, but in the majority of instances is either a multi-disciplinary ward round, or a case conference, or a meeting held at varying intervals at which each patient is discussed.

Any of these may involve two-way visiting. Community based staff, social workers, district nurses, health visitors, home-help organisers and general practitioners, come into the hospital; while occupational therapists undertake home visits with community staff and make assessments of their patient's capabilities and rehabilitation needs. Most important, whenever feasible, the patient and his family form part of the planning team.

WHO

As has been pointed out in the literature, frequently the geographical proximity of individual health workers does not create an instant team. It is not always easy to work as a team member and doctors and nurses are often strong individualists. There are also differing ideas about who actually constitutes a community or social health team. Is the patient's home-help a member? How about the W.R.V.S. meals-on-wheels server, or the volunteer visitor, or the immigrant who keeps the corner shop open seven days a week for these elderly people without deep freezes and refrigerators? What of other tradesmen, and the church? Now, as never before, there is a need for all members of the health and social service teams to work *with* as well as *for* the community.

Certainly the patient and his family are team members, for the success of most discharges depends in the end on the abilities of the patients themselves, and of their families and friends, or others, who care for them. All the treatment and help provided by the hospital can be wasted if those who are to provide care on discharge are not well-informed and supported. The nature and timing of information passed to relatives and patients and their comprehension of it are factors which influence recovery and future cooperation. They must be confident that back-up support will be available to them from community teams when and where it is required. A return to community participation, to self-reliance and to essential support, rather than indiscriminate bestowals of largesse from the welfare state, could make continuity of care for discharged hospital patients an attainable goal.

In order to make the most of his capacity for self-care, professionals must use their patient's adequacies and abilities rather than concentrate on their deficiencies. Similarly the community to which they are discharged should be encouraged to use its own local resources and develop self-reliance. If, for instance, it is identified that a need of the patient is at least one meal prepared for him, it does not necessarily have to be provided by the meals-on-wheels service: the liaison nurse may often be able to organise a neighbour to provide this for the short period it is required. Likewise, a patient who lives alone and is unable to shop does not necessarily need a home-help. He may be visited by a voluntary worker who will get his shopping when she does her own.

No one person can completely identify and adequately meet the multiple and often complex needs of many of our patients. Collaboration and cooperation must replace the fragmented approach to the development of discharge procedures; agreed procedures must supercede the hit-or-miss approach of today's practice; and finally, only coordination will ensure that agreed procedures, through liaison, are carried out efficiently and effectively to provide continuity of patient care.

REFERENCES

Age Concern 1973 Care is rare (out of print)
Betjeman John Executive (Poem)
Binks F, Allen 1978 Changing the subject. Lancet July 1
Cang Stephan 1977 Why not hospital-at-home here? Age Concern, London
Continuing Care Project: 1975 Going home?
1979 Getting better?
1979 Nobody told me
1979 Help! I need somebody
1979 It would be nice to feel someone cared
Isaacs Bernard, Neville Yvonne 1972 The measurement of need in old people. Scottish Home and Health Dept, Edinburgh
Kipling Rudyard 1865–1936 The elephant child (Poem)
National Corporation for the Care of Old People 1979
National Corporation for the Care of Old People 1980
1979 Organising aftercare
1980 Rights and risks
Orr J G 1977 Care of the elderly patient in hospital. Nursing Times. 73, (27): July 7
Pitkeathley J, Gay P 1978 When I went home. Pitman Medical, London
Raphael W, Mandeville J 1979 Old people in hospital. King Edward's Hospital Fund, London
Royal College of Nursing/British Geriatrics Society 1973 Improving geriatric care in hospitals
Reynolds M 1978 No news is bad news. British Medical Journal, Vol 1
Roberts I 1975 Discharged from hospital. Royal College of Nursing, London
Skeet M, Crout E 1977 Health needs help. Blackwell Scientific Pubs, London
Skeet M 1979 Home from hospital, 5th edn. McMillan Journals, London
Williams I 1979 The care of the elderly in the community. Croom Helm, London

FURTHER READING

Organising Aftercare — An examination of ways in which aftercare arrangements for elderly hospital patients could be improved in order to ensure their fullest recovery and maintain their independence. National Corporation for the Care of Old People for the Continuing Care Project 1979.
Rights and Risks — A discussion document on civil liberty in old age from the National Corporation for the Care of Old People written by its Assistant Director, Alison J. Norman. 1980.
Old Age: A Register of Social Research 1977–78. Over 160 current or recently completed research projects. The register is arranged in subject order and extensive detail is provided on each project. National Corporation for the Care of Old People.
The Care of the Elderly in the Community. A description of some of the problems encountered by members of the community health and social teams looking after old people at home and some of the ways in which these problems may be solved. Croom Helm 1979.

28

Counselling

Gaynor Nurse

The word counselling is increasingly used in professional circles and this chapter is concerned with what exactly is meant by the term, how the skill is exercised, and what part it has to play within the role and function of those who work in the community.

Most people would agree that the overall aim of community care is to enhance the health potential of individuals. In order to achieve this end many avenues are followed and many agencies are set up, both statutory and voluntary. Differing tools are used, and a variety of methods employed, ranging from trying to change the environment to working in depth with one individual.

The background training of many community health workers is geared towards *doing* things for people, towards being the individual with the knowledge and expertise, delivering information, providing facilities. All these attributes are essential, but often not enough attention is paid to creating an environment in which people can be helped to help themselves, with the aim of eventually making the helper redundant in a particular situation. As human beings we are all interdependent, and at times the greatest help we can give another is to narrow the gap between the all-knowing, all-powerful, all-adequate professional and the uninformed, powerless, dependent patient or client. This is where the method of helping called counselling may be appropriate.

DEFINITION

What do we mean by this word? Considerable mystique still surrounds it. Vaughan (1976) has collected together a useful selection of definitions ranging from those who see counselling as mainly a problem-solving approach to those who see it as helping individuals towards maturity and the meaning of life. He suggests that amongst the many schools of thought three elements of the definition usually recur:

1. The concept of person-to-person form of communication marked by the development of a subtle emotional understanding, often technically described as rapport or empathy.
2. This communication is centred upon one or more problems of the client.
3. It is free from authorative judgements or coercive pressures by the counsellor.

A useful comprehensive definition was compiled over ten years ago by the Steering Committee of the Standing Committee for the Advancement of Counselling (now called the British Association for Counselling), which stated that counselling is 'a process through which one person helps another through purposeful conversation in an understanding atmosphere. It seeks to establish a helping relationship in which the one counselled can express his thoughts and feelings in such a way as to clarify his own situation, come to terms with some new experience, see his difficulty more objectively, and so face his problem with less anxiety and tension. Its basic purpose is to assist the individual to make his own decision from among the choices available to him.'

So it is an enabling process, helping the individual towards growth, whether through an immediate problem that is concrete and explainable or through a situation which has a broader scope to do with the meaning of life, with wholeness and integration.

Where does this fit into the work of the community care worker? Counselling is not the whole answer to the ills of the world, and the professional skill is to assess what is the most appropriate form of help for this particular individual at this particular time. Hopson (1978) identifies four types of helping strategy:

1. *Direct action* — taking action yourself to provide for someone else's needs.
2. *Giving advice* — making suggestions about courses of action another person can and possibly should take, looking at it from your position.
3. *Teaching* — helping someone acquire knowledge and skills that you think they need.
4. *Counselling* — helping someone to explore a problem so that he or she can decide what to do about it.

These categories often overlap, and any one individual, for example a stoma patient or a new mother, may need two or more types of help. So counselling is one of a range of skills which can be used by the practitioner, and is gradually coming to be recognised as being an important aspect of caring. It is also a skill which those whose professional background is often based on knowledge, authority and power may find difficult to learn.

THE CLIENT

What kind of person needs the type of help which comes under the broad definition of counselling? Before identifying specific individuals it is useful to think about the needs of each and every human being, which are as much a part of those of us who call ourselves professional helpers as of those whom we call patients and clients. One of the clearest categorisations of these needs is given by Maslow (1970) who places them into broad hierarchical bands:

a. Physical needs, such as food and water
b. Safety needs, such as protection from injury and pain
c. Social needs, such as affection, approval, identification
d. Esteem needs, such as prestige, self respect, success
e. Need for actualisation.

The first and second needs would not be met by counselling as defined in this chapter, except perhaps in the basic form of helping a person to provide answers for himself. But in the provision of the last three the process of counselling has an important part to play. Most nurses have at some time met the pregnant woman who has all the outward signs of a comfortable home and loving husband and yet who is fearful and apprehensive about her coming motherhood; or the only daughter looking after an aged parent who has woven her life around this care and in consequence lives in a narrow and restricted environment; or the young girl living in one room with an active toddler; or the mother with a large family who finds herself pregnant yet again; or the father about to be made redundant; or the middle-aged woman who can find no purpose in life now that the children have grown up. These and many others are met with day after day by those working in the community.

In counselling, the word client, although still an unsatisfactory term to many, is usually used as distinct from patient, for the latter concept carries associations of illness, whether mental or physical. It also implies being passive and letting others, either doctor or nurse, make decisions for him. In counselling, the client has an active part to play in the therapeutic process, and the client and counsellor, although in different roles, are a partnership, working, seeking, and exploring together.

Mention must also be made, not only of the clients with whom we are in a professional helping relationship but also of us the carers who try to help them. We too are very human, with all the physical and psychological needs common to all living persons and yet we are expected to meet the demands of others. As well as the stresses of our ordinary lives, there are additional stresses which are specific to people who work in such situations, for example concern over the inadequate social conditions of many patients and clients, ethical problems such as euthanesia and abortion where clear-cut guidelines often do not exist, problems presented by different cultures and backgrounds, being at the receiving end of both the positive and negative feelings of others, unsatisfactory working conditions and organisational structure. The helper too needs support and needs to feel cared for, within what can loosely be called a counselling environment.

THE COUNSELLOR

What sort of person should the individual be who wishes to fulfill the counselling part of her professional role? She will see herself primarily as a midwife or district nurse, health visitor or community psychiatric nurse, social worker or auxillary helper, or whatever her occupation is. She will hopefully be as expert in her particular role as it is possible for her to be. Is this alone sufficient for the counselling aspect, or does the ability to counsel vary with the kind of person the helper is? If one asks any group of people what they see to be the important qualities looked for in a counsellor, the suggested adjectives are likely to include: tolerant, accepting, self aware, available, non judgemental, caring, mature . . . the list is endless and one is left at the end feeling that if all these attributes *were* to be found in any one individual then that person would be pretty impossible to live with! From the increasing research and evaluation undertaken, it is being found that the most important ingredient in the helping relationship is the person of the helper herself. Combs (1974) shows continually that the use of self is the most effective instrument we have, and that *how* we use ourselves 'makes the interaction whatever it is to become'. Rogers (1961) also equates 'the degree in which relationships can be created which facilitate the growth of others to the measure of growth which the helper has achieved in himself'.

Carkhuff (1969) identifies three essential ingredients which need to be present in the helper, and these have been emphasized and reinforced by many others as well. 'The three necessary and sufficient qualities' as they are often called are:

1. Non-possessive warmth
2. Genuineness
3. Empathy.

1. Non possessive warmth, or 'unconditional positive regard' to use a jargon phrase, is to do with warmth and caring; with valuing the other individual as a worthwhile person; with accepting the other as he is, a quality which can only be realised when we are first able to accept ourselves — easy to say, difficult to do. It specifically excludes such attitudes as condemnation, exhortation and judgement. These latter aspects can be right and proper in some other categories of helping — but not in counselling.

2. Genuineness, or self-congruence. It is important to be one's real self and not to hide behind a role, which it is all too easy to do. A counsellor needs to be spontaneous and open, to be her authentic self. In order to do this a certain amount of self awareness is necessary, and the readiness to disclose a little of herself when this is appropriate. Authenticity allows the helper to forget herself and to concentrate on the client, instead of being too concerned with how she is being seen by the client, and being overpreoccupied with strategies and techniques.

3. Empathy is firstly to do with perceiving the feelings and meanings of the other person, to see things from his point of view. It is to do with accurately understanding not only the other's thoughts but more particularly his feelings. It does not mean actually having the same feelings as the other, but rather with recognizing and accepting that someone else's feelings are real to him at this moment. The second important part of being an empathic person is to communicate your understanding back to the client, so that he too recognizes your perception and acceptance of his feelings, and that you are tuned in to him as he is, here and now.

THE COUNSELLING RELATIONSHIP

What are some of the characteristics in which a meeting between two people becomes a relationship which can be called counselling? Obviously it has to do with the personalities, attitudes and expectations which both the counsellor and the client bring to the situation.

Community health workers will bring not only their professional expertise but also themselves as people, and clients will bring the specific difficulty or problem together with all that makes them the particular individual they are.

Tolbert (1972) identifies seven criteria necessary to form an effective counselling relationship:

1. Helper and client are both 'themselves', or congruent. There is some spontaneity, and the situation is real rather than forced.
2. Acceptance of the client as a unique and valued human being. 'Warm', 'friendly', 'caring for' are descriptive terms.
3. What the client is saying and experiencing is understood. There is empathy, not sympathy.
4. The persons involved 'communicate'. They understand each other.
5. 'Trust' is present. The client trusts the helper to accept him, to keep confidences, to be deeply concerned. Thus he can be himself without fear of judgement, ridicule or punishment.
6. Concern for the client is the focus of attention. This can be shown in many ways, but especially by the helper's complete attention to the client.
7. What the client is exploring is important; manipulation, resistance, superficiality are not present.

Thus the district nurse who makes a home visit primarily to give some form of medication may find herself with a patient who really wants to talk of his concern about the future quality of his life. The professional relationship must then not only include the necessary technical skills and knowledge but also be one where the nurse does not know the answers, is not the dominant person, but creates an atmosphere in which the patient is able to explore those feelings and to feel heard and accepted.

Once more Rogers (1961) has some very pertinent comments. He says: 'If I can create a relationship characterized on my part by:

1. A genuineness and transparency in which I am my real feelings;
2. A warm acceptance of and prizing of the other person as a separate individual;
3. A sensitive ability to see his world and himself as he sees them; then the other individual in the relationship will:
    a. Experience and understand aspects of himself which previously he has repressed;
    b. Find himself becoming better integrated, more able to function effectively;
    c. Become more similar to the person he would like to be;
    d. Be more self-directing and more self-confident;
    e. Become more of a person, more unique and more self-expressive;
    f. Be more understanding, more acceptant of others;
    g. Be able to cope with the problems of life more adequately and more comfortably.'

COUNSELLING SKILLS

What are some of the important skills which the counsellor employs in order to help the client? It has already been stated that to concentrate too much on techniques can be a barrier to creating a truly helpful relationship, and can inhibit the use of the counsellors own, genuine self. Nevertheless some of the component skills of the counselling process are so basic and essential that it is as vital to use them appropriately as it is the more technical nursing skills such as performing an aseptic technique or administrating drugs.

1. Attending. Just because we are in the same room as someone or even talking with him does not mean we are necessarily really giving him our full attention. Egan (1975) suggests a model of helping, consisting of three stages in which the client is helped to:

a. Explore his feelings and his behaviour;
b. Come to a degree of understanding about himself and his difficulties;
c. Act in some way on this understanding, perhaps by making decisions or coming to terms with the situation.

He states that before this process can even start there has to be what he calls 'the prehelping stage', that is, Attending, without which none of the other stages can take place. This means both a physical and psychological presence, so that we can truly 'be with' the other, and he in his turn feels he really has our presence in a whole way. Two aspects of attending are particularly important:

(i) *Environment* — the actual practical surroundings in which counselling takes place can help or hinder the way in which the client perceives our attention, our concern for him as a person. Whether the setting is formal, for example a clinic or an office, or very informal such as the street, launderette, or kitchen in the client's home, it is essential that notice is taken of the external framework. So far as is possible distractions such as the telephone, other people, children, television, are kept to the minimum; the position and level of chairs, removal of artificial barriers, comfort — all these and others are important adjuncts to really being *with* the other person, and often considerable ingenuity has to be employed to that end.

(ii) *Posture* — our body gives many cues about our feelings, and plays a large part in communication of which we are often unconscious. Some of the skill in attending lies in being aware of the signals our body is giving to the other person. Ordinary things like whether we are sitting in a relaxed manner or perched nervously on the edge of the chair; what our hands (and feet) are doing; whether our arms are tightly crossed in front of us as if we were defending ourselves, or are placed in an open, accepting position; how much eye contact is taking place between us; whether we are leaning slightly towards the other or half turned away. In many human contacts what our body says is at variance with what our tongue in saying, and in an interaction such as counselling this can make or mar the outcome.

2. Listening. This is an activity we have all been engaged in to a greater or lesser extent since the day we were born and recent experiments show that it probably takes place *in utero* as well! It is a daily activity and one we take for granted — yet how often do we stop to wonder about the quality of our listening? For some of us it can be very salutary to recognise that, although we may stop talking and allow the other person to speak, we often do not really hear what they are saying and are primarily waiting for them to stop so that we can then give our own point of view. Many barriers get in the way of effective listening, including:

- preoccupation with someone or something else
- trying to remember what has been said previously
- hearing what we expect/want to hear
- anxiety over what is being said
- desire to terminate the session because of length of time or busyness.

It is frequently said, when faced with someone in distress or difficulty: 'I didn't know what to say, I could only listen.' To have or give the experience of being really listened to can be healing in itself, and the skill of listening may be the most useful therapeutic activity we can engage in.

3. *Responding* — Non-verbal cues, previously mentioned, are important ways of letting the client know how we are responding to them. Eye contact, body posture, facial expression, movement — all give clear indications about our own interest or boredom, approval or disapproval, irritation, concern, etc. Silence too has a very real place in communication, and using it appropriately can be of much value. Most of us need to practice the skill of 'letting silence be', being comfortable with its use and aware of its meaning within the counselling relationship.

Verbal responses are of many kinds. A useful categorization is that given by Clinebell (1966) of the five main types of response used in conversation:

a. Evaluative — one which carries the value judgement of the helper.
b. Interpretive — one which tends to teach or explain the dynamics of the others behaviour.
c. Supportive — one which seeks to reassure, encourage or inspire another.
d. Probing — one which asks questions.
e. Understanding — one which reflects the other persons feelings and attitudes.

Each has its place and value in different professional relationships, but it will be noticed that four out of the five take the onus away from the other person, and we need to be aware that this is so.

Self disclosure, challenge, reflection, feedback — these are some other forms of responding which may have a place in the counselling process. To aid the other person in his self-exploration and understanding and then come to a decision, demands recognition of the type of response which is the most appropriate one for the particular place that the client has reached at that particular time.

4. *Decision-making.* Much counselling in the community is to do with a specific problem or difficulty, and it may be that another category of helping i.e. physically doing something for the client, advising, guiding or teaching is the most appropriate way (we always need to ask the question appropriate for whom? Is it because it is really in the best interest of the client, or is it because it makes the helper feel more comfortable and satisfy his own need to *do* something?) When a health visitor, for example, is in touch with a family where the mother is finding it difficult to cope with the demands of her toddler as well as the new baby, and the mortgage repayments are in arrears — this type of situation calls for a multiplicity of helping techniques, and the skill is to know which one is appropriate when.

If in counselling one of the main aims is to help the client to help himself, then we need to enable him to decide and put into practice his own steps in problem solving and decision-making. Stages which have been found valuable in this part of the counselling process include helping him to:

- identify and clarify the problem in as concrete a way as possible
- establish priorities, so that not too much is attempted at one time
- set specific goals which are realistic and obtainable
- work out possible means for achieving these goals
- build some method of evaluating whether these goals have/have not been achieved
- follow up and review progress.

Sometimes it will be found that the means chosen or the decisions made originally were too difficult to implement. The client may then need further help in deciding on different methods, concentrating on another issue first, or maybe facing the reality that some situations just cannot be changed. The counselling skill here lies in enabling the client to utilise his own resources, take responsibility for his own actions and decisions, and finally to become as independent as possible.

CONCLUSION

If, as has been suggested in this chapter, it is accepted that: (1) health is not achieved once and for all at any one time but is a process which varies according to the demands of life (2) counselling is one way of helping the growth of the individual (3) the needs of the client are also common to all of us (4) the person of the counsellor is of critical importance (5) the relationship is the enabling factor which makes growth possible and (6) counselling skills are an essential part of the process. How then can the community health worker be helped to achieve and practise this particular form of promoting health? Some people appear to be natural counsellors; but, as with 'born nurses', the good become even better with education and training. Three ways are therefore suggested for achieving a greater awareness of the potential for and use of counselling:

1. In all types of basic training, methods of teaching elementary communication and interpersonal skills should be developed in order to increase deliberately the amount of such learning that takes place.

2. Community health workers should be encouraged to attend recognised courses in counselling skills. Whether it is possible to 'teach' counselling is debatable, but it is certainly possible to enable inherent skills to be improved and enhanced, and to give opportunities for the helper to develop greater self-awareness and growth.

3. Learning does not cease once a course is finished, and all persons involved in this type of helping need continuing support and encouragement. This is one of the recommendations of the Counselling in Nursing Report (1978) which states that support is an essential provision for anyone engaged in counselling situations, and suggests it can be provided in a variety of ways according to differing needs and the availability of resources.

If quality of life is an essential component of the health of the community, then counselling is one of the ways towards this achievement.

REFERENCES

Carkhuff R 1969 Helping and human relations. Holt Rinehart and Winston, New York
Clinebell H J 1966 Basic types of pastoral counselling. Abingdon Press, New York
Combs A W, Avila D L, Purkey W W 1974 Helping relationships — basic concepts for the helping professions. Allyn & Bacon, Boston
Corey G 1977 Theory and practice of counselling and psychotherapy. Wadsworth, California
Egan G 1975 The skilled helper. Brooks Cole, California
Hopson B 1978 Counselling. Nursing Times 74 (12 January): 50–51
Kalisch B J 1973 What is nursing? American Journal of Nursing 73 (9)
Maslow A H 1970 Motivation and personality. Harper & Row, London
Rogers C 1961 On becoming a person. Constable, London
Royal College of Nursing 1978 Counselling in nursing. Working Party Report
Tolbert E L 1972 Introduction to counselling. McGraw Hill, New York
Vaughan T D (ed) 1976 Concepts of counselling. Bedford Square Press, London

FURTHER READING

Bridge W, Clark J M (eds) 1981 Communication in nursing care. HM&M/John Wiley, Chichester
Jourard S 1971 The transparent self. Van Nostrand Reinhold, New York
Kennedy E 1977 On becoming a counsellor. Gillard MacMillan, Dublin
Nurse G 1980 Counselling and the nurse, 2nd edn, HM&M/John Wiley, Chichester
Proctor B 1978 Counselling shop. Burnett Books, London
Speck P 1978 Loss and grief in medicine. Balliere Tindall, London
Wallis J H 1973 Personal counselling. Allen and Unwin, London
Wilson M 1971 The hospital — a place of truth. Department of Theology, University of Birmingham

29

Talking with clients

Kathleen Robinson

One of the most welcome facets of recent developments in nursing education and research has been the increased emphasis on personal interaction rather than on task performance. Some branches of nursing, notably health visiting and psychiatric nursing, have always been concerned with social events rather than physical tasks, but in all specialities from intensive care to midwifery there has recently been an increased interest in how nurses and clients interact. This development mirrors the earlier focus of attention on G.P./patient interaction and parallel interests can also be found in other health care areas, such as health education.

The interest is generated by a growing awareness of the inadequacies of patient care, and criticisms of existing practices have come from both the professional and consumer lobbies. The consumer lobby has been concerned to counter the tendency to dehumanise the client and has exphasised the positive role of the client in decision making and self-help. The professional lobby too has been concerned with the existing status of client as object, but has also been concerned to explain the failure of medical care to effect great changes in the health status of individuals by focusing attention on the relationship between professional and client as the weak link in the system of health care provision. Without being unduly cynical, it might also be supposed that nurses and other paramedical workers are interested in establishing a claim to expertise in the area of interpersonal relations as a counter to the dominance of the medical profession which is based on the doctor's monopoly of expertise in clinical diagnosis and prescription. This is particularly true of health visitors, who are of course open to the charge that they 'just' talk, and who therefore feel the necessity to elevate talking with clients to the status of a professional skill.

Because the interest has been fired by the desire to solve some of the apparent problems of health care, there has been a tendency to impose the status of 'problem' on the whole area of interpersonal relations. This has, of course, the advantage for professional health workers of settling the question of the *problem* and concentrating on the *solution*, in which we then claim exclusive expertise, thus avoiding any searching examination of health care goals and processes. It assumes, for instance, that 'patient non-compliance', which is jargon for patients not doing what we tell them to do, is caused by an interpersonal 'problem' and is not a reflection of patients' needs and choices.

Thus the process of interaction between worker and client is labelled as a problem, and because health workers are traditionally seen as acting *on* the client, who remains essentially passive, the problem is seen to be related to the health worker's actions. Obviously we must assume that the motives and aims of the worker are correct, (after all, when we ask her she says she wants to help the client) so the problem must lie in how she communicates with the client. Somehow her speech must be failing to communicate adequately her aims and intentions. The problem has become a technical one of communication.

This theme of communication failure fits well into the nurses' existing mode of practice. Although it may be promoted as an attempt to destroy the traditional, task-centred, nurse-dominant mode of practice, communication has become just another task to be performed on the patient. Just as the nurse can be taught a sterile dressing technique, so she can be taught the supposedly precise skill of communication.

This theme of communication as a skill has been taken up by the nursing press. During 1981 both the Nursing Times and Nursing Mirror included a series of articles on Communication. Indeed 1981 was designated by the Nursing Times as 'the year of communication' and they also ran a regular interesting and instructive feature on communication skills which concentrated on natural examples of nurse/patient talk and was called, appropriately, 'Talking Points'.

However, I want to show that the prevailing view of communication as a problem is based on an inadequate view of the nature of language in social life. My use of the term language here follows that of Harold Garfinkel. Filmer defines this as 'a much wider sense than the purely verbal, as comprised of common vocabulary, grammar and syntax, not only of words but of symbols, gestures, expressions, deportments and so on of all kinds' (Filmer et al, 1972). Both researchers and teachers have concentrated on using language studies to offer evaluative and prescriptive explanations. This focus has neglected the description of language use; a description which could tell us a great deal about how both workers and clients go about deciding what, in practice, health care is all about.

To those whose reaction to the previous paragraph was to say that you are not interested in the place of language in ordinary life, but only in the nature of professional communications, I would suggest that health care *is* a part of ordinary life. Being a nurse of therapist or doctor or patient is only one facet of anybody's life. Moreover, the social relationships in health care proceed by the same processes as those in any other social system. That is not to say that they do not have particular and peculiar problems, but that they are constructed and maintained in the same way as other social relationships. Although health workers tend to think of their problems as unique, this view is rather an introverted one for there are many other facets of life which present equally difficult and distressing episodes and require equally delicate handling. A few health care problems are probably unique and I am not concerned here with the technical problems of communicating with sense-impaired patients. In general it is important to concern ourselves with the abilities of ordinary people and to remind ourselves that that is what health workers and clients are — simply ordinary people in a particular setting. We have no reason to suppose that we all leave our advanced social skills, and in particular our ability to talk, at the door when we arrive at a hospital or clinic or surgery, and even less reason to suppose we forget them in the course of a domiciliary visit. We must, therefore, look at the use of language in social life in general before assuming that any problems encountered in health care settings are attributable to poor social skills and particularly to poor language use.

Two interlinked points are basic to an understanding of our practical use of language. Firstly, it is important to realise that behaviour cannot be viewed as distinct from thought. The desirable qualities in interaction can be characterised as dispositional concepts (Ryle, 1963). That is, for example, to say that someone is 'caring' is not a statement about their inner state of mind but is a statement about their actions, and in particular about their talk. This is in direct contrast to the prevailing view that would imply that one could have 'caring' thoughts but lack the capability of displaying 'caring' behaviour.

Secondly, we must realise that the meanings given to language are public meanings, arrived at through social agreement. The meaning of all my actions, including my speech, is dependent on the interpretations given them by others.

These meanings are not constructed in a vacuum; they are available to us in any social context. This context is composed of many facets — of history, of the particular biographies of the participants, their previous shared experiences, the material context, and many more. The contribution of the past is particularly important in the construction of the meaning of any social act. The understanding of the meaning of things which has been arrived at in the past has become institutionalised, and these past ways of agreeing on how the world was ordered have come down to us as social rules. For instance, we now take it as self-evident that certain physical or mental states are abnormal and can be labelled and treated by a doctor; we understand that if a nurse punctures our skin with a needle we should not regard it as an assault and strike back.

Thus in order to make sense of the words uttered by our co-participants in interaction we must have available a set of generalised ideas about how people act in certain situations. Moreover, we must assume that our co-participants have access to the same set of ideas or understandings.

Thus the meanings of social acts are seen to be given by existing social structures through the medium of language which defines the typical features of the world. They would appear to be reflections of the apparent order of society. But of course society is not 'given'; it is itself a construct of everyday people going about their everyday discourse.

Social rules do not dictate our actions. Indeed they have no substance or life apart from the demonstration of them in our actions, primarily talking. In order for common understandings of how the world is ordered to be sustained we must continuously cooperate to demonstrate that they are still true.

Thus while we appear to be acting in the way in which, for instance, the institution of nursing demands, we are by our very actions recreating and sustaining that institution which is dependent on our reaffirmation for its existence. Meaning is given to us by society, but we in turn construct that society, through the process of interaction.

However, the frameworks in use in any society do not specify what any utterance will mean. Speech use can be likened to another complex activity — playing games. We do not play games by following rules but rather play inside a framework of rules and understandings that make the game possible. For instance, there is (probably) no rule that says that footballers do not play with parrots on their left shoulders, although pirates can, but we know that this should not happen. Similarly we have an understanding of what sort of things should and should not happen in different sorts of talk. Inevitably, given the complexity of interaction and the uniqueness of each piece of talk, these things happen all the time, so it is encumbent on the participants either to interpret them as permissible in this context or to redefine the context as different from the original interpretation. Thus the participants in talk do not just recognise the context and produce appropriate talk, rather they proceed with the interaction and try to demonstrate that their actions are reasonable according to some frame of reference which they believe the other participants share. This is a mutual and continuous exercise.

How can we relate this discussion of language use in everyday life to language use in health care settings? The way we use language everyday is, of course, the same as that use in particular health care settings, from patient's home to hospital theatre. Our speech as health care workers will contain our definition of what sort of setting it is and what sort of interaction is appropriate. The client will interpret the words in accordance with his or her view of the context and together they will build a picture of, for instance, what nursing is in this context. Their creation will be unique but will build on, refer to, and reaffirm an institutionalised version of nursing. They will manage this primarily through their talk.

In practice this means that any attempt to manipulate the talk of one of the participants to an encounter from outside that encounter is a misguided enterprise. Firstly, any artificial attempt to use, for instance, open-ended questions, would appear strange in the talk. It would ignore part of the context i.e. what had just been said, and possibly go against the grain of the encounter. Thus the nurse would not appear to be more skilful but would apparently be paying less attention to the utterances of the particular patient. Proponents of language manipulation may believe, as do Byrne and Long who analysed G.P. talk (Byrne and Long 1976), that the clients' talk is not causative of the health workers next action, and that the doctor acts independently of what the client has just said, but this is clearly not so.

Secondly, the client would attempt to interpret any new utterance, such as an open-ended question, in the light of the context and might place a particularly closed interpretation on it. Think for example, of the schoolteacher's 'open-ended' 'what are you doing, boy' towards a pupil caught smoking.

Transcripts of tape recordings of health visitors' home visits which were collected as part of a research project include the example of a question asked of a client by a health visitor:

'How have things been?'

On the surface this question would appear to be as open-ended as a question can be, but the question was asked by the health visitor in the context of a professional visit to a family with a young baby so 'things' was interpreted rather precisely, and the client answered.

'Well, they haven't. He's been absolutely ravenous. I've had to start him on solids . . . '

The point to emphasise is that the client did not make a free choice of what to reply in a vacuum but in a context of expectations and experiences which appeared as social rules. She made the interpretation, probably quite reasonably, that health visitors are not interested in 'things' such as how the dahlias are blooming, the state of the nation's economy, or the conversation the client had with the milkman that morning, but they are interested in how well babies feed. Moreover, she also understood that clients are seen by health visitors primarily as mothers and attempted to demonstrate that the problems of mothering were at the forefront of her concerns.

Such interpretations of any utterance are not permanent, once and for all defintions. As the context changes so interpretations may change, and of course the context of any utterance is continually changing as new utterances are produced. The research data includes another example of talk between health visitor and client which illustrates this. The opening sequence is:

HV Hello there, how are you? Were you feeding?
Client Yes.
HV Fine, how's it going?
Client All right.

It would perhaps be difficult to summarise this if the conversation ended there — as well it might in a hurried hospital or clinic consultation. We could say that the mother was asked about her general health and the feeding of her child. Although she did not specifically say that she was well, she had an opportunity to discuss it and she did specifically say that the feeding was going well.

What happens when we add further utterances to the conversation?

HV How have the other two been with him?
HV Is he feeding quite well?
HV And is he fairly regular with feeding?

Each subsequent utterance changes our perception of the opening sequence. If another question has had to be asked then it is no longer understood to have been contained in the opening sequence.

Ascription of meaning is essentially a joint enterprise, requiring *mutual* work. The acts of working which constitute conversation are meaningful because members of a social group share a sufficiently similar system of relevancies or understandings about the nature of social life.

It is more likely that dissatisfaction with nurse/patient communication arises from disparity in the system of relevances than from technical difficulties. It is also more likely that the patient thinks of herself as a person while the nurse sees her as object, than that the nurse cannot manage to address the patient as a person. The fact that on the following day the nurse can talk about the patient as a person to her tutor does not invalidate this analysis, for the conversation with the tutor progresses in a different context, for different purposes and with a different set of expectations. It is important to remember that the nurse is not deliberately lying in either context; she was merely trying to negotiate different realities in individual situations.

This negotiation is an active and continuous process. MacIntyre's study of interactions in an ante-natal clinic show how it works in practice. In the clinic, standard data had to be collected on each patient but the relevent information was elicited by an interview in which the staff would use various questions in relation to the same information. For instance the patient could be asked: 'Have you ever had any urinary tract infection?' or 'Have you ever had any trouble with the water works?'

MacIntyre states that the choice rests on typifications of the patient built largely on a categorisation of the husband's occupation which was assumed to be reflected in the competence of his wife to organise her experience and answer questions. However, these typifications, although built on past cultural experience and expectations, are open to negotiation in the present. Thus for one working-class patient who to the question 'Have you ever had anything wrong with the water works?' replied 'Yes, I had a urinary tract infection in 1969 which responded to treatment on sulphonamides,' subsequent questions were phrased to take account of her newly defined competence.

We must conclude that any strategy which aims to label, count or manipulate talk at the level of the individual utterance is essentially inappropriate. Consequently, any strategy which aims to judge any sequence of talk by criteria external to that talk is also inappropriate. Because we cannot say definitely what any sequence of words means except by reference to our system of relevences then it is not possible to say that a participant in a conversation has 'missed the point' or 'missed a cue' because their judgement of what was meant inside the context of the conversation must be superior to ours. They were there and we were not. It is a strategy akin to that of the football supporter on the terraces who inevitably knows better than the players what they should have done with the ball.

Moreover, the system of understandings used by the tutor or researcher as the basis of her critique of another's communications is basically derived from the expectations and agreements of the past, which have come to have the status of social facts: of what nursing really is. Thus we are using an institutionalised version of reality to criticise what is happening now, and neglecting the opportunity available to us in our study of language to produce a version of what nurses and patients today believe nursing to be. If we look carefully at the utterances nurses and patients are producing rather than setting them against an abstract model of social skills we will be able to map with some accuracy the negotiation and production of nursing practice. We may then see that the problems lie not in inadequate skills but in the differing purposes and expectations of the different participants, and this sort of critique could form the basis of a much more fundamental review of our relationship with the patient.

REFERENCES

Byrne P, Long B 1976 Doctors talking to patients. HMSO, London
MacIntyre S Some notes on record taking and making in an ante-natal clinic. Sociological Review 26 (3)
Ryle G 1963 The concept of mind. Peregrine Books, London

FURTHER READING

Anderson D C 1979 The classroom as a context for health education. In: Anderson D C (ed) Health education in practice. Croom Helm, London
Filmer P et al 1972 New directions in sociological theory. Collier-Macmillan, London
Wootton A 1975 Dilemmas of discourse. Allen and Unwin, London

30

Problems of evaluation in preventive health care

June Clark

The demand for evaluation nowadays falls heavily upon all nurses, practitioners as much as managers.

For the practitioner, evaluation of nursing action is an integral part of planned care. At the level of the manager or policy maker, the demand is made because economic pressures require that expenditure must not only be accounted for, but justified. At the same time, however, there is considerable confusion about what evaluation means, and expectations about how it can be done and what it will achieve are often hopelessly unrealistic. In particular, it is insufficiently appreciated that approaches and techniques which have been found useful in one field may be neither useful nor possible for another. The evaluation of health care is a notoriously difficult task; the evaluation of a preventive service such as health visiting is especially difficult because it presents a number of special conceptual and methodological problems.

The literature on the evaluation of health care includes a number of definitions; one of the most useful is that of Williams (1974) who has defined evaluation as 'when a person assesses an object on dimensions of value'. The definition is useful because it stresses the subjectivity and relativity which is inherent in the concept of evaluation, and identifies the three elements which must be carefully specified. In the evaluation of health care none of these three elements is unequivocal or readily defined.

THE PERSON

The 'person' may be, among others:

a. the person receiving care (the patient or client)

b. the person giving care (the health visitor, the nurse, the doctor)

c. the persons responsible (e.g. in managerial or financial terms) for providing care (e.g. a district nursing officer, a health authority, government)

The perceptions and, more importantly, the values of these persons will certainly differ and may conflict. Conflicting values introduce serious problems for the determination of criteria by which worth is to be judged; in particular different values produce different goals, and therefore different criteria for success. Congruence of values and goals is likely to be greater in the presence of an evident problem which is a source of concern to all parties, for example where a patient, suffering from a particular illness or symptom has actively sought or been referred for professional help, although, as considerable research in the field of medical sociology has shown, it is by no means certain. While lack of congruence may occur in any medical or nursing field, it is particularly common in health visiting which is intrinsically and inevitably a 'moral activity' (Dingwall, 1978).

THE OBJECT

In the evaluation of health visiting, definition of the 'object' is particularly difficult. The object to be evaluated is frequently defined simply as 'health visiting'. However one cannot evaluate 'health visiting' any more than one can evaluate 'hospital nursing' or 'medicine' or 'education'; formulated in these terms the object is too global. The object to be evaluated must be operationalised, i.e. it must be closely specified in terms of a particular activity or aspect of practice as it is applied by the particular agent to the particular recipient in particular circumstances. It is for this reason that description must precede evaluation. Adequate specification of the independent variable (i.e. the object to be evaluated) is essential and this presupposes the availability of detailed descriptive information. At present the available descriptive information about health visiting activity is woefully inadequate. One reason for the dearth is the conceptual and methodological difficulty of obtaining such information; it is difficult to isolate the specific techniques or procedures in an activity which consists of interpersonal social interaction (which is one reason why it is easier to evaluate a technical nursing procedure than nurse-patient communication), and it is extremely difficult to observe or to record — much less to control — the behaviour of the agent or the recipient in the private setting of the client's home.

THE DIMENSIONS OF VALUE

The dimensions of value in health care are numerous; they differ from person to person and different people accord different weights to different dimensions. Attempts are sometimes made to define the dimensions of value in health care in unitary terms by using the word 'quality'. Quality is not, however, a unitary concept; it includes many dimensions and components. Although quality cannot be quantified, it is likely that some of its ingredients can. If we are to evaluate the quality of health care, health professionals must use their professional judgement, and patients, clients, or consumers, must use their subjective experiences to spell out which ingredients should be examined on this basis. Three seem to have an obvious importance: effectiveness, efficiency, and satisfaction.

While these three dimensions can be related to one another, perhaps as components of an index, it is important to recognise that they are nevertheless quite distinct and that the relative weights attached to them vary with the person making the evaluation. For the therapist, the most important dimension in the evaluation of health care is probably effectiveness, i.e. that the therapy improves or cures the condition being treated. Yet in the evaluation of a particular form of treatment, for example, although effectiveness may be the most important dimension for the therapist, the patient may place a higher value on convenience and the service planner on cost. Quenzer (1974) has noted that when patients are asked to evaluate the nursing care which they have received they rarely mention effectiveness at all.

Sometimes it is the balance between the various dimensions which is important. For example, just as the patient may be willing to sacrifice a certain amount of effectiveness for the sake of comfort or convenience, so a health authority or a manager may for the sake of cost. Williams (1974) has described this problem as the 'trade-off' between ends; he argues that the classical evaluative model is too limited because it concentrates on the achievement of 'one stipulated end', and suggests that while we are now beginning to tackle the next level of complexity by considering the 'two stipulated ends' model (e.g. cost benefit analysis and operational research techniques) a much more complex model must be developed to consider three or more stipulated ends.

Once the dimension of value has been selected some means of measuring it must be established. For example, to measure length, we require the establishment of a standard or criterion such as the inch, which we operationalise as the interval between two marks on a ruler. Although the dimension (length as opposed to weight) and the standard or criterion (e.g. inch as opposed to centimetre) are subjectively chosen, the measure itself must be objective, and must satisfy the requirements of validity, reliability, and sensitivity. The choice and development of criteria which meet these requirements is a central problem in evaluation research.

EVALUATIVE RESEARCH STRATEGY

Suchman (1967) distinguishes between 'evaluation' which he defines as 'the social process of making judgements of worth' and 'evaluative research' which he defines as 'the utilization of scientific research methods and techniques for the purpose of making an evaluation.' How then can the concepts and problems so far discussed be translated into an evaluative research strategy?

A useful framework for evaluating the quality of health care has been developed by Donabedian (1966, 1968). Donabedian suggests three components to be considered, each of which requires its own approach and methods. The three components are structure, process, and outcome. *Structure* includes all the factors associated with the setting in which care is given — the physical facilities, equipment, staffing levels, organisational structure, characteristics of care givers. *Process* means the performance of care, and in particular (in the evaluation of nursing care) what the nurse does and how she does it. *Outcome* is the result of care, defined in terms of the patient's condition or welfare. The difference between the three approaches can be shown by the picturesque example of the task of evaluating the flight of a bird: the structural approach would involve study of the number, length and arrangement of its wing feathers; the process approach would involve counting how often it flapped its wings; and the outcome approach would measure how far it had flown. The critical factor is the relationship between the three components, in particular the relationship of structure and process to outcome. The discovery of a beneficial outcome is of limited practical value unless one know what factors are necessary for it to happen (structure) and how it was actually achieved (process).

The 'structure' approach

The 'structure' approach has been used in this country in evaluative studies of primary medical care (Office of Health Economics, 1974) and also in nursing. In nursing the best known example (although it is rarely recognised as such) is the list of specifications laid down by the General Nursing Council for the recognition of hospitals for nurse training. This heading would also include some of the many kinds of management audit, and the great body of work on staffing ratios. In health visiting, work which would fall under this heading includes most of the early attempts to evaluate attachment to general practice (e.g. Abel, 1969), and the first line management audit forms used for health visitors by South Tyneside A.H.A.

As Jelinek has pointed out: 'the measurements of structural characteristics are important as indicators of predisposition for or constraints against high quality care' (Jelinek, 1974). The main strength of the structural approach lies in the fact that it deals with fairly concrete and accessible information which should be relatively easy to obtain. It should not be too difficult to find out, for example, how many health visitors in a district have access to telephones, clerical help, a private interview room (e.g. Sidwell, 1979) or whether they have access to 'consultative' support, adequate professional up-dating etc. and on the basis of this information to make a judgement, for example, that if most of them have none of these things the quality of the health visiting service in that locality is likely to be poor.

The weakness of this approach lies in its basic assumption: that if the structure is good, good care will follow — that if there are enough nurses, of the right kind, organised in the right way, the quality of nursing care will be high; that if health visiting caseloads are small, or if all health visitors are attached (or not attached) the quality of the practice or care given will be high. This assumption cannot be accepted at face value; in order for it to be tested, a link must be demonstrated between the structural indicators and relevant outcome criteria.

This weakness, however, ought not to lead to its complete rejection. Expressed in another way the assumption is that certain factors, while not *sufficient* for good care, are nevertheless deemed to be *necessary*. Given our present lack of almost any criteria on which to assess quality of care or standards of practice, the development of an agreed set of structural criteria against which practitioners and managers could compare their service would be a very useful first step.

The 'process' approach

The 'process' approach focuses upon the actual performance of the giving care. This approach has been the one most widely used in attempts to evaluate nursing, and a number of instruments have been developed for this purpose in the U.S.A., e.g. the QUALPACS scale, (Wandelt & Phaneuf, 1972), and the CASH scale (Commission for Administrative Services in Hospitals, 1965). This approach also includes most of the work which is generally subsumed under the heading 'nursing audit' (Phaneuf, 1976) although some audit tools are based on structural factors as already mentioned.

Process evaluation is attractive because it is related to the day-to-day management of nursing activities, which are susceptible to control and if necessary to change. Process measurement provides useful and practicable indicators for corrective action.

The process approach does however have several weaknesses:

1. The choice of questions (i.e. the criteria) depends upon agreement about what 'ought' to happen; such consensus is not easy to achieve.

2. If the criteria are too simply task oriented, nurses quickly learn how to get a high score, so that if repeated measurements are made, the score may improve without any change in quality.

3. A simple yes/no response can easily be made to the question 'did the nurse do so and so?'; it is more difficult to answer the question 'did she do it well or badly?'.

4. Unless the process criterion is linked with an outcome criterion the approach gives rise to the 'so what?' phenomenon i.e. whether the nurse did so and so or not, did it make any difference?

There are four major difficulties in using the process approach for the evaluation of health visiting:

1. We have no accurate descriptions of what health visitors actually do in their practice i.e. descriptions of the process of health visiting.

2. There is little consensus (at least there is nothing written either as the result of research, or even in prescriptive textbooks) about what health visitors ought to do in specified circumstances from which a list of audit criteria might be compiled.

3. Health visiting records are inadequate for use in retrospective audit; in particular they do not record what the HV did, but usually record aspects of the situation (e.g. child development milestones, immunisational state etc.).

4. Concurrent audit is virtually rendered impossible by the difficulty of direct observation of dyadic interaction in a private setting.

Nevertheless, there are some areas which have been explored (on the whole not very successfully) and some which I think might be developed into something useful.

1. *Allocation of time*

Several studies have been undertaken of the HVs allocation of time of various activities (Clark, 1981). These are not useful for evaluative purposes because:

a. the method of recording (self recording using diaries or work records) makes the data itself highly suspect; (self-recording is always suspect, but self-recording of work time is particularly suspect);
b. the categories of activity recorded are unrelated to purpose;
c. there is no consensus about how health visitors *ought* to distribute their time among the various activities.

2. *Number of visits*

This forms the basis of official statistics. Quite apart from the accuracy of the data, which is questionable, there is no consensus about how many visits ought to be undertaken, and in any case the use of the number of visits as a criterion leads to the 'so what?' phenomenon already mentioned.

3. *Clientele*

A number of studies have attempted to record the HV's clientele (Clark, 1981). The data is suspect and not by itself useful for evaluative purposes. However, the relationship between recorded clientele and demographic indices of 'need' (the construction of which is a difficult task, but not immpossible) could possibly form a basis for evaluation. Wiseman has developed a tool which could be used for this purpose, and which is described later in this book.

4. *Subject matter*
Two studies (Marris, 1969; Clark, 1973) have recorded in some detail the subject matter which health visitors discussed with their clients. While both of these studies suffer from considerable methodological weaknesses, they show that subject matter discussed may be relatively easier to record than other aspects of health visiting activity and I believe could possibly be developed into something which could be used as an evaluative criterion at least at the microscopic level of evaluation. This was suggested by Clark at the time of her descriptive study: 'It would certainly be valuable in an evaluation of standards of care to be able to compare the recorded frequency of certain topics which postulated a priority of topics important in certain situations.' (Clark, 1973 p. 36). Further work on the development of a valid and reliable category system for the analysis of subject matter is in progress.

5. *Development of audit criteria*
Research is urgently needed to try to discover whatever consensus there is among health visitors about what health visitors 'ought' to do in specified circumstances. This is an essential prerequisite for the development of any kind of audit instrument.

6. *Peer group review*
Peer group review is a system whereby a group of professionals critically review one another's practice, usually on a retrospective basis, comparing it with standards or criteria which they have agreed among themselves to be 'desirable' as 'good practice'. This is usually much more acceptable to the practitioners than an external audit and the criteria chosen can be much more specific to the particular field of practice. Most field-work teachers and tutors, and many nurse managers already undertake this kind of activity, usually on a one-to-one basis rather than in peer groups, as part of their teaching of managerial role. I believe, however, that this approach could usefully be developed as an evaluative tool, both at the microscopic level of the individual health visitor's practice, and as a first step in the development of criteria which could then be tested and used on a wider scale.

The 'outcome' approach
Outcome evaluation focuses on the results of care; it therefore involves an assessment of whether or not a previously stated objective has been achieved. This is the classical model of evaluation, the one which is central to medical research, and the one which nursing and health visiting is under great pressure to follow. The model is conceptually very simple:

Stated objective ⟶ *Care given* (to be evaluated) ⟶ *Result of care*

Evaluation is the comparison between the stated objective and its achievement.

The model also fits well with the conceptual framework which we have come to know as 'The Nursing Process' (N.B. not to be confused with process evaluation).

Assessment	→	*Plan* (stated objective)	→	*Implementation* (care given)	→	*Evaluation* (achievement of stated objectives)

The advantages of outcome evaluation are obvious; the validity of outcome as a dimension of quality is seldom questioned.

There are, however, three major problems which must be tackled for outcome evaluation to be of any use:

1. choice of outcome criteria
2. the attribution of a particular outcome to a particular intervention
3. the relationship of outcome to process.

1. *Choice of outcome criteria*

To be of use, any criterion must be appropriate and measurable.

(*a*) *Appropriate.* In the evaluation of medical care the outcome criterion which has most commonly been used is survival. That is, effectiveness (which is the dimension of value most commonly chosen) is measured in terms of mortality rates. Examples include studies of surgical fatality, survival rates following various forms of treatment, and the use of perinatal or maternal mortality rates as indicators of the effectiveness of maternity care. Even in medical research, however, the appropriateness of survival as the goal or criterion is debatable; it may not be an appropriate criterion, for example, for an evaluation of the care of the elderly or the management of the congenitally abnormal neonate.

A second criterion commonly used in the medical research is morbidity. For example, a particular surgical technique may be evaluated in terms of infection rates, a drug in terms of relief of symptoms. Preventive health programmes (e.g. immunization programmes) may be evaluated on the criterion of the prevalence of a disease.

Both mortality and morbidity, however, derive their relevance as outcome criteria from the medical model in which disease is perceived as a problematic abnormality which is susceptible to change by means of medical intervention, i.e. the stated objective against which achievement is measured is the removal or reduction of the abnormality. Such a model is, in my view, not appropriate to health visiting, in which the intervention (i.e. health visiting activity) is applied not to abnormality but to normality, and in which the stated objective is something which is, in WHO terms 'not merely the absence of disease'. In other words, I believe that if they are to be relevant and appropriate, outcome criteria for the evaluation of health visiting activity must be defined in terms of 'health'.

(*b*) *Susceptible to measurement.* A concept (mortality, morbidity, or health) is not susceptible to measurement; it has to be approached via an indicator. For example, the length of a piece of string can be measured by the interval between two marks on a ruler; mortality is measured by the number of people who die in a specified period of time. The indicator which is used to measure mortality (i.e. whether the patient is alive or dead) and most of those used to measure morbidity are measurements of a patient's 'state'. Some 'states' are difficult enough to measure, especially mental 'states' (e.g. anxiety) but it is easier to measure a 'state' and to demonstrate a change in 'state' (i.e. by comparing 'before' and 'after' measurements) than it is to measure behaviour or to demonstrate the change in behaviour which is the object of health education. Even within the limited framework of morbidity, therefore, the search for indicators is especially difficult for health visiting. The choice of 'health' as the appropriate outcome criterion raises enormous problems of definition and measurement. As Turner (1978) has remarked:

> While illness, disease, and fitness can be measured by socially agreed and testable parameters, health is an abstract concept which is more than a physical measurement and cannot be assessed solely by BP, peak flow, trait measurement and so on.

Note, however, that while the sentiment is sound, the detail of Turner's argument is not valid. It is not the fact that health is an abstract concept that causes problems, (so are mortality and morbidity) but the fact that unlike mortality and morbidity the concept is so difficult to define that it is difficult to choose indicators through which to approach it.

Some work has been carried out on the development of a 'health index', i.e. a collection of indicators which together might constitute a reasonable and measurable approach to the concept of health. Two attempts are reviewed by Hicks (1976). Williams (1974) has argued the need to develop a multi-dimensional index based on functional definitions in which a before and after scoring system would supply the measure of effectiveness. The task is not easy, but it should not be dismissed as impossible.

Meanwhile there is great danger in choosing criteria simply because they are measurable. Some measurable criteria are available in health visiting; they might include, for example, completion of immunization programme, increased use of preventive services (e.g. family planning clinics), reduced use of other services (e.g. casaulty departments). But it is important to recognise that even these are value laden (they may be objectively measurable, but they are subjectively chosen on the basis of value judgments). Moreover, they are difficult to interpret (e.g. reduction in G.P. consultations may be due to reluctance to consult in the presence of need as much as to a reduction in need), and in any particular case the objective chosen as the criterion (e.g. change in smoking behaviour) may have to be sacrificed in order to achieve some other more highly valued objective (e.g. maintenance of a relationship with a hostile family in which children are thought to be at risk of non-accidental injury). Attempts to assess the effectiveness of health visiting on the basis of these criteria alone, when others, not used because of difficulties of measurement, are much more important or relevant, would be highly misleading and potentially dangerous.

2. *The difficulty of attributing a particular outcome to a particular intervention*
Donabedian (1968) has pointed out that 'outcomes depend on a host of antecedents, including the nature and magnitude of need, provider and client behaviours, and the capabilities of medical science. For this reason, particular health outcomes

cannot be attributed to any one factor (for example, physician performance) unless all other significant factors are held constant'.

In a laboratory experiment the outcome (dependent) variable can be directly attributed to the experimental (independent) variable because all other (intervening) variables can be controlled. In most medical research (e.g. where a new drug under trial or a new treatment is in effect the experimental variable) control is achieved by careful selection of subjects and precise specification of the intervention, and conclusions are based on probability theory. The classic method is the randomized controlled trial, and this method has come to be accepted by many influential authorities (e.g. Cochrane, 1971; Suchman, 1967) as *the* appropriate method for evaluative research.

However, Karaper-Jorgensen (1978) has pointed out the difficulties of applying the RCT method to the evaluation of long-term outcomes and to preventive health programmes. He argues that the validity of the RCT approach depends on the existence or creation of two identical, homogeneous, and well-defined groups, on the assumption of a mono-factorial disease model (i.e. one factor is responsible for the disease and a specific intervention produces a specific effect on the individual) and on the assumption of stability of attributes of the individuals as well as the environment.

He rejects the use of the RCT method for long-term outcome evaluation, and particularly for long-term outcome evaluation of preventive programmes on six grounds:

1. Conventionally used tests of the effectiveness of random allocation are ineffective since the mean and standard deviation of the two groups, compared on one variable at a time, may be similar while the multi-variable distribution (e.g. age, sex, socio-economic status) of the constituent individuals may be very different.
2. The mono-factorial disease model is inadequate for describing the majority of illness states, and certainly chronic states.
3. The RCT can evaluate only mono-factorial intervention whereas most preventive programmes have several components, and a mono-factorial long-term preventive trial is unrealistic because society and human beings very often change more than one factor at a time in interventions towards health.
4. It is socially unacceptable; the denial of a treatment to one group, even where the efficacy of the treatment is as yet unproven, raises ethical problems, and may be impossible for political reasons.
5. It assumes stability of attributes of individuals, and it assumes that environmental change, and the passage of time, produce equal change in the two groups.
6. It is expensive; running a control group costs money, sometimes almost as much as running the experimental group.

All of these difficulties apply to the evaluation of health visiting. The health needs and problems with which health visitors are concerned are complex, multi-factorial, and mediated by different individual responses. The problem of intervening variables is exacerbated because the outcome is widely separated in time from the intervention (e.g. the effect of mothercraft classes in schools on future parenting) and behavioural rather than physiological. Health visiting is a universalist service which it would be politically impossible to deny or to withdraw.

A further problem is the attribution of a health outcome to a specifically nursing intervention instead of to, for example, a medical intervention. This is particularly difficult for health visiting because of the great number of determinants of social behaviour.

Perhaps the most difficult problem of all, however, is the relationship between a positive intervention and a negative outcome i.e. a 'non-event'. It is logically impossible to prove causation for an event which did not happen; the best one can do is to replace proof by an estimate of probability. The whole concept of prevention implies an outcome which 'does not happen'.

3. *The relationship between outcome and process*
Attention has already been drawn to the critical importance of the relationship between outcome and process. It is possible to demonstrate a beneficial outcome without knowing why or how it was achieved. One reason for this may be the difficulty of attributing a particular outcome to a particular intervention; a second may be inadequate understanding of the intervention itself (i.e. of the process). In certain circumstances (e.g. in the face of life-threatening disease) such understanding might be regarded as an unessential, although perhaps desirable, luxury. But the demonstration of an outcome is by itself of limited value because without an understanding of its antecedants the outcome cannot be replicated or translated to other situations.

One study concerned with health visiting where a beneficial outcome has been demonstrated in terms of a reduction in the number of 'cot deaths' is the work of Emery in Sheffield. The design of the study enables the outcome to be attributed with a high degree of probability to the activity of the health visitors, but until the process of the 'health visiting activity' is specified and described it is impossible to know whether the same outcome would have been achieved by sending each family a weekly postcard, and it is impossible to use the research findings to achieve the same outcome in other areas.

CONCLUSION

It is clear that, as Bloch (1975) has suggested, the ultimate goal for the evaluation of professional practice must be the 'process related to outcome' type. For this to be achieved, she suggests, five preliminary steps are necessary (I have adapted the wording from nursing to health visiting):

1. Development of a set of measurable outcome criteria specific to health visiting.
2. Development of valid and reliable methods for measuring these outcomes.
3. Development of a set of measurable process criteria.
4. Development of reliable and valid methods for measuring the process of health visiting in all its various forms.
5. Testing of the various aspects of health visiting practice in relation to patient/client outcomes.

Bloch points out that neither nursing nor any other professional group has yet completed all these steps and suggests that the goal in nursing should be to work steadily and resolutely towards their achievement. In health visiting we have not yet begun them, and are possibly not yet ready to begin. We have not yet established consensus on what are the relevant dimensions of value, let alone developed criteria or standards against which they can be measured. We have not yet made sufficiently explicit the goals of the activity which we call health visiting (although most health visitors can define their goals in relation to specific activities with specific clients), nor the means by which we try to achieve them. We are as yet unable to describe or analyse our activity in such a way as to specify it (or any aspect of it) as an object for evaluation. In such circumstances, present attempts to evaluate health visiting, certainly in global terms, must be regarded with considerable scepticism.

A great deal of work needs to be done, and the sooner it is begun the better. There are a number of areas, particularly at the microscopic level of individual health visiting practice, where research which can and should be undertaken might not only produce information which is badly needed for the maintenance and improvement of individual standards of practice, but might also lay the foundations for larger scale evaluative strategies. Some suggestions have been made in this paper. In particular we need much more information about health visiting objectives, what they are and how they are achieved; about what consensus there is about what constitutes good health visiting activity. The use of peer group review — even on the small scale of a small group of health visitors working with a nursing officer — could be used not only for the evaluation of individual practice but also to suggest criteria (particularly process and outcome criteria) which could be developed and tested by research. Publication of small trials and even of detailed case studies would greatly help in the specification of dependent and independent variables for research. As yet we have barely begun.

REFERENCES

Abel R A 1969 Nursing attachments to general practice. DHSS Social Science Research Unit Study No 1. HMSO, London

Bloch D 1975 Evaluation of nursing care in terms of process and outcome. Nursing Research 24 (4): 256–263

Clark J 1973 A family visitor. Royal College of Nursing, London

Clark J 1981 What do health visitors do? A review of research 1960–1980. Royal College of Nursing, London

Commission for Administrative Services in Hospitals 1965 CASH: A quality control plan for nursing service. (mimeograph)

Dingwall R 1982 Community nursing and civil liberty. Journal of Advanced Nursing 7: 4

Donabedian A 1966 Evaluating the quality of medical care. Millbank Memorial Quarterly 44 (2): 166–206

Donabedian A 1968 Promoting quality through evaluating the process of patient care. Medical Care 6: 181–202

Emery J 1981 Health Visitor 54 (8): 318

Hicks D 1976 Primary health care. HMSO, London

Jelinek R C, Houssmann D, Hegyvary S, Newman J F 1974 A methodology for monitoring quality of nursing care. (DHEW Publication No HRA 74–25). US Government Printing Office, Washington D.C.

Karaper Jorgensen F 1978 Scandinavian Journal of Social Medicine Supplement 13.

Marris T 1969 The work of health visitors in London. (Research Report No 12). Greater London Council, London

Office of Health Economics 1974 The work of primary medical care. Office of Health Economics, London

Phaneuf M 1972 The nursing audit. Appleton Century Crafts, New York

Quenzer R 1974 The development of patient centred behaviour patterns in nurse training. M. Ed thesis University of Manchester

Suchman E A 1967 Evaluative Research. Russell Sage Foundation, New York

Turner V 1978 Health visitors? Health Visitor 51, (3): 82–83

Wandelt H S, Phaneuf M C 1972 Three instruments for measuring the quality of nursing care. Hospital Topics 50: 20–29

Williams A 1974 Measuring the effectiveness of health care systems. British Journal of Preventive and Social Medicine 28 (3): 74

31

Goal attainment: One approach to evaluation

Karen Luker

The Concise Oxford Dictionary defines the word goal as an 'object of effort' and this may be interpreted as what the nurse and patient/client are working towards. Nurses, and in using this word I include health visitors, have in the past been reluctant to define the object of their effort in terms of the patient or client. Goals, if they have been mentioned at all, have usually been described in terms of what the nurse does. For example a district nurse may visit a home to do a general care or to do a dressing and injection. The health visitor may visit to carry out a routine developmental check or health education and to all intents and purposes regardless of the outcome of the visit in terms of benefit on the patient/client, the goal can be said to have been achieved when the visit is completed.

The emphasis upon what the nurse does rather than on the effect of the nursing action on the patient or client can be partially accounted for by looking at the type of information community nurses are required to record. To make their activities accountable monthly or weekly statistical returns are filled in by all community nurses and although they may vary from area to area they commonly require the nurse to classify her visits in terms of the reason why she visited and the age grouping of the patient/client. The statistics collected by community nurses in this way are complied centrally and used to illustrate the work of both district nurses and health visitors. It would seem however that if we shift the emphasis away from what the nurse does towards what the patient/client achieves or more specifically to the effect of the care upon the patient then we may learn a little more about the effectiveness of community nursing care.

Talking about goals is rather like putting the cart before the horse in that there has to be a reason or purpose for setting a goal. It is suggested here that district nurses and health visitors should set goals for each patient problem which they identify. Health visitors are sometimes rather reluctant to consider themselves as dealing with problems; they pride themselves in their uniqueness because they claim to visit families with no apparent problems. Problem is a word health visitors may easily associate with the term 'problem family'; here the word 'problem' is used in a different context. A health problem is something which concerns the nurse or the patient/client about the patient's/client's health at the time of assessment. Problems may be either actual or potential. Actual problems are present at the time of assessment or reassessment, whereas potential problems are not present. However there are indicators or cues present which point to a potential problem which in time may become actual if no nursing action is taken. An example of an actual problem at a health visiting assessment may be a baby with a sticky eye, a baby who refuses to suck at the breast or a child who has regressed to soiling himself. Health visitors are often more concerned with potential problems, that is with preventing actual problems from occurring, and hence with more long-term health goals. An example of a potential problem for a couple expecting a baby who already have a three-year-old child might be jealousy on the part of the three-year-old after the baby is born. The health visitor would be keen to prevent the problem occurring and would therefore discuss ways in which the family might prepare the three-year-old for the arrival of the baby. Arrangements would also be discussed regarding the management of the child during his first separation from his mother which is inevitable in a hospital delivery. By intervening before there is an actual problem, the health visitor hopes to promote the well being of the whole family.

District nurses, unless they are involved in case finding, are usually only referred a patient after an actual health problem has been identified such as varicose ulcers or incontinence. Patients with actual problems may also have potential problems, for example an incontinent patient may have the potential problem of developing pressure sores or dehydration or both.

The health visitor's clients are not usually put through any test of eligibility; this means that that they do not need an actual problem in order to receive the service. On the other hand all the patients visited by the district nurse will usually have been put through some test of eligibility. For example if the patient is already in hospital the ward sister will decide if he needs the services of a district nurse on discharge; similarly if the patient is ill at home it is the general practitioner who decides. Since health visitor clients are not put through any test of need some clients will have no actual health problems but almost all will have at least one potential health problem. Health visitors are sometimes described as nurses who who visit families from conception until the grave. When looking at life across a developmental time span one can see that the younger one is, the more potential problems one has and the fewer actual problems and the older one is, the more actual problems one has and the fewer potential problems. For example a child of six months of age may have attained his expected developmental milestone and may have no actual health problems but he will have a lifetime ahead of potential health problems. However, a potential problem is usually only considered by the nurse if it has a higher than average probability of becoming actual. For example all babies may become obese, but the infant whose siblings or parents are obese would be considered by the health visitor to have a potential problem in this area. Similarly all elderly people could be said to be at risk of falling in the home. However, the district nurse would record this as a potential problem only if there were indicators to suggest that there was a greater than average risk of the old person falling such as if the elderly person had failing vision due to cataracts and dizzy spells due to hypertension.

Now let us look a little more closely at goal setting. Goals are usually set after a problem has been identified, hence goal setting takes place after the assessment stage of the nursing process. It was stated earlier that goals should be patient or client specific and should make explicit what the end result of nursing care is to be. In short the goal is a statement of the expected outcome of care. The goal statement should be written wherever possible to convey exactly what the outcome of care is thought to be so that any nurse would interpret it in the same way. In evaluation language, inherent in the goal statement should be the criterion or standard against which the nurse is to measure the effect of her care. The criterion may take the form of new knowledge acquired by the patient/client as a result of teaching by the nurse, or a change in behaviour such as a visit to the dentist, or an improvement in a physical problem such as incontinence. Whatever the criterion is to be, it should be clearly stated so that any nurse would understand what constitutes improvement or deterioration. Now let us consider an example:

All new born infants are at risk from developing gastrointestinal infection. This risk could be said to be increased if for example the infant is bottle-fed, if the bottle is made up for two feeds and reheated and if the mother has little understanding of the need for sterilisation and the way in which to sterilise bottles. In such circumstances the health visitor may list gastrointestinal infection as a potential problem and intervene accordingly.

Goal statement 1

The mother will *demonstrate* that she understands about the preparation of bottle feeds and sterilisation.

This goal statement has limitations because it does not tell us how the mother will demonstrate her understanding and we have no time limit, will it be at the next visit or the next baby? The second statement gives us this additional information:

Goal statement 2

The mother will discuss the way in which she makes up the bottle feeds and the way in which she sterilises the bottles and will give a practical demonstration at the next visit. *The next visit should be made at feed time.*

Community nursing is more complex in some respects when it comes to evaluation than hospital nursing. In the community we are dealing with families and not individuals, although this is not to say that hospital nurses do not consider the family. When visiting patients/clients in their own homes we are directing our care at each family member. The initial reason for the visit of a district nurse may have been precipitatd by the incontinence of an elderly family member but, despite the fact that the elderly person is the 'patient' in the usual sense of the word, it may well be that the district nurse focuses her care equally upon the daughter who feels she cannot go on indefinitely caring for her mother. In hospital a nursing care plan is usually made only for the patient and the patient is easily identified since he is the one who occupies the bed on the ward. Goals are written which usually relate directly to the patient. In community nursing it is not always clear who is the patient/client and it may be necessary to make more than one care plan. Similarly goals may on occasions be in conflict with each other and many compromises will need to be made. If, for example, a mother feels that she can no longer care for her mentally handicapped child at home because she is getting no support from her husband, then there are three individuals to consider and three different people against which to evaluate the effect of district nursing or health visiting intervention.

District nurses are involved in giving a more practical type of care to their patients than health visitors. District nurses may from time to time visit patients who have been discharged from hospital after having had an operation resulting in a colostomy. Although patients share the same condition they may in fact have different problems. For example an elderly man may have adjusted psychologically to life with a colostomy but may be unable to change his own bag and care for his stoma due to arthritis of his hands. In other cases it may be the patient or relations who have difficulty in adjusting socially or psychologically to the colostomy. In all cases goals should be set for individual patient problems rather than specific conditions.

Here is an example of possible goal statement relating to the actual problem of inability to care for colostomy.

Ultimate goal

The patient will care for his own colostomy and will demonstrate this by discussing care of the stoma and surrounding skin; and by giving a practical demonstration of a bag change by a certain date.

Although this is the ultimate goal for most patients who have a colostomy, it will probably be necessary to set more short-term goals which will be specific to individual patient problems.

Examples of short-term goal statements

1. The patient and carer will talk about the effect that the colostomy has had on their lives.
2. The patient and carer will look at the stoma when the nurse is changing the bag.
3. The patient and carer will assist the nurse and will ask questions about the stoma.

Once these short-term goals have been attained it may be necessary to set additional short-term goals until the ultimate goal is reached. These additional goals may relate to such matters as diet, smell and bag disposal. The goals will vary for each patient since it is anticipated that not all patients will experience the same problems.

Evaluation involves the collection of information which is specific to the problem in question. The patient goal statement dictates the information to be collected. Evaluation can only be carried out after nursing care has been given and involves a comparison of the patient/client problem before and after intervention. Goal setting in the context of the nursing process occurs in the first instance after assessment and identification of patient problems and thereafter are continually reassessed. Care should be planned in order to achieve the desired patient outcome or goal. Nurses at present are not in the habit of writing down patient/client goal statements; the emphasis still tends to be placed on the intervention stage of the nursing process and lack of time is often the reason given for not documenting goal statements and patient/client progress away or towards the goal. Unfortunately assessment, planning and intervention without evaluation cannot provide nurses with the information they need to improve their practice and hence the quality of patient/client care. Broadly speaking evaluation is concerned with estimating the effectiveness of nursing care and this incorporates the concept of change. Nurses are constantly involved in assessing changes in patient's/client's problems but rarely document their findings and it is this failure to document that prevents nursing records being used retrospectively for evaluative purposes. When nurses claim that they are using the nusing process it is usually the beginning of the process which they have formalised, namely assessment. However assessment does have some similarities with evaluation in that both involve the collection of information about a patient/client or family. Information collected during the assessment is usually directed by a predetermined format. Similarly information collected for evaluative purposes is predetermined by the goal statement. The procedure for collecting both types of information/are the same since the skills of interview and observation are used and records and charts are consulted. Both assessment and evaluation are ongoing processes and can occur wherever and whenever a nurse is in contact with a patient/client.

Evaluation of patient/client nursing care has implications on an individual level for nurses because it gives them feedback about the effectiveness of the care which they give. It also affords an opportunity to change care which is ineffective in solving the patient/client problem and this can only serve to benefit the patient/client.

Evaluation by means of goal attainment also has implications for nursing as a profession. If nurses can be encouraged to use this approach and record the care which they give in a systematic way, then it may become possible eventually to predict with some degree of accuracy the outcome of certain nursing interventions.

32

Post-natal support groups

Gwen Hiskins

The development of self-help groups has for a long time been recognised as a means of providing support for individuals facing particular problems. Different organisations have been formed by and for people suffering from particular diseases or coping with social or personal problems ranging from agarophobia to widowhood. During the past decade in particular groups run by parents providing support in the problems of parenting have sprung up all over the United Kingdom and the United States. Probably the oldest and best known of these is the National Childbirth Trust which runs post-natal support groups in addition to its perhaps better known ante-natal classes and breast-feeding counselling service. In Southampton the 'Scope' scheme aims to create a neighbourhood support service for families, with training aimed at increasing group members' self confidence and awareness. 'Homestart' in Leicester, aims at forming friendships in the home, on a one-to-one basis, to give help and encouragement before members feel safe in a group situation. 'Home Plus', a more recently established group in Bristol, operates in a similar way, training experienced parents as one-to-one visitors.

The relatively new organisation, M.A.M.A. (Meet a Mum Association) has highlighted the isolation of young mothers in the community, and their need for the company of other mothers with babies and small children, the sharing of ideas and problems, and the forming of new friendships. The Federation of Self Help Groups for Parents Under Stress (O.P.U.S.), organised by parents and professionals in partnership, includes Parents Anonymous, an emergency phone-in service for parents, which developed from ideas started in America.

Several other organisations including The London Voluntary Services Council and the Church of England Children's Society, have been instrumental in starting groups for mothers with babies and small children. Many researchers are investigating facilities available for parents with a young family. For example Bristol University, requested by the Social Science Research Council, are involved in a pre-school evaluation project in health and education and an examination for ante-natal and post-natal facilities. This will include, among other considerations, an examination of the use of post-natal support groups, including those run by health visitors, social workers or community workers, as well as those where the schemes are based on a partnership between parents and professionals. Another example is the current work being carried out at the Thomas Coram Unit, which is investigating support available for first time parents and which will help to show the necessity for schemes such as post-natal support groups.

THE START OF AN INNOVATION

About 12 years ago, while I was working as a health visitor in Harrow, Middlesex, I was approached by the young mother of a new first baby, who told me that she and some other young mothers she had met in the maternity ward, felt they would like to belong to a small post-natal support group. They all appeared to come from middle class backgrounds, and had the common problems of having worked in interesting jobs until about the seventh month of pregnancy, little experience of babies or small children, and having families some distance away (Sprott, 1969). When I suggested they join groups already organised from clinics or church halls, some of the mothers indicated that they preferred smaller, more intimate groups, and felt lost in large groups of people. Several came from small families themselves, and were only children, or perhaps had one sibling. I soon found that their knowledge of the needs of babies and small children was minimal, and they appeared to feel devalued in their new role of motherhood, having felt confident and capable in their previous employment. Although they all attended Child Welfare Clinics with their babies, and were in touch with their Health Visitors, they felt they needed a small, safe group, where they could exchange information, and try out new ideas (Durham, 1972). As the mother who had first approached me had experience in a professional capacity and some knowledge of group work, I suggested we should work together in setting up a simple framework for small, post-natal support groups, where the mothers and children met in each other's homes.

At first, we decided to have eight to ten mothers in each group, as the houses were fairly large, and, at that time, all the mothers had only one baby. We chose the group leaders from the mothers who were interested in the work, who were calm, tactful, sensible people, who had some knowledge of working with people, and, if possible, had some experience with children. We tried to have people in each group within walking distance of each other, and each member took turns in having the meeting in her own home.

The groups started as friendship groups, meeting every two or three weeks; they chatted about their homes and babies, their husbands joining in when they were at home. The system appeared popular and soon we were having referals from other health visitors, general practitioners and social workers, who knew of lonely mothers in the area. After trying children between the ages of two to four years in the groups, we decided to have only babies and children up to the age of two years when starting, as older children, not yet at school, proved too disruptive for the groups, and these children were bored. If the children grew with the group, they became like 'adopted' cousins, and played happily together; the parents becoming like 'adopted' aunts and uncles. Although husbands could usually not be present at day time meetings, but only at evening socials, they were usually happy for their wives and children to attend group meetings, and would enquire what had taken place. In this way, husbands too were getting more experience and knowledge of child care (Seymour, 1977). In many ways we were trying to replace the lost extended family.

RESEARCH PROJECT 'HOW MOTHERS HELP THEMSELVES'

In 1976, I was fortunate to be awarded a Maw's Health Visitor research scholarship, and therefore, I was able to investigate the possibility of extending this group system. With this assistance, and the help of a tutor who was a health visitor, researcher and sociologist, I was able to undertake a small research project to study the small group system with a cross-section of the population of mothers with babies, and small children, in the area where I worked.

The hypothesis which formed the basis of the research was that small post-natal supportive groups of mothers with babies from both manual and non-manual culture, would benefit from these groups by:

a. being able to meet mothers with babies or young children.

b. being less lonely than if they did not join a group, as the groups endeavour to combat inexperience, lack of support and isolation.

The study was designed to describe, through a series of interviews, how members of post-natal support groups react to the group situation; the support they had from their families and friends, and the degree of isolation they encountered.

The study was undertaken in an outer London Borough, which was a largely residential suburban area, with a mixture of owner-occupied and rented property, and several council estates. Mobility of population made maintaining members within the groups difficult at times. The mothers interviewed were those who were part of the stable population. The mobility within this small number is illustrated by the fact that the number of members within groups dropped from 32 at the first interview, to 28 in the second, and 26 in the third.

Four research groups of mothers and small children were established:

Group A consisted of mothers whose husbands were in non-manual occupations

Group B consisted of mothers whose husbands were manual workers

Group C included mothers from all social classes

Group D also included mothers from all social classes who all attended the same ante-natal group.

A fifth group of mothers, who all attended the same ante-natal class, but were not formed into a group, acted as a control group.

The five groups were set up between July 1977 and February 1978. Three interviews were carried out, in February 1978, August 1978 and June 1979. The numbers in each group and the numbers who were interviewed are shown in Table 32.1.

Table 32.1 Group membership and times of interviews

		February 1978	August 1978	June 1979
Group A	Non-manual	9	8	7
Group B	Manual	7	7	6
Group C	Mixed social class	9	7	7
Group D	Formed of mothers from an ante-natal class	7	6	6
Group E	Controls. Mothers Attending the same ante-natal class, but no group formed	11	10	10
		43	38	36

The groups meet regularly, and they decide the frequency of the meetings.

Group A Meets once a month. At the time of the third interview, the group had existed for 23 months. All the members said they attended meetings regularly.

Group B Meets once every two weeks. At the time of the third interview, the group had existed for 17 months. All but two members attended regularly. One of these explained that this was because the children had been ill, and the other said she had not attended regularly as her husband was on shift work, and it was sometimes difficult to go to meetings.

Group C Also meets every two weeks. At the time of the third interview, the group had existed for 19 months. All but two members attended regularly and these two said that they attended less than usual recently because they had been working part-time.

Group D Meets once a month. At the time of the third interview the group had existed for 16 months. All but one mother said they attended every month. This mother explained that the meetings were too far away, and she had no means of transport.

The purpose of the first interview was to establish base line information for two of the areas of concern, namely the help and support the mothers received from their relatives and friends, and the amount of contact with other people.

The second interview investigated the help and support received, whether or not they still attended the group meetings, and the contact they had with other people.

The third interview again looked at the help and support, contact with others and the value of the group to the mothers.

The Mothers

Of the 43 mothers interviewed at the beginning of the project, 16 had had some experience with other people's children, 27 had not. Twenty four had lived in the area for less than two years, nine for less than a year, and, except in Group D, few had relatives living nearby. Although most (29) of the mothers telephoned their relatives from time to time, only 18 visited or were visited by relatives as often as once a week. Contact with friends was greater: 35 visited friends at least once a week, although six mothers said that they did not have any friends living near. The mothers' main support at this time came mainly from their husbands. Nineteen husbands had been present at the birth of the baby, and 35 had been at home with their wives for at least some time after the birth. All but six of the mothers said that they were able to go out with their husbands occasionally in the evening, and almost all said that their husbands helped with the care of the baby.

By the time of the second interview, the mothers' social isolation was less because the group itself was providing a means of social contact. By this stage 10 mothers had jobs, and by the time of the third interview 15 were working. Some mothers (24 of the 38 mothers who were asked in the second interview) also belonged to other groups in addition to their post-natal groups; working class wives belonged to baby sitting clubs, young wives groups, a rifle shooting club and a cub-scout committee, while middle class wives belonged to the National Childbirth Trust, a tennis club, a handworkers' guild and an operatic society.

The Group Meetings

At the time of the second interview, when the groups had been established for between six and thirteen months 27 of the 38 mothers said that they were still attending the meetings. The reasons most commonly given were to help their children to mix with other children, to meet other mothers to form friendships, and to share problems. The following comments were typical: 'For my little girl, she is an only child; it helps her to mix. It is good for me, so I see other people's difficulties too.'

The fact that most of the mothers continued to come to the meetings and found them enjoyable did not mean that they were entirely satisfied. Satisfaction was less in the 'manual workers' groups than in the 'non-manual' group; all the members of Group A described themselves as satisfied or very satisfied, compared with only half of Group B (manual), although satisfaction was also high in Groups C and D where the members came from all social classes. It would however be too simplistic to explain this difference solely in terms of social class; in this group the leader said that she did not enjoy the meetings and was moving away from the area shortly, and these feelings must have had some effect on the other group members. In my view the criticisms expressed and the positive suggestions made for improvement must be interpreted as a healthy sign of the groups' potential for growth and their ability to adapt to their members changing needs.

Table 32.2 Showing if mothers were or were not satisfied with the post-natal support group meetings

Mothers satisfied or not satisfied	Group A Non-manual	Group B Manual	Group C Mixed classes	Group D Ante-natal class	Totals
Very satisfied	1	0	2	1	4
Satisfied	6	3	4	3	16
Not satisfied	0	2	0	0	2
Don't know	0	1	1	2	4
Totals	7	6	7	6	26

THE PRESENT POSITION OF C.H.A.T. GROUPS

The name C.H.A.T. (Contact, Health and Teaching) was chosen by the group members themselves. We now have 35 active groups covering a cross-section of social classes in our area. In a further ten groups, which have now lasted longer than five years, some people have moved away, but many keep in touch with each other. The groups have no fixed life-span; they continue just as long as the group wishes.

The framework of the groups remains as originally planned except that the size is limited to between six and eight mothers with small children in each group. Six groups form a unit, and join together for some activities so that the parents and children have the chance to make a large circle of friends. Experienced leaders help new leaders to form groups, and they become group advisors.

Each group has a deputy leader and treasurer, chosen by the group, and we have a monthly newsletter to which all groups contribute ideas. News is also circulated on activities for parents and children in the area. An eight week course on aspects of health, education and the community, is organised from a clinic in the autumn, using outside speakers; the parents choose the subjects. In conjunction with this, a creche is arranged with the help of a nursery nurse tutor and students from a college of higher education, and sixth formers from a local college.

We have a library of 140 books covering all aspects of health, education and community life, and this was made possible by raising funds within the groups. The expertise of willing group members is also used in giving short talks within the groups, for example, an ex-hairdresser has spoken on the care of children's hair, and an ex-teacher on various aspects of education.

Each year C.H.A.T. designates a special project, which the individual groups can support if they wish. Some groups will choose to support particular charities at home or abroad, and will raise funds any way they wish, such as Spring fetes, Autumn fairs, nearly new sales to which all C.H.A.T. members are invited.

In the past, some C.H.A.T. members have taught parentcraft to teenagers at a comprehensive school, where the students were taking a 'Family and Community' course. Immigrants are welcomed into all groups, and the exchange of knowledge on child-rearing patterns is valuable. Our referal system is still the same; we do not advertise and membership is still by invitation. We now find that each group can support one member with deeper problems, such as a depression, or rejection of baby, and the supported member usually improves rapidly; in such cases, the coordinator will keep in close touch with the member's general practitioner.

Many ideas and activities have been tried out in different groups over the past years, for example: baby sitting, outings, parties for the children, social evenings for husbands too and swimming lessons for babies. Some pressure groups have also formed to improve local facilities, for example, more creches for babies in local colleges where mothers attend day time classes.

When a group has been established for about six to twelve months, the members often wish to try some specific work in the community, such as starting a toddlers group, or adopting elderly people. The group library helps to give information on most activities, and practical guidance is offered too.

The groups are intended as growth groups, and to be creative, so the whole system is parent orientated, allowing the parents and child to experiment and use their talents, as well as learning in the traditional form.

We are now holding quarterly evening meetings of group leaders, to explore new ideas and to discuss policy for the future. It would appear that this group system is adaptable to the needs of different areas, and that it is low in cost, time and manpower to the professional worker involved.

REFERENCES

Durham E 1972 The role of self-help in service provision. Journal of Applied Behaviour Science. Social Services Review 435–443

Katz A, Bender E 1976 The strength in us. Franklin Watts

Killilea M Mutual help organisations support systems and mutual help. Grune & Stratton, London

Research Project 'How mothers help themselves' available from King's Fund Centre and The Health Visitors Association
Seymour R 1977 Developing aspects of fatherhood. Midwife, Health Visitor and Community Nurse 13 (12): 390–391
Sprott W 1969 Human groups. Pelican, London, ch 4, p 63

FURTHER READING

Bion W R 1977 Experience in groups. Tavistock Publications, London
Perkins E 1979 Defining the need. International Journal of Nursing 16: 275–282
Seymour R 1974 An experimental group for mothers of young children. Midwife and Health Visitor 10: 6154–6158
Stranik M, Hogberg B 1979 Transition into parenthood. American Journal of Nursing: 1, 90–93
Thompson S, Kahn J 1973 The group as a helping technique. Pergamon, London
Tyler R Social policy and self help groups. The Journal of Applied Behavioral Science: 445–447

33

Needs infinite: resources finite

Joyce Wiseman

INTRODUCTION

A health visitor's perspective

To those within health visiting, and those without, the role of the health visitor is open to many interpretations. It was only during participation in the health visitors' training course that I, personally, became aware of the potential value of this professional worker.

Prior to the course, my actual knowledge of the work of the health visitor was limited to the vision of a rather middle class, middle aged, country type lady who usually drove round in a car, but occasionally used a bicycle, to visit homes where there were babies and young children. When not on her rounds she could be found sitting behind scales, dressed in a white coat, in an 'infant welfare clinic' weighting babies, and providing kindly and appropriate professional advice to young mothers.

I look back on the learnings and teachings from the course as one of the most enjoyable and valuable experiences of my life. It is only after qualification that one recalls a series of collective impressions, occurrences and reactions of a negative response to health visiting, by clients and the general public at large based in the origins of a dried-up source of general knowledge.

Clients referred to the health visitor as 'the lady from the welfare' or 'the woman from the town hall'. Husbands asked how wives (with no nursing qualifications at all) could obtain 'a job like yours', and for a period in the late 1960s, I remember performing an informal mini-type survey by asking various friends, acquaintances and professional workers what sort of duties they thought a health visitor carried out, or indeed what exactly a health visitor was. Responses varied from vague comments on health, or frank 'don't knows'. Frequently, if the question was not asked of them, it was directed to myself as health visitor. This vagueness of role has been fully expressed by Clark (1973), Hunt (1972) and many others. Dingwall (1976) again states in his paper: 'Innovatory thinking in schools of health visiting can have relatively little impact on health visiting practice unless there are corresponding reforms in work situations.'

Despite these awakening experiences to the fact that the community at large did not appear to place too much importance on the health visitor and health visiting as the health visitor training course had advocated, one did carry on, with the light somewhat diminished, but not completely extinguished. Occasionally, an actual 'glow' would occur because of an apparently high regard and attitude of a client or fellow worker to one's health visiting knowledge and expertise.

'Carrying on' of course meant performing home visits, the traditional activity of the original health visitors of the Salford Ladies Sanitary Reform Association of 1862 (McEwan, 1962), attending schools, child welfare clients, maternity and various other clinics, as well as performing group health education teaching sessions.

In all these activities, the greatest difficulty encountered in 'carrying on' occured when endeavouring to perform 'selective' health visiting. This, of course, usually meant looking through the client record cards and attempting to ascertain which clients would most benefit from a health visit. It was difficult to gauge from records and known clients and I could not help wondering how many people there were, out there in the community, silently crying out and requiring a preventive health visiting service of whom the health visitor had no knowledge. Discussions on this problem with many and various other health visiting colleagues never revealed a satisfactory answer to the problem. Individual health visitors had a variety of methods to help them to become aware of clients requiring visiting, together with an apparently satisfactory relationship and liaison service with fellow field workers from other agencies.

Another death-knoll to the dedication of the cause is a succession of 'no access' visits and, quite illogically, the health visitor may feel snubbed at the apparent disregard for her worth when not finding clients at home. She will also be aware of the waste of working hours and the economical implications of the lost hours and travel times.

It could be said that frequently the health visitor has to perform her health visiting responsibilities in a randomised and totally unscientific fashion. Her one source of systemised referral is from the Notification of Births procedure, which ensures that she is informed of all new births occurring within the community to which she is ecpected to provide a health visiting service. Other health visiting referrals originate from a diversity of sources such as general practitioners, other health care workers, social services, schools, the clients themselves and neighbours. The only other official notifications of potentially existent clients stem from such sources as notifiable diseases, and even the reliability of these is questioned by health visitors in many instances.

A manager's perspective

What about the health visitors' managers? How are they assisted towards determining their health visitor establishment levels? Their decisions must take into account the health visitor's potential visiting requirements and the community's preventive health care need? Guidelines are to be found in a Department of Health and Social Security. Circular (1972) entitled 'Aids to improved efficiency in the local health services deployment of nursing teams', of which Paragraph 9 is headed, 'Health Visiting' and quotes in full:

> The Jameson Report in 1956 recommended a national average of one health visitor to 4300 population. In terms of health visiting only (i.e. excluding school nursing) this represents one health visitor to 4600 population approximately. While subsequent experience confirms this estimate as reasonable to some areas, a ratio of one health visitor to 3000 population may be desirable in others, e.g. those with a highly developed system of attachments to general practice or with a high immigrant population. Such provision would be exclusive of supporting ancilliary staff.

However, the validity of the department's guidelines could be questioned. The Jameson Report (Ministry of Health, 1956), from which they have taken their recommendations is now nearly thirty years old. A research study of that age could be said to be irrelevant and outdated as circumstances are superceded by subsequent events. Since the Jameson findings and recommendations, new 'care groups' have emerged as a result of social change such as immigrants, especially those from Asia, who have come to the United Kingdom in large numbers during the last twenty years.

The problems of drug dependency and obesity have only been highlighted during the last 10 to 15 years, whilst the number of elderly people in the population continues to increase. Changes in the divorce laws have increased the number of family break-ups since the 1960s.

Hicks (1976) in his book *Primary Health Care* questions the method of estimating the ratio of health visitors to population, both by the Jameson Committee and the DHSS, who have taken their recommendations from the Jameson Report (1956). Hicks suggests that it is time to have a re-examination of the ratios, and further recommends that this is done by some good operational Research!

It is within this background that a research study was carried out with the objective of developing a management tool to assist nurse managers with their allocation of health visitor resources.

The methodology was first developed by formulating estimations of the numbers of clients existent within respective care groups. This approach helps to establish a concrete base of knowledge, both to the health visitors and their managers, of a community's preventive health care needs. From this knowledge-base managers can be assisted towards formulating health visiting target objectives, allocating health visitor responsibilities, and determining the health visitor manpower establishment required in the local organisation of health visiting.

The management tool also endeavours to measure the health visitors' activities to the health visitors' own perceived view of priorities, which again can be compared to their managers' own judgement of health visitor responsibilities and community need. The following section, defines and describes the management tool.

DEVELOPING A MANAGEMENT TOOL TO ASSIST NURSE MANAGERS WITH THE ALLOCATION OF HEALTH VISITOR RESOURCES.

There are three essential component parts related to health visiting practice:

- the client
- the health visitor
- the organisation.

The focal point is, of course, the client, and both the health visitor and the organisation, to be effective, must orientate and revolve their activities and development so that they contrive to respond to the required needs of the client. The client is a member of a community as a whole whose circumstances and subsequent demands of service vary, depending upon such variables as, health, environment, ethnic origins and culture.

The health visitor is a professionally qualified preventive health care worker, whose perceptions and interests are influenced by life's experience and the conditioned learning brought about through her training. Her health visiting practice is affected by the constraints of the community needs and the organisation.

The organisation can be regarded on the two levels of national and local organisation. The national organisation of the health service is influenced by a variety of factors, such as political strategies, changing national priorities and current resources. This eventually has an effect upon the local organisation of health visiting through governmental policies, directives and memoranda.

Local organisation of management is further affected by local conditions of geography, environment and resources.

Fayol (1848–1925) stated that for an organisation to succeed a purposeful system of management is required which contains the five essential elements of planning, organising, coordinating, controlling and communicating, and the degree of success of all five elements is very dependent upon the ability of managers to motivate staff.

Managers should be able to relate these criteria to their own organisational circumstances so that it is possible to interpret and discuss the implications of these managerial systems and skills in the health visiting context. Planning and successful forecasting for health visiting resources is dependent upon managers receiving knowledge of present and future community trends and needs.

Organising gives the manager a responsibility for specifying health visiting workloads and for the setting of short term and long term objectives for improving the organisational service. This involves staff development and motivating staff to achieve the objectives.

The coordinating activity of health visiting management gives the manager a responsibility to synchronise the health visiting service with other disciplines in the hospital and community field. This will provide a coordinated health service which will contribute towards continuity of patient/client care, which must be beneficial to the community.

A control cycle of management is necessary to regulate the organisation so that its activities are in accordance with the supply and demand for service. This helps to maintain a quality and quantity control of service standards. Communication is the common denominator and binding factor which makes the organisation a cohesive whole. It is, therefore, essential that a reliable communication system exists throughout the organisation of health visiting.

In this research study data is gained from the three sources of community, health visitors and nurse managers, (the latter regarded as the representatives of the organisation). By combining the use of the data in a variety of ways, a management instrument has been developed which is intended to assist nurse managers with their organisational responsibilities.

The Community

A sector, the 'research sector', of a health district was selected as 'a community' which is defined in the context of health visitor 'care groups', which are referred

Table 33.1 Data sources from which estimations have been made of the annual numbers within the research care group population.

Ante natal mothers	Numbers estimated from the vital statistics issued by the Area Health Authority's Epidemiology Unit.
Post natal mothers	This care group was entered after a request by the health visitors themselves. Data obtained as for Ante Natal Mothers
0–1 year (routine)	Vital statistics obtained from the Area Health maintained by the health visitors themselves.
0–1 year (at risk)	Numbers estimated from the sector's "At Risk" Register maintained by the health visitors themselves.
1–5 years (routine)	Numbers gained from the 1971 census and then adjusted to the estimated sector population.
1–5 years (at risk)	Numbers within this group obtained from the sector's "At Risk" Register.
5–16 years (healthy) i.e. School Children.	The 1971 census was used to formulate calculations on this care group, and then adjusted to the sector population.
5–16 years (mental handicap)	Numbers for this group obtained from the sector's Handicapped Register.
5–16 years (physical handicap)	As Above.
16–65 years (healthy)	Numbers obtained from the 1971 census and then adjusted to the estimated sector population.
16–65 years (mental and physical handicapped)	The Disablement Register maintained by the Disablement Resettlement Officer supplied the required information.
65 years plus (routine) i.e. 65 years — 75 years.	Numbers obtained from the 1971 census then adjusted to the sector population.
65 years plus (at risk) i.e. 75 years and over	The 1971 census provided basic information on which estimations for this care group were made.
Infectious diseases	Estimations of the annual numbers falling within this care group category were made from the sector's Notifiable Disease Register.
Problem families	Estimations based from the records maintained by the health visitors' managers.
Metabolic disorders	Estimation of numbers within this category made from information gained from the International Classification Disease Code maintained by the Regional Health Authority.
Psychiatric disorders	Estimations made from the International Classification Disease Code maintained by the Regional Health Authority.
Drug dependents Alcohol, cigarettes, etc.	Care group numbers estimated from various sources:- ALCOHOL — National Council on Alcoholism. CIGARETTE SMOKING — A.S.H. and Population Trends No. 7 DRUG ABUSE — (i.e. Cannabis and Misuse of Controlled and Narcotic Drugs) Home Office Statistics (1974).

Table 33.1 (*cont'd*)

Obesity	Calculation of the number of persons categorised within this group were made from the D.H.S.S. (1976) book — "Research on Obesity".
Bereavement	Estimations were based on the Death Rate Statistics issued by the Area Health Authority's Epidemiology Unit.
Immigrant families	The 1971 census provided the basic information from which estimations were made to establish number within this care group in the sector.
Terminally ill	This care group number was estimated from the Death Rate Statistics issued by the local Epidemiology Unit.
Acutely ill (*Other than infectious diseases*)	It is accepted that this care group cuts across all the care group categories, and any may fall within this category for a transient period.
Single parent families	Numbers within the sector provided by the Social Services Department and which originated from the 1971 census.
Marital visits	Assessment made for this care group from Population Trends No. 6 and No. 7.

to by The Council for the Education and Training of Health Visitors as vulnerable groups in the community. A total of 25 care groups have been identified in the study, and the list can be seen in Table 33.1, together with the data sources which were used to formulate estimations of the approximate annual care group membership existent within the care group populations.

Figure 33.1 presents in histogram form the estimated distribution and structure of the community's care group populations. The care group estimations should help to provide the nurse managers with some tangible evidence of care group client membership. This should assist them towards determining a community's preventive health care need, which will include the allocation of health visitor resources and manpower requirements.

The nurse managers also need to be informed of the health visitors' activities, as well as the health visitors' self-perceived view of the community's health care need.

The health visitor

Data is gained from the health visitor on the two aspects of activity and priority. Knowledge of the health visitors' activities is gained through self-completion questionnaires (see Fig. 33.2), which are given to the health visitors, together with clear guidelines for their completion, including definitions of the meanings of the listed functions.

Twenty five health visitors participated in the research study, and completed the activity questionnaire over an eight week period. The questionnaire attempts to determine the level of health visitor contact to the respective care group client membership, the functions carried out to the care group clients, the source of

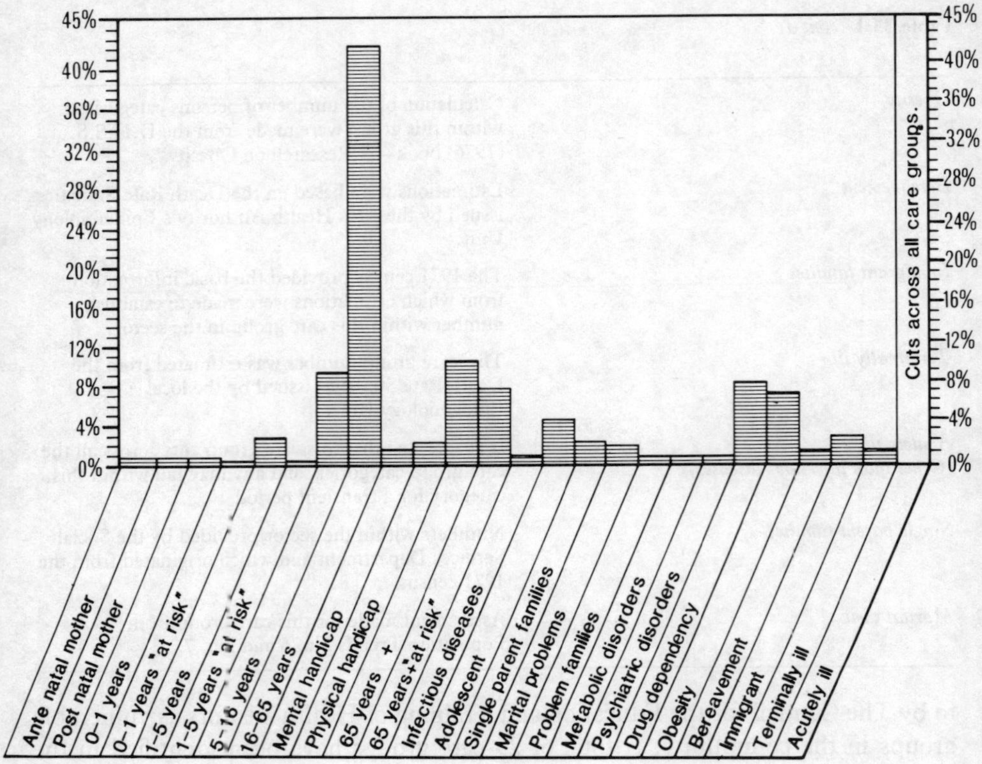

Fig. 33.1

referral to the health visitor and the influence of the referral source on the health visitor working pattern.

After analysis, the computer data can be cross-referenced and compared in a variety of ways, which can be useful for managerial discussion and decision-making.

However, to help the managers formulate any conclusions on the work direction of the health visitors, they will need a yardstick to help them compare the current health visitor activity with their own perceptions of community needs. The nurse managers should estimate ideal target health visiting contact levels to the various care groups, together with their estimated lower bound contact levels. The ideal target contact levels to a care group would be taken to be the idealistic model for care group contact, whilst the lower bounds would be the lowest contact seen to be acceptable for a preventive service to be existent to the client care group.

Because the managers have an estimated care group population for the community, it is possible for them to quantify their upper and lower health visitor contact visits. This is illustrated in Figure 33.3 where the reader can compare the health visitors' activity from the survey data, together with the managers upper and lower estimated required contact levels.

How does the current health visitors' activities and the managers' recommendations of upper and lower contact levels to the care groups compare with the

Health visitor's name. ____________________

Day of week ____________________ Date ____________________

HEALTH VISITING RESEARCH STUDY – ACTIVITY QUESTIONNAIRE

(Please use one questionnaire for each contact)

(Tick appropriate boxes)

What is client's AGE GROUP?	What is client's CARE GROUP?	What was YOUR FUNCTION in this contact? (PRIMARY / SECONDARY)
☐ First year	☐ Ante natal mother	☐ ☐ 1. Medical diagnosing
☐ 1–4 years	☐ Post natal mother	☐ ☐ 2. Social diagnosing
☐ 5–15 years	☐ Child (routine contact)	☐ ☐ 3. Comprehensive appraisal
☐ 16–64 years	☐ Child regd. "at risk"	☐ ☐ 4. Monitoring observation of services to clients
☐ 65 years +	☐ Adolescent	☐ ☐ 5. Monitoring observation of client (s) condition
	☐ 65 + (routine contact)	☐ ☐ 6. Health education advice
	☐ 65+ "at risk"	☐ ☐ 7. Prophylaxis prevention
	☐ Infectious diseases	☐ ☐ 8. Screening programme
	☐ Physical handicap	☐ ☐ 9. Psychological supportive
	☐ Mental handicap	☐ ☐ 10. Liaison and co-ordination of services
	☐ Psychiatric disorder	☐ ☐ 11. Non-routine recording
	☐ Metabolic disorder	☐ ☐ 12. Research data recording
	☐ Unmarried mother	☐ ☐ 13. School health medical inspection
	☐ Illegitimate child	☐ ☐ 14. Hygiene inspection
	☐ Marital visits	
	☐ Problem family	
	☐ Drug dependence alcohol, cigarettes, etc.	
	☐ Obesity	
	☐ Bereavement	
	☐ Immigrant	
	☐ Acutely ill	
	☐ Terminally ill	

Who requested this contact?	Where was this contact made?	Where a relative of the care group was the main focus of attention WAS IT,
☐ G.P.	☐ School	mother? ☐
☐ Hospital	☐ Home	father? ☐
☐ Social Services	☐ Clinic/Health Centre	son? ☐
☐ Schools	☐ Clinic/Hospital	daughter? ☐
☐ Police	☐ Telephone	grandmother? ☐
☐ Client's family	☐ IF NO ACCESS	husband? ☐
☐ Client herself		other? ☐
☐ By your own initiative		
☐ Other eg. neighbour		

Fig. 33.2

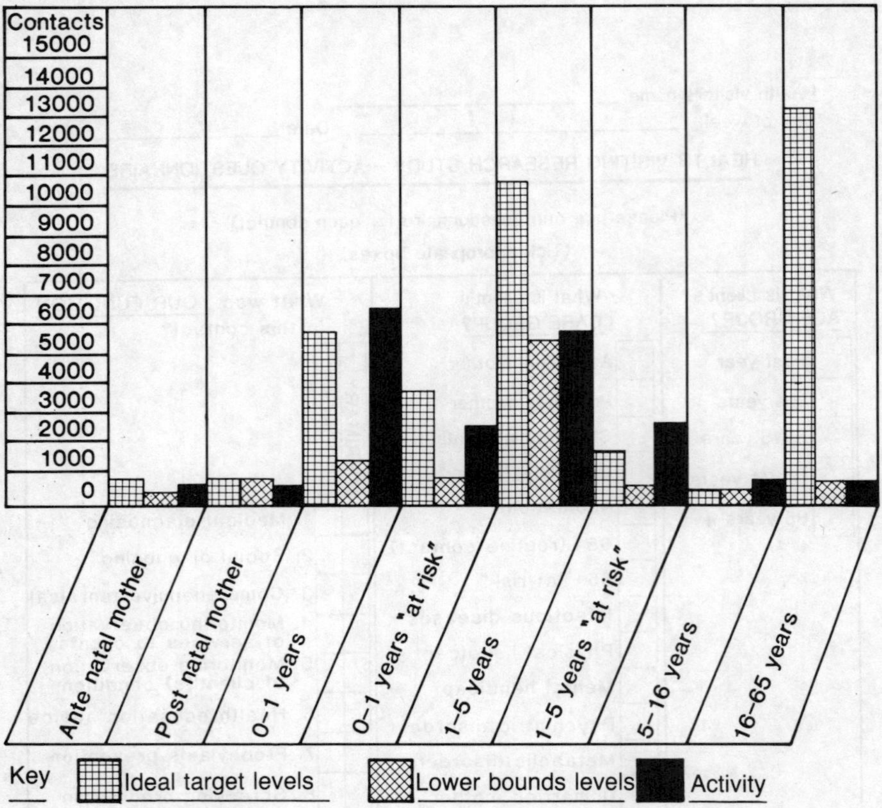

Fig. 33.3 (i)

health visitors' own self-perceived community care group needs and direction for health visiting?

In the study, the researcher held structured interviews with each of the respective health visitors which lasted from two to four hours. The purpose of the interviews was to gain from the health visitors, themselves, their own subjective judgements of health visitor care group priorities. The study piloted and tested this approach to investigate the viability of this type of interview between nurse managers and their health visitor staff. It would appear to be a useful tool for nurse

Table 33.2 Health Visitors' 'top ten care group selections'

0–1 year 'at risk'
1–5 years 'at risk'
0–1 year 'routine'
1–5 years handicapped
Problem families (with young children)
1–5 years 'routine'
The single parent family
Ante-natal mothers
5–15 years, mental or physical handicapped
65 years plus 'at risk'

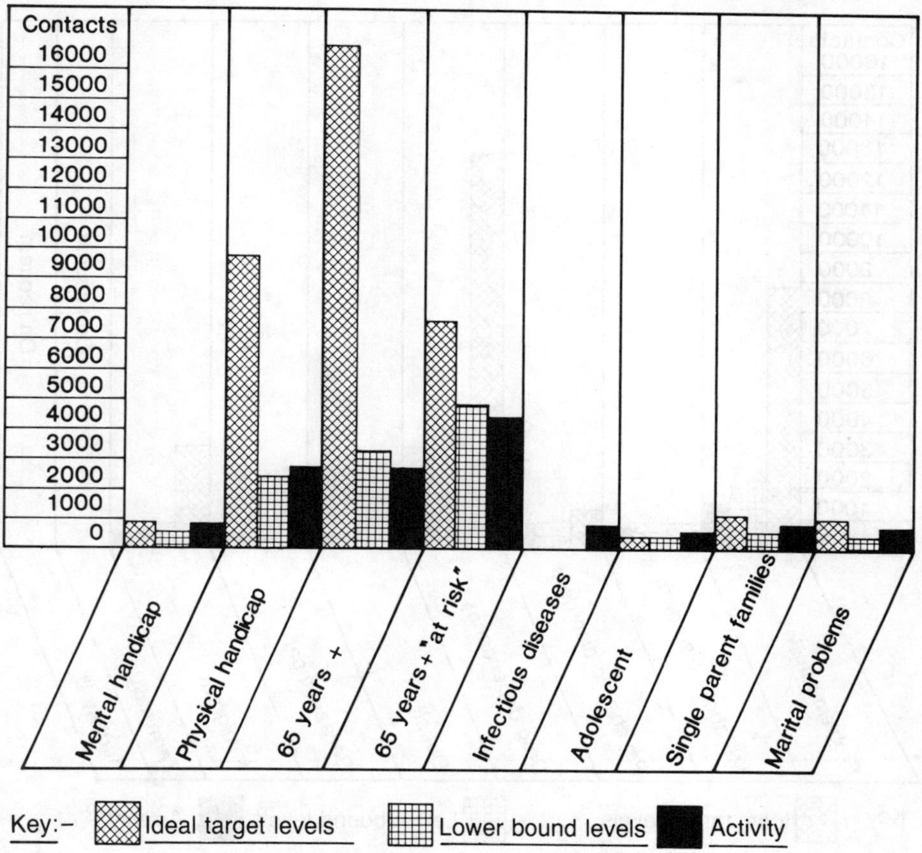

Fig. 33.3 (ii)

managers to gain an insight into health visitors' interests and views of health visiting priorities.

In the study the health visitors indicated a strong interest and health visiting belief in the ante-natal mothers, the 0–5 age group, the handicapped school-child, the single parent family, the problem family and the elderly 'at risk' (see Table 33.2).

The comparison with health visitor activity, shown in Figure 33.3, would indicate that, on the whole, the health visitors do follow through their own professed interest of priority in their health visitor practice. The managers will have to determine if they wish this pattern of health visiting to continue, or if they wish a change of emphasis to take place in their health visiting practice.

POTENTIAL VALUE OF THE COMBINED DATA TO NURSE MANAGERS

The nurse managers are now in a situation where they can perceive the distribution of the community's care group population. This can be compared with the

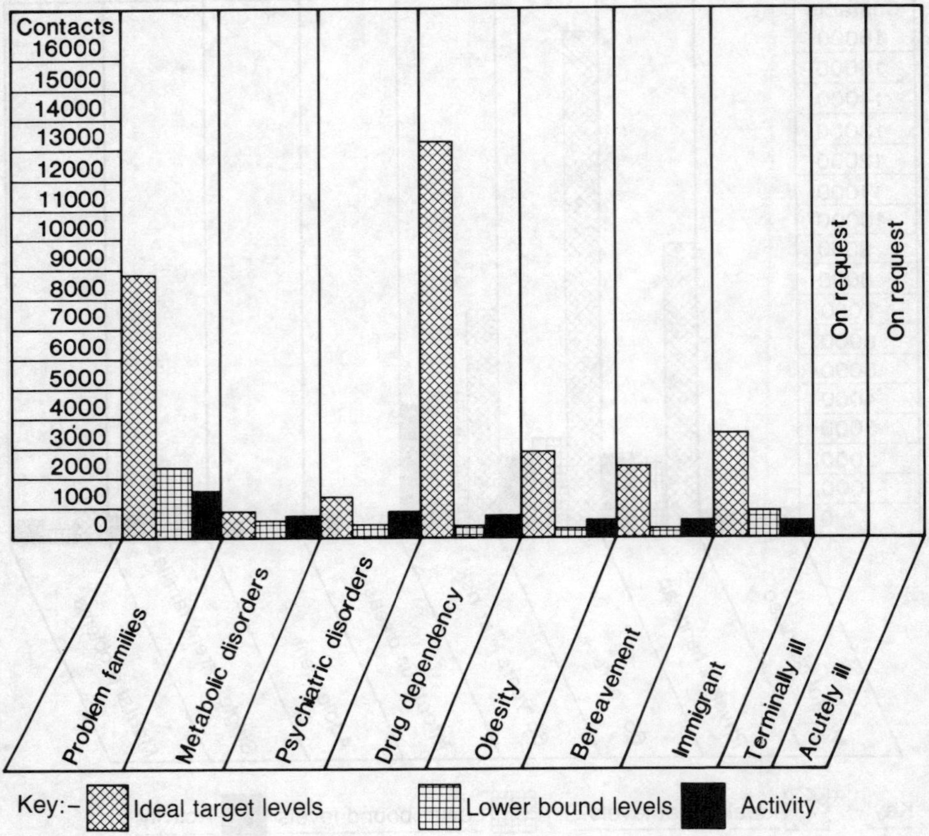

Fig. 33.3 (iii)

managers' recommended 'ideal target' and 'lower bound' health visiting levels, together with the health visitors' activity data analysis and the health visitors' subjective views of priority.

The managers may wish to proceed cautiously with the analysis of the data, and refrain from drawing too many conclusions from the findings. However, there is potential for its use to improve the preventive health care delivery to the community. Similarly, it can assist with the staff/career development of the individual health visitor, and hopefully, improve her job satisfaction.

Where short-falls to the client care group are observed, the nurse managers can refer to the priority search interview data of each health visitor. In some instances she could be recommended for specialist health visiting where her particular interest appears to lie. Alternatively, where care groups are perceived to be of low health visitor priority by both managers and health visitors alike, it could become policy for this care group to be accepted as a low priority care group for health visitor responsibility.

The ratio of health visitors in the study per head of population was lower than the recommendations laid down by the Jameson Report (1956) and the relinquishing of health visitor responsibility to certain care groups could be one way of directing health visitor resources to places of perceived priority.

The study also showed varying numbers of home contacts to the clients by the health visitors. Some health visitors made an average of approximately one dozen home contacts per day, whilst others made only three or four home visits a day. The manager will need to investigate if the work organisation itself is preventing a health visitor performing home visiting, e.g too many clinics?, or does the health visitor need counselling so that she re-organises her work more effectively?

Advantages to this approach for health visitor service planning are, briefly, threefold:

- Practical use is made of information systems and statistics;
- Health visitor job satisfaction and career development is assisted;
- Health visitors and managers together can make target health visiting objectives, determine health visitor priorities, and so help to shape their own profession of health visiting.

REFERENCES

Clark J 1973 A family visitor. Royal College of Nursing, London

Department of Health and Social Security 1972 Aids to improved efficiency in the local health services deployment of nursing teams. Circular 13/72. HMSO, London

Dingwall R 1976 The social organisation of health visitor training. 26th February, Nursing Times Occasional Paper

Hicks D 1976 Primary health care — a review. HMSO, London

Home Office 1975 The 1974 statistics of the misuse of drugs in the U.K. HMSO, London

Hunt M 1972 The dilemma of the identity of health visiting. 3rd February, Nursing Times Occasional Paper

International Statistical Classification 1975 International classification disease code, 8th edn. World Health Organisation, Geneva

McEwan M 1962 Health visiting: A textbook for health visitor students, 4th edn. Faber and Faber, London

Medical Research Council 1976 Research on obesity. HMSO, London

Ministry of Health 1956 An inquiry into health visiting. Report of a working party on the field of work, training and recruitment of health visitors (The Jameson Report). HMSO, London

National Council on Alcoholism 1977 Report of the working party on alcoholism (The Braine Report). National Council on Alcoholism

Office of Population, Census & Surveys 1971 The Census, 1971. HMSO, London

Office of Population, Census and Surveys 1976 Alcoholism and mortality. Population trends no 6, 36–40. HMSO, London

Office of Population, Census & Surveys 1977 Population, age & sex. Population trends no 7, 39. HMSO, London

34

Primary health care in Britain and abroad

Barry Reedy

Until some 20 years ago, relatively few people in the National Health Service had any idea of the way in which health services were provided abroad, even in countries as close to us as Europe. Since then the development of cultural, scientific and other kinds of international exchange have increased our knowledge of the methods by which other countries maintain the health of their people and provide for the five elements of a health service: the diagnosis and treatment of illness, the prevention of illness, health maintenance, bed-side nursing and rehabilitation.

At first the exchange of visits by health professionals was almost confined to clinical specialists and most of those from Britain were made to the United States of America. In recent years this commerce has become worldwide and it now involves workers in many other health service disciplines and professions. Their experiences and the consequent development in their thinking and outlook have already enabled us to see our own health service more knowledgeably and dispassionately than before. In return, the National Health Service has attracted many visitors from abroad and some have imitated it in varying degrees according to their own requirements. Understandably some of the visitors from Third World countries have been cautious about the tendency for doctors trained in Western medical schools to be evangelists for scientific medicine as if it was the only system for the diagnosis and treatment of illness. Particularly in the Far East, Africa and South America there are other systems of medical intervention (such as acupuncture) and some of these appear to be as valid as our own in certain circumstances.

Because there is also a close similarity between clinicians of different nations in the medical language which they use, there tends to have been an assumption that they also use the same methods for providing health services. Whilst there are similarities, there are also many differences in this respect and it is a frequent and sometimes disturbing experience amongst those who visit health services abroad to discover that a common medical language is of little avail when poverty, drought, lack of sanitation and the vastness of the terrain are the real imperatives.

Surprisingly, even the Americans have these problems and in our own mountainous and tural areas, conditions sometimes call for expedients such as the so-called 'triple-duty' nurse — the combined health visitor, nurse and midwife. Furthermore, many societies retain a system based on traditional healers which cannot be ignored when elements of a westernised health service are introduced, often to be available only to the wealthy who can pay for this kind of care. Nevertheless these paradoxes can be used constructively by students of the organisation of health services and some take the magniloquent view that the whole world is a laboratory for experiments in designing systems to provide health care (Roemer, 1977). Certainly the description and, when competently done, the evaluation of alternative systems ought to become as important for developing our own health service as clinical research is for the development of nursing or medical practice. Furthermore, patients ultimately benefit from the knowledge and insights of such diverse people as the sociologists, anthropologists, geographers and economists who are often involved in this kind of research.

All this assumes that it is possible for politicians and social administrators to make free choices about the kind of health service which is most suitable for their country. In fact this is rarely possible and only occurs under special circumstances, as for instance in Tanzania (Gish, 1978), where there were previously almost no services at all, or in Cuba (Ministry of Public Health, 1973) where a political revolution allowed the creation of a completely new system based on polyclinics and health centres. The wealth of a country is also of crucial importance and whilst rich nations can afford to build more medical schools, train more doctors and conduct expensive scientific research, poor nations may decide to base their health services on sanitarians and medical assistants, or other so-called 'mid-level' workers (Fendall, 1972)

Much of what is available, particularly in developed countries, also depends on historical precedents. Americans are at present anchored to a system based on the individual states at least partly because of a mistrust of federal government which dates from the American revolution. In many parts of the world, nursing is still carried out by religious organisations but in Britain we have a secular nursing service which owes its existence mainly to the Crimean War and the influence of Florence Nightingale. In France, the nursing and health services are fragmented both by the legacy of an administration based on 'departements' and by the multitude of religious, voluntary and state agencies which act independently of each other (Cornillot & Bonamour, 1973).

In modern times, perhaps the two major constraints on the development of health services are high birth rates and the isolation of quite large populations in both a geographical and a social sense. These, together with poverty, are probably also the major contemporary determinants of the emphasis which is given in different countries to the division between primary or 'first contact' care and care based on institutions such as hospitals. Historically, the latter have existed in various forms for many centuries in the western world. Throughout their existence they have been associated with all the concomitants of power, prestige and wealth, but they are also exceedingly expensive, both to build and to run. Although their intervention at a technical level may be decisive or life-saving for patients, the contact that they have with individual patients for any other purpose is often minimal and, at least in Britain, is becoming progressively shorter on average. Behind the hospitals since historic times, there have been lay figures such as the herbalist and the midwife to whom people could turn for immediate advice or assistance in illness, their most effective point of 'first contact'. In many Third World countries these may still be the only resources for care but in Europe a more formal system of primary care, stemming from the function of first contact, grew through the late 18th and 19th centuries. This has developed 'par excellence' in Britain, Scandinavia and Holland and an eclectic account of our own system of so-called 'general practice' will make subsequent comparisons with other countries clearer.

In Britain the function of healing with plants has in past centuries lain between the unqualified herbalists and those more expert and ambitious who became apothecaries and, (by examination), members of the Society of Apothecaries. Whilst they were popularly regarded as tradesmen by the community there were also surgeons who were treated as craftsmen and whose expertise was often based on military experience. Finally there were physicians, members of a learned profession, trained and qualified in the university medical schools of the time. Any of these could act as the point of first contact in illness but the physicians tended to work in the larger towns and centres of learning whilst the surgeons and apothecaries were more widely distributed and were the main providers of care in the rural areas. Today's agent of primary care, the general practitioner, emerged as a complex amalgam of all three types but most saw themselves predominantly as surgeons, hence the term 'surgery' used even now for their premises. By the middle of the 19th century an early form of professional licensing had developed but considerable confusion was caused by the diversity of licensing bodies for the three groups of practitioner. The first Medical Act in 1858 was therefore mainly designed to simplify this position and to protect the public by establishing a register of all those practitioners who were considered to be qualified to practise medicine in one form or another. In 1919, the Nurses Act fulfilled a similar purpose for the nursing profession. Indeed, the latter half of the century saw similar acts with the same intention for a number of other professions quite unconnected with medicine or nursing.

The Medical Act did not distinguish between specialists and general practitioners. At that time any registered doctor could practise in the community or in hospital, but as medicine itself developed, the more able or ambitious doctors became more specialised and began to be consulted by their colleagues about difficult cases. The status that this conferred enabled them to charge higher fees to patients and as scientific medicine developed and became centred on the hospitals, a crucial distinction grew between the two classes of doctor. Those who worked in hospitals and were called in as consultants by colleagues tended also to be sought out by the wealthy urban middle class to provide them with primary care. The less expert and the country doctors, whether having a hospital appointment or not, became, in fact, the physicians of the poor and were thus less able in justice to be selective about the kind of cases they saw. This distinction has become firmly rooted in our system but nowadays many G.P.s welcome the absence of selectivity and find it a challenge to cope with the wide variety of patients and conditions which present to them in their practice.

During the latter half of the 19th century the out-patient departments of the hospitals took over the function of the old poor law dispensaries and became the main providers in the towns of first contact care for the indigent. These low cost facilities were sometimes also used by the middle classes, and thus by undercutting fees, the hospitals came into direct financial competition for patients with the urban G.P.s. The problem was resolved by an agreement that consultants would see no-one in the out-patient department without a letter of referral from a G.P. This system has remained a cornerstone in relations between G.P.s and hospital consultants ever since, with certain exceptions such as venereal disease clinics and accident departments where patients may attend on their own initiative. Thus began the unique separation which exists virtually only in Britain between hospital services and primary care services.

At the turn of the century, some G.P.s received a small regular income by committing themselves to provide medical services for the members of friendly societies and trade unions. This was similar in principle to present day insurance systems in many other countries, including America, but in 1911, this principle was formalised and extended by Lloyd George's National Insurance Act. In return for a secure income in the form of a capitation fee, G.P.s contracted to provide regular primary care services for manual workers of all ages and for the very poor. Thus the scheme covered only part of the population and at first was not extended to cover the remainder of the population or the hospital and local authority services. It was not until the inception of the National Health Service in 1948 that everyone had the right to register with a G.P. for the full range of services. The 1911 Act set up Insurance Committees to administer the scheme and these committees eventually became Executive Councils under the National Health Service (N.H.S.) Acts, and then Family Practitioner Committees with the reorganisation of the N.H.S. in 1974. Each area health authority has one of these committees to administer the general practitioner and certain related services such as pharmacy. They are remarkable for their evident historical continuity since 1911, even to preserving the form of the G.P.s' early record system, and their loyalty to the tradition of general practice is very high. Collectively these committees have helped to ensure the preservation and administrative independence of the G.P.s from the hospital and local authority services.

The general practitioners' status as independent contractors to the National Health Service is highly valued by most G.P.s because they genuinely believe that, for a number of reasons, it is in the best interests of their patients. However, independence is also linked with other developments which have tended to isolate the G.P.s from former sources of power such as hospital appointments. Senior hospital appointments were virtually closed to G.P.s at the inception of the N.H.S, although part-time and supervised clinical assistantships in out-patient departments remain and are claimed to assist the manpower problems of the hospitals. Outside the conurbations there are still a number of small 'cottage' hospitals, nowadays called 'community' hospitals, and these contain the only beds which G.P.s can control for their own patients. Even so, the type of case they can admit is limited and regional health authorities try to ensure that at least the operative surgery, midwifery and casualty work is referred to district hospitals under consultant control.

Nevertheless, preservation of the cottage hospitals can easily be justified by the care they provide for the many cases of temporary illness or disability in patients of all ages which require nursing care rather than technological excellence. Cottage hospitals also have the advantage, particularly for the elderly, of keeping patients close to their relatives and other sources of social support.

Unfortunately the number of cottage hospitals is very small and it is probable that fewer than 10% of G.P.s have any access to them. Neither do G.P.s have access to district hospital beds, (save through the referral process), although an increasing number have direct access for their patients to pathology and X-ray investigations and these enable the younger G.P.s in particular to do far more for their patients without referral to a specialist. This lack of hospital beds was a major source of low status and morale during the 1950s and early 1960s and it was compounded by other factors such as low salaries and poor working conditions, including a 365-day, 24-hour 'on-call' responsibility.

Following threats to resign from the N.H.S, the government agreed with the G.P.s in 1966 on a so-called 'charter' for the reform of general practice. Their terms of service were amended in order to allow the delegation of work to nurses and others and to lay staff in their practices. A monetary award was linked conditionally with the formation of group practices consisting of three or more doctors, the employment of administrative staff and the improvement of buildings and equipment.

In 1968, the Health Services and Public Health Act encouraged concessions from the local health authorities by increasing the development of government-built health centres and establishing the principle by which nurses and other professionals employed by the local authorities could work more closely with G.P.s on the basis of the so-called 'attachment' relationship. This was a basic step towards the creation of inter-disciplinary health care teams for which the precedents had already been set abroad, notably in America and Scandinavia, and foreshadowed in Britain as early as 1920 in the report of the Dawson Committee (Consultative Council on Medical and Allied Services, 1920).

These were all organisational changes but equally important were the changes made earlier by the General Medical Council in professional training and practice. As from 1953, medical graduates were unable to register for independent practice, regardless of their career intentions, until they had completed a further year as house officers in approved hospital posts. This far-sighted step was the preliminary to developing programmes of in-service training for G.P.s, for long a *sine qua non* for doctors specialising in hospital work. Since then, doctors intending to make their careers in primary care now have the additional option of training programmes which involve them in three years of hospital work in the key specialties affecting general practice, such as paediatrics, psychiatry and medicine. Many of these posts lead to higher qualifications but the additional hospital experience by itself has been sufficient to create a cadre of younger G.P.s who are far more knowledgeable and experienced clinically than their older colleagues were at the same stage in their careers. Much of this progress has occurred under the influence of the Royal College of General Practitioners which was established in the early 1950s to encourage high standards of general practice. The College has also been closely associated both with the creation of academic departments of general practice, now established in the majority of medical schools, and with much of the research currently undertaken in both clinical and behavioural aspects of primary care.

Although this brief account of the evolution and present form of general medical practice in Britain may appear to have ignored the concurrent and parallel developments in the other caring professions, such as nursing and health visiting, their progress has been extremely important and it is arguable that the development of each profession has ultimately depended on the progress of the others. Despite our own misgivings about some of the shortcomings of our health service, it seems clear that in world terms, we now have a sophisticated system for providing primary care. Whilst there are differences in some respects (and notably in certain vital statistics such as perinatal mortality rates) our health service and our primary care services in particular bear a generic resemblance to those of all the other countries with a welfare state economy.

Thus in Western Europe, Japan, New Zealand and Australia, most of the population is covered by government-owned or sponsored health insurance which inevitably evokes a system for government control of expenditure. In most of these countries the hospitals are also mainly controlled by government institutions or by local authorities and their personnel are usually salaried. Nevertheless the medical providers of care are professionally independent and tend, as in Britain, to be divided into specialists and generalists, that is general practitioners, whilst the public health and preventive services form a separate tier and carry out their functions separately from the curative services. In general, only highly trained specialists are permitted to work in hospitals and when G.P.s transfer their patients to specialist care there is also a complete transfer of responsibility for the patient. Britain and the Scandinavian countries provide typical examples of this pattern, whilst countries such as Germany, France, Italy and Spain vary from it in some respects.

Amongst the major industrialised nations, only the Americans have no system of compulsory health insurance and although there are signs of change, the provision of health care is essentially still a matter of pluralism and free enterprise. This may seem surprising when the main causes of morbidity, heart disease, malignancy, cerebrovascular disease and accidents, are the same in America as in Europe, but much of the explanation lies in the history and ethical values of the American people.

In 1911, the year in which British general practice became established, a radical change in the American system of medical education led in the opposite direction and within 30 years, to the virtual disappearance of the G.P.s in America, particularly in the rural areas and the urban ghettos. Instead the emphasis was placed on scientific research and medical specialism with the consequences, amongst others, that the system for delivering health care became hospital-based and the increasing numbers of doctors lived almost exclusively in wealthy suburbs. This relocation of doctors is becoming a problem in our own conurbations but in Britain, government planning has at least ensured that overall, a more or less adequate number both of G.P.s and specialists practise in each region and area. In the U.S.A the total number of doctors is more than adequate for the population as a whole but they are seriously maldistributed between urban and rural areas and one-third of all American doctors practise in only 3 of the 52 States, New York, Pennsylvania and California.

The predominant ethic of Americans and of their doctors is that of freedom to choose the best that can be afforded and those patients who can afford it refer themselves to doctors without constraint in the belief that the more specialised the doctor, the more likely he is to solve their problem. Thus first contact care is provided by any of the 70% or so of doctors who have practice premises (called an 'office') in the community as well as in hospital. In contrast with Britain, only about a quarter of these call themselves 'generalist' or 'family physician' and the majority specialise in medicine (the so-called 'internists'), obstetrics and gynaecology, or paediatrics, and patients are often referred within the same practice from one to another of these specialists.

Primary care is also provided by even more specialised doctors such as dermatologists and cardiologists who may spend more of their time on their hospital work than in their 'office'. In fact there is no barrier to any doctor admitting his own patients to any hospital which has granted him admitting rights on the basis of his specialty qualifications, and very few American doctors are without these rights. With the demands of this dual role in hospital and community it is not surprising that recently two kinds of assistants have emerged as so-called 'mid-level' practitioners, the physician's assistant and the nurse practitioner (Reedy, 1978). The latter tend to be more independent and to work in rural areas and public health clinics rather than in doctors' offices. In some respects their work is not unlike that of our health visitors.

British G.P.s are increasingly grouping themselves so as to share their resources and responsibilities but whereas these groups usually consist of three or four doctors, in America there is a growing number of extremely large groups consisting of 50 or more specialists, often with their own pathology laboratories, X-rays and other facilities. Together with the smaller groups and single-handed doctors these are the forms taken by private practice (which has almost disappeared amongst British G.P.s) and they deal with most of the first contact work in America. Apart from the emergency departments in urban hospitals, which account for some 10% of first contacts, there are a number of other facilities for primary care which were created by the federal government. They include the 'health maintenance organisations' which employ salaried doctors and operate their own insurance schemes to give comprehensive cover to their members; 'neighbourhood health centres' which concentrate on prevention and health education in urban ghettos (and are stigmatised by American doctors as manifestations of 'socialised medicine') and the 'community mental health centres' which provide out-patient care for the mentally ill.

From the patients' point of view the greatest difference between the British and American systems lies in methods of payment. In Britain government health insurance is compulsory for all, but in America, one half of all the contacts for primary care are paid for directly by the patient. Apart from this, about equal proportions of patients have private health insurance from organisations such as Blue Cross or Blue Shield or else they qualify for the federal and state systems such as Medicaid (for the very poor) or Medicare (for the elderly). There are other sources of assistance as well but all these insurances tend to be selective and people who can afford insurance for primary care may not be able to afford the higher premiums for accidents or prolonged care in hospitals. As the emergency rooms of hospitals may be the only care available for indigent populations and racial minorities, particularly in inner urban areas, there is a serious gap in the provision of health care in America which has been estimated to affect as many as a quarter of the population and for which there is almost no parallel in Britain.

Thus at the level of scientific and technological achievement in medicine, the Americans have no equal but their delivery system is relatively ineffective by our standards and the root of their dilemma is well summed up by Stephen (1979) when he says that: 'Health care is a product of social and political environment, constrained and influenced by the mentality and philosophy of both patients and doctors'. This is something of a truism, but in the third major group of systems for providing health care, the socialist systems, their present form has in the first place been dictated by a political philosophy and mediated by a political revolution.

The two earliest and still the major examples of this form are the U.S.S.R. and China whose present systems date from 1917 and 1949 respectively. Since then, countries such as Cuba, North Korea and Angola have followed suit, but their pre-revolutionary systems all shared the characteristic that they were modelled on Western medical technology and delivery systems which were quite inappropriate for agrarian economies with vast populations outside the urban areas. The main problem is that of the proportionate distribution of health manpower and this is common to all Third World countries regardless of their political system.

It is often the case that whereas more than four-fifths of the population live and work outside the towns, only a quarter or less of the physicians (and a similar proportion of nurses) do so. The usual solution has been the development of a medical auxiliary grade of personnel of which the archetypes are the 'feldsher' in the U.S.S.R. and the very similar 'physician's assistant' in the U.S.A. and elsewhere. These archetypes both had military origins but the largest scale development of this kind, and the one which has caught the popular imagination, is that of the so-called 'barefoot doctor' in China, whose origin and deployment truly reflects the socialist philosophy in health care.

Characteristically, socialist systems have been modelled on that of post-revolutionary Russia where health care is a public utility in which all personnel are civil servants and all facilities are owned by the government. As the responsibility for this totality of care is centred in the U.S.S.R. in a unified and monolithic ministry of health, it is not surprising that the system is claimed to be extremely hierarchical and bureaucratic. In China, the changes that were required to provide for 800 million people in 25 provinces and 2000 counties were clearly incompatible with a rigid administrative system and the abandonment of the Russian model of centralisation was encouraged by the break in relationships between the two countries in 1960 and the subsequent proletarian cultural revolution in China. Under Mao Tse Tung, three general principles emerged for health care: the need to retain and assimilate both the Western and the traditional forms of medicine; to lay stress on health care in rural areas and to concentrate on the prevention of illnesses such as cholera, plague, schistosomiasis and kala-azar, all of which were endemic.

Thus the decision was made to provide a minimal but widely available level of health care for the rural populations by rapidly training a grade of medical auxiliary who would be selected and paid from within each community by its members. These auxiliaries are the famous 'barefoot doctors', now said to number approximately one million (Roemer, 1977). They are deployed in relation to each of the rural 'production Brigades' which number between 500 and 3000 people, approximately the same number as those registered with the British general practitioner, and their emphasis is on immediate practical skills rather than theoretical knowledge. They receive their formal training in the nearest hospital or health centre from the numbers of 'mobile medical teams'. These consist of doctors and other medical and related personnel who are outposted for periods of up to one year from the teaching and other large hospitals in the major towns.

Barefoot doctors have their own village consulting rooms and are the point of first contact in their communities, treating minor illnesses with drugs or herbs and referring obscure or serious problems to a health centre or hospital. They are particularly important for immunisation and other preventive work and play a major part in the drive to provide birth control. Financial arrangements vary between communities from the fee for service to payment through local health insurance schemes which may be voluntary or compulsory. The public also has free access on a fee-paying basis to the traditional healers, herbalists, acupuncturists and bonesetters, who are widely used in the community and to a lesser extent in the hospital services.

Although the Chinese have adopted what appears to be the most logical expedient for their primary care services, the urban teaching hospitals continue to train doctors in the Western medical tradition inherited partly from European religious missionaries. During the Cultural Revolution of 1966 to 1970 and the drive to train the rural auxiliaries, orthodox medical training was reduced to three years but is now expanding again, if not yet to the eight years which some prestigious hospitals offered in the early 1960s. There is already some suggestion that, as with the feldshers in the U.S.S.R, the best of the auxiliaries could become eligible for a full medical training in an orthodox medical school. This raises a commonly voiced question about all kinds of medical auxiliaries and particularly the better-educated ones in America and Russia.

For a variety of social, psychological and intellectual reasons, some of these auxiliaries undoubtedly develop an aspiration to qualify fully as a doctor and the question is to what extent should the truly able ones be allowed and encouraged to progress in this way. The question seems unlikely to affect the nurse practitioner stereotype because it appears that their motivation is in general towards the development of what is generically a nursing rather than a medical role and the evidence for the generalisation 'once a nurse, always a nurse' is fairly strong.

At present the Russians accept the most able of their feldshers (about 20%) for medical training whilst the Americans may yet find that their assimilation of the osteopaths into the orthodox medical profession in the mid-1960s constitutes an irresistible precedent for their own physician's assistants. The problem in the Third World seems to be a marked lack of medical schools for training anyone at all and there seems little prospect of many more schools under present economic conditions. There is also the deterrant that a market for primary care has been created in many countries although few, if any, have a historical tradition and supply of motivated doctors for this purpose as there is in Britain and other parts of Europe. Fortunately it is likely in practice that many auxiliaries have a natural limit to their confidence and capacities (Reedy, 1978) and that the number of high-flyers will always be small.

Perhaps the more important question for the Chinese, as for everyone else, is to know whether the present system will be able to cope with the more intransigent problems such as those connected with old age, malignancy, affluence and anomie when the diseases due to infection, poverty and underdevelopment have been controlled and are reduced to negligible proportions.

REFERENCES

Consultative Council on Medical and Allied Services 1920 Report on the future provision of medical and allied services. HMSO, London

Cornillot P, Bonamour P 1973 France Health service prospects: an international survey. The Lancet and Nuffield Provincial Hospitals Trust, London, p 55

Fendall N R E 1972 Auxiliaries in health care. Johns Hopkins, Baltimore

Gish O 1978 Planning the health sector: the Tanzanian experience. Croom Helm, London

Ministry of Public Health 1973 Cuba Health service prospects: an international survey. The Lancet and Nuffield Provincial Hospitals Trust, London, p 157

Reedy B L E C 1978 The new health practitioners in America: a comparative study. King Edward's Hospital Fund for London

Roemer M I 1977 Comparative national policies on health care. Marcel Dekker, New York

Stephen W J 1979 An analysis of primary medical care — an international study. Cambridge University Press, Cambridge

FURTHER READING

Blanpain J, Delesie L, Nys H 1978 National health insurance and health resources: the European experience. Harvard University Press, Cambridge, Massachusetts

Pritchard P 1978 Manual of primary health care: its nature and organization. Oxford University Press, Oxford

Stevens R 1966 Medical practice in modern England: the impact of specialization and state medicine. Yale University Press, New Haven

Fry J (ed) 1977 Trends in general practice. Royal College of General Practitioners and British Medical Journal, London

Watkin B 1975 Documents on health and social services 1834 to the present day. Methuen, London

Index